Joanne

Geriatric Care and Research Organisation
GeriCaRe

In association with

Quality of Life
Research and Development Foundation

✳✳

Handbook of
DEMENTIA

Editors
Nilamadhab Kar
MD, DPM, DNB, MRCPsych
Consultant Psychiatrist
Wolverhampton City Primary Care Trust,
Wolverhampton, UK

David Jolley
MSc, FRCPsych
Professor of Old Age Psychiatry,
University of Wolverhampton,
Director of Dementiaplus,
Penn Hospital, Wolverhampton, UK

Baikunthanath Misra
MD, DPM, LLB
Professor of Psychiatry
Mental Health Institute
SCB Medical College
Cuttack, India

Paras Medical Publisher
Hyderabad, India

Handbook of Dementia

First published in the UK by

ANSHAN LTD
In 2006

6 Newlands Road, Tunbridge Wells,
Kent. TN4 9AT. UK
Tel/Fax: +44 (0) 1892 557767
e-mail: info@anshan.co.uk
Web Site: www.anshan.co.uk

Published in arrangement with
Paras Medical Publisher, 5-1-475 First Floor
Putlibwoli, Hyderabad - 500 095, India.
E-mail: parasmedpub@hotmail.com

© N Kar, D Jolley, B Misra

ISBN 10: 1 904 79889 6
ISBN 13: 978 1 904798 89 7

British Library Cataloguing in Publication Data
A catalogue record for this book is available from the British Library

PREFACE

The number of people affected by dementia grows as the absolute number and proportion of older people in the world increases. This phenomenon has massive implications for personal, family and societal economics. Early identification and initiation of management of dementia offers a better chance of improving the quality of life for patients, of increasing the support to their caregivers, and using shared resources to the best effect. It is important that health professionals and the general public should be sensitive to the presence of this disease, its nature, prospects for treatment and optimal patterns of care.

Geriatric Care and Research Organisation (GeriCaRe) is trying to bring into focus these issues by a range of educational programmes. 'Handbook of Dementia' is one such initiative of GeriCaRe, which aims to provide, within one volume, a user-friendly review of current knowledge and thinking on dementia.

The need for such a book has been expressed in various forums. It is the humble wish of GeriCaRe that the Handbook of Dementia will meet this need and become adopted as a resource book, which is used with confidence in everyday practice.

It is expected that this book will be useful for the physicians, psychiatrists, neurologists, geriatricians, general practitioners, nurses, occupational therapists, clinical psychologists, social workers, caregivers and family members of dementia patients. We hope that it will also be read and used by policy makers and researchers.

We acknowledge with gratitude the help of many individuals in the preparation of this book: Professor Mary Ganguli, MD, MPH, Professor of Psychiatry, and Epidemiology, Division of Geriatric and Neuropsychiatry, University of Pittsburgh School of Medicine, Pittsburgh, USA for the permission to print Cognitive Screening Battery, Hindi Geriatric Depression Scale and Everyday Activity Scale of India; Professor PSVN Sharma, MD,

DPM, Department of Psychiatry, Kasturba Medical College, Manipal, 576119, India; Dr K Jacob Roy, of Alzheimer's and Related Disorders Society of India, Kerala, India, who is also advisor of GeriCaRe; Murali Narayan Reddy, DPM, DNB, Consultant Psychiatrist, Old Age Psychiatry, New South Wales, Australia; Sudha S Bhat, MD, Department of Pathology, KMC, Manipal, Vivek Pattan, MD, Gwent Health Care NHS Trust, Newport, South Wales. In addition we also thank Sasmita Kar for considerable help in coordination; Naveen Kumar, Ganesh Prasad for assisting Ravikala Rao with the computer work, Alison James, for secretarial help in preparation of the manuscript and Saroj Ballav for the publication activities. Shri Harish Chandra Kar, President, GeriCaRe, and his team have been extremely helpful.

We have been greatly helped by all the authors by their support and cooperation. Their interest and contribution towards the dementia care have made this book possible.

✳✳

CONTRIBUTORS

❑ **Susan M Benbow**, MB, ChB, MSc, FRCPsych, ·Diploma in Family Therapy, Professor of Mental Health and Ageing, University of Wolverhampton; Fellow in Mental Health and Ageing, National Institute of Mental Health in England; Consultant Psychiatrist (Old Age Psychiatry) Wolverhampton Primary Care Trust, Penn Hospital, Penn Road, Wolverhampton, United Kingdom.
Email: susan.benbow@wlv.ac.uk

❑ **Srikala Bharath**, MD, DPM, DCAP, MRCPsych, Additional Professor of Psychiatry, National Institute of Mental Health and Neurosciences, Bangalore, 560029, India; and Consultant Psychiatrist, Mental Health Unit, Lister Hospital, Stevenage, Herts, SG1 4AB, United Kingdom.
Telephone: 01438 781079; Email: shrikalabharath@hpt.nhs.uk

❑ **Raveesh BN**, MD, PGDMLE (Postgraduate Diploma in Medical Law And Ethics), LLB, MSc (Forensic and Legal Psychology). Assistant Professor of Psychiatry, Department of Psychiatry, JSS Medical College and Hospital, Mysore, India. Email: raveesh6@yahoo.com

❑ **Alistair Burns,** MBBS, FRCPsych, Professor in Old Age Psychiatry, School of Psychiatry and Behavioural Sciences, Education and Research Centre, Wythenshawe Hospital, Manchester, M23 9LT, United Kingdom. Email : A_Burns@fs1.with.man.ac.uk

❑ **Soumitra Shankar Datta**, MD, DPM, DNB, Department of Psychiatry, Christian Medical College, Vellore, 632 002, India. Email: sdatta@nhs.net

❑ **Sandip Deshpande**, MD, Senior House Officer, Psychiatry, Cefn Coed Hospital, Cockett, Swansea, SA2 0GH, Wales.
Email: docsandy2004@yahoo.co.uk

- **Anthony James Elliott**, MBChB, MRCPsych, Msoc Sci (Dist), FRSH, Consultant Old Age Psychiatrist, Clinical Director, Services for Older People, Shelton Hospital, Shropshire, West Midlands UK, SY3 8DN; Associate Director, Dementia Plus; Senior Lecturer, Department of Psychiatry, Wolverhampton University, Tel: 01743 492097 or 492209; Fax: 01743 492292; Email: t.elliott@which.net

- **Jenny La Fontaine**, MA, DPSN, RMN, Cert Ed Fahe, RNT, PGCert Integrative Counselling, Consultant Nurse, Birmingham Working Age, Dementia Service, Birmingham and Solihull Mental Health Trust, Rubery Lane, Birmingham B45 9AY, UK. Email: LaFontaine@bsmht.nhs.uk

- **Mary Ganguli**, MD, MPH, Professor of Psychiatry and Epidemiology, Division of Geriatrics and Neuropsychiatry, Department of Psychiatry, University of Pittsburgh School of Medicine, 230 McKee Place, Room 405, Pittsburgh, PA 15213-2593, USA. Email: gangulim@upmc.edu

- **Ian Greaves**, MBChB (Hons), BDS (Hons), BMSc, Fellow of the Royal College of General Practitioners, Honorary Associate Professor at the University of Kentucky USA; Honorary Senior Lecturer Wolverhampton University; General Practitioner, Wharf Road Surgery, Gnosall, ST20 0DB, Stafford, UK, Tel: 01785 823916 Email: drgreaves@drgreaves.fsnet.co.uk

- **KS Jacob**, MD, PhD, Professor of Psychiatry, Christian Medical College, Vellore, 632002 India. Email: ksjacob@cmcvellore.ac.in

- **Jagadisha**, MD, Assistant Professor of Psychiatry, National Institute of Mental Health and Neuroscience, Bangalore, 560029, India. Email: jagatth@yahoo.com

- **David Jolley**, MSc, FRCPsych, Professor of Old Age Psychiatry, University of Wolverhampton; Director of Dementiaplus, Penn Hospital, Wolverhampton WV4 5HN, United Kingdom. Email: Dementiaplus.wm@wolvespct.nhs.uk

- **Rosie Jenkins**, MBChB, MRCPsych, Consultant Psychiatrist, Old Age Psychiatry, Wolverhampton City Primary Care Trust, Penn Hospital, Penn Road, Wolverhampton, WV4 5HN, United Kingdom. Email: dr.jenkins@wolvespct.nhs.uk

- **Nilamadhab Kar**, MD, DPM, DNB, MRCPscyh, Consultant Psychiatrist, Wolverhampton City Primary Care Trust, Corner House Resource Centre, 300 Dunstall Road, Wolverhampton, WV6 0NZ, United Kingdom. Honorary Medical Advisor, Geriatric Care and Research Organisation, Email: nilamadhabkar@yahoo.com

- **Salman Karim**, MBBS, FCPS, Lecturer in Old Age Psychiatry, School of Psychiatry and Behavioural Sciences, Education and Research Centre Wythenshawe Hospital, Manchester, M23 9LT, United Kingdom. E-mail: SKarim@fs1.with.man.ac.uk

- **Sudhir Kumar**, MD, DM (Neurology), Department of Neurological Sciences, Christian Medical College, Vellore, 632002. India. Email: drsudhirkumar@yahoo.com

- **Baikunthanath Misra**, MD, DPM, LLB, Professor of Psychiatry, Mental Health Institute, SCB Medical College, Cuttack, Orissa, 753009, India. Email: baikuntha.misra@rediffmail.com

- **Jisu Nath**, MD, Senior Resident, Department of Psychiatry, All India Institute of Medical Sciences (AIIMS), New Delhi. Email: jisunath@hotmail.com

- **Vivek Pattan**, MD, Department of Psychiatry, Gwent Health Care NHS Trust, Newport, South Wales, UK

- **P Ravikala V Rao**, MD, Professor of Pathology, SDM College of Medical Sciences, Sattur, Dharwad, 580009, India. Email: ravikala_rao@hotmail.com

- **Shovan Saha**, BOT, MSc, OT, Associate Professor, Department Of Occupational Therapy, Manipal College of Allied Health Sciences, Manipal, 576104, India. Email: shovansaha@yahoo.com

- **Ravi Samuel**, MA (SW), M Phil, PGCARM (Lond), Cognitive Behaviour Consultant, K Gopalakrishna Department of Neurology, Voluntary Health Services, Medical Centre, Taramani, Chennai, 600113, Tamil Nadu, India. Email: rsam_67@yahoo.co.uk

- **Somnath Sengupta**, MD, Associate Professor, Department of Psychiatry, Institute of Human Behaviour and Allied Sciences (IHBAS), Dilshad Garden, Delhi. Email: sn_sengupta@hotmail.com

- **KS Shaji**, DPM, MD, Assistant Professor of Psychiatry, Department of Psychiatry, Medical College, Thrissur, 680596, Kerala, India. Phone 0091-487-361755, Fax 0091-487-361097, Email: shajiks@vsnl.com / shajiks@md4.vsnl.net.in

- **S Shaji**, MBBS, DPM, Consultant Psychiatrist, Urban Community Dementia Services, Kochi, India. Email: sdrshaji@rediffmail.com

- **Shanthini V**, MA, K Gopalakrishna Department of Neurology, Voluntary Health Services, Medical Centre, Taramani, Chennai, 600113, India. Email: V_Shanthini@yahoo.com

- **Krishnamoorthy Srinivas**, DM, FRCP, Chairman, TS Srinivasan Dept of Clinical Neurology, Public Health Centre, West Mambalam, Chennai, 600033, India. Email: tssn@giasmd01.vsnl.net.in

- **Sunitha Thomas**, BOT, Assistant Lecturer, Department of Occupational Therapy, Manipal College of Allied Health Sciences, Manipal, 576104, India. Email: garnets05@yahoo.co.in

**

CONTENTS

1

Introduction: Dementia– The Challenge

Nilamadhab Kar

A Growing Concern

As more and more people live to advanced age, with the increasing life expectancy, prevalence of dementia will increase because it is primarily the illness of old age. For example, between 1985 and 2025, Canada is predicted to experience a 135%, USA 105%, UK 23% increase in size of the over-65 population. The changes in developing countries, where recent progress in public health has extended longevity, the increase will be even more striking; for instance, Guatemala, will have 357%, Mexico 324%, and India 264% increase in their elderly individuals (Cummings, 1995).

Prevalence of dementia doubles every 5 years starting from 1% at age 60 to about 30–40% by 85. The economic cost of dementia is huge and includes the expense of caring for the disabled individuals for a long time. Dementia is no doubt a major public health issue (Cummings, 1995), a threat to the well being of older people, and a tragedy both for its victims and for their families.

Invisible Agony

Even if dementia has a major presence, often these patients are not identified at all or at least not so initially. While most of the patients in the community are not identified, in many who attend hospitals for treatment for various physical problems, dementia is missed. Either the symptoms are passed off as age-related or they receive less or no attention in the presence of pressing concerns of physical ailments or sensory impairments, which most of the elderly at that age suffer. One of the many reasons for which this happens is that there is not only lack of awareness in the community but also a lack of orientation among health care professionals.

Multifaceted Problem

Dementia is a multifaceted disorder and its management requires attention to the underlying disorder, cognitive impairment, behavioural and psychiatric symptoms, consequences of disability and associated conditions, and care of the caregivers.

It has multiple causes ranging from genetic, metabolic, infective, to exposure to various toxins (Lishman, 1987). While the core clinical features remain same, the symptoms present in various combinations and in different rates of progression. Often this makes clinical diagnosis a puzzling task, at least initially (Kar et al., 2000).

A therapeutic nihilism is encountered often amongst clinicians in the management of dementia. Though there are many medicines available for the cognitive impairment, the response to these, the stage of illness, cost-benefit ratio and affordability (especially in developing countries) are many issues that weigh heavily in the process of clinical decision-making. Besides the cognitive impairment, the behavioural and psychological symptoms associated with dementia come as a major concern not only for the caring family members but also for the professionals. Most of the dementia patients in their advanced age are so vulnerable to side effects (Cheong, 2004) that it often becomes difficult to balance between benefit and risk. Behavioural interventions appear time-consuming; improvements, if any, seem so minimal and that fade so quickly that it often tests the patience of the caregivers. In addition, there are other management issues like capacity for decision making especially for specific treatments and legal matters.

Challenges Ahead

Dementia robs all that makes someone a unique being. With the cognitive capabilities gradually drained, the person behind the human form gradually fades. Yet, so much remains intact, though in bits and pieces, in a disordered frame. While more and more human beings are living longer, and more and more people falling prey to dementia the blank stares of the victims tell that there is so much to be done.

More research to understand the aetiologies, and the risk factors, development of newer molecules and methods to treat the pathology receive main impetus now. However, issues of care of these patients and their caregivers are also to be looked at systematically as these issues bring in real challenge before not only the families and professionals but also the state. Predicting accurately, and identifying those at definite risk, and methods to delay the onset of illness are also research issues now. Reversing the pathological process and prevention may sound ambitious aims at present, but these demand research; and who knows what might be achieved!

REFERENCES

- Chandra V, Ganguli M, Pamdav R, Johnston J, Belle S & DeKosky S. (1998) Prevalence of Alzheimer's disease and other dementias in rural India: the Indo-US study. *Neurology,* 51 (4), 1000–1008.
- Cheong JA. (2004) An evidence-based approach to the management of agitation in the geriatric patient. Focus: The Lifelong Learning in Psychiatry, 2, 197–205.
- Cumings JL. (1995) Dementia: the failing brain. *Lancet,* 345, 1481–1484.
- Gopinathan VP. (1998) Alzheimer's disease – A commoner cause of senile dementia. *Journal of Indian Medical Association,* 96, 5, 149–150.
- Kar N, Sengupta S & Sharma PSVN. (2000) Diagnosing dementia due to Alzheimer's disease: Clinical perspective. *Indian Journal of Psychiatry,* 42, 267–270.
- Lishman WA. (1987) *Organic Psychiatry, The Psychological Consequences of Cerebral Disorder.* Oxford: Blackwell Scientific Publication.

- Rajkumar S, Kumar S & Thara R. (1997) Prevalence of dementia in a rural setting: A report from India. *International Journal of Geriatric Psychiatry,* 12 (7), 702–7.
- Rajkumar S, Kumar S. (1996) Prevalence of dementia in the community: a rural-urban comparison from Madras, India. *Australian Journal of Ageing,* (15), 9–13.
- Shaji S & Roy KJ. (2001) An epidemiological study of dementia in an Urban Community, in Kerala, India. Book of Abstracts, Alzheimer's Disease International Conference. Christ Church, New Zealand.
- Shaji S, Pramodu K, Abraham R, Roy KJ & Varghese A. (1996) An epidemiological study of dementia in a rural community in Kerala, India. *British Journal of Psychiatry,* 168 (8), 745–9.

2

Clinical Features of Dementias

Soumitra Shankar Datta, Sudhir Kumar, KS Jacob

INTRODUCTION

Dementia is defined as a progressive loss of intellectual abilities of sufficient severity to interfere with social and/or occupational functioning. "Dementia" is a descriptive term, not a specific disease or condition. Dementia is produced by more than one underlying pathophysiological processes. The essential feature is the development of multiple cognitive deficits, which include memory impairment and at least one of the following cognitive disturbances: aphasia, agnosia, apraxia or a disturbance of executive functioning.

CLINICAL FEATURES

The deficits seen in dementia affect multiple domains of cognitive function. They cause significant impairment in social and occupational functioning. These deficits suggest a decline from a previously higher level of functioning.

Memory Impairment

It is the central feature of dementia. It usually occurs early in the course of the illness. New learning ability is impaired and patients forget previously learned material. They may lose their wallets and keys and forget about food being cooked on the stove. They can get lost in unfamiliar neighbourhoods. Personal information (e.g., occupation, schooling, birthday, details of family member) may not be recalled in advanced stages of the condition.

Formal testing of memory should include tests for registration, retention, recall and recognition. The ability to learn new information is assessed by asking patients to learn a list of unrelated words. The patient is then asked to repeat the words in order to assess registration and repeat the list after several minutes to check for recall. They can be asked to recognise the words from a written list, which is provided. Patients with difficulty to learn new words are unable to recall the information despite prompts and clues. Those who have problems in retrieval are able to make use of the clues. Remote memory is tested by asking the individual to recall personal information and past materials, which are of interest (e.g., politics, sports, movies, music, etc.) to patients. It is also necessary to determine the impact of the problems in memory on the person's day-to-day functioning. Ability to do different activities of daily living, ability to work, shop and the ability to return home should be ascertained from the patient and his family.

Memory impairment, the hallmark of dementia, is said to go through various stages and is not necessarily dependent on the type of dementia. These stages are not discrete. They are briefly described:

Stage I: Mild Memory Impairment
Mild memory lapses occur, but cause only a few problems for the person and are often attributed to other factors, such as the effects of normal aging, stress, or depression. Forgetting errands, failing to pass on messages, becoming disoriented in unfamiliar surroundings usually suggests the onset of memory impairment. Recall of episodes in the near distant past may be impaired. Conversations with other people are often forgotten. However, such memory problems do not necessarily indicate a progressive neuropsychological impairment.

Stage II: Mild to Moderate Memory Impairment
Memory impairment slowly becomes more pronounced and starts to have a significant impact on the activities of daily living. The person may seek medical help, often prompted by a relative or friend, and is likely to become reliant on a caregiver. Failing to recognise friends,

becoming disoriented even in familiar surroundings, confusing the time of the day or day of the week and becoming increasingly unable to keep track of daily events are commonly seen.

Stage III: Severe Impairment
The failure to recognise close relatives suggests severe impairment. The problems in memory become severe. Manifestations like wandering, forgetting to turn off the gas stove can increase the concern for the person's safety. The person is not able to recall personal details. Confabulations can also be present in this stage (Miller and Morris, 1993).

Aphasia

Aphasia is an acquired disorder of language due to brain damage. The patients with dementia may develop aphasia. Patients may lose the phonetic production of speech, the ability to comprehend speech, to repeat, and to hear or read words. In *motor aphasia*, the word output is reduced, the speech may be telegraphic and prosody of speech may be lost. This occurs due to involvement of inferior frontal gyrus (Broca's area). In *sensory aphasia*, comprehension to verbal or written commands may be impaired. This occurs due to involvement of superior temporal gyrus (Wernicke's area). *Global aphasia* may have features of both the above. *Alexia* refers to difficulty in reading, whereas *agraphia* refers to difficulty in writing. In *nominal aphasia,* patients may find it difficult to name objects or remember the names of people. With advanced stages, the individual may become mute, or have deteriorated speech patterns such as *echolalia* (i.e., echoing what is heard) or *palilalia* (i.e., repeating sounds and words over and over again).

Apraxia

It is defined as inability to execute learned motor activities to command despite intact motor functions, sensory functions, and comprehension of the required task. Dominant parietal lobe involvement can give rise to ideomotor and conceptual (formerly called ideational) apraxias. *Ideomotor apraxia* refers to patients who make errors when asked to pantomime movements . This could include buccofacial commands (blow out a match, protrude your tongue, drink through a straw), limb commands (salute, use a toothbrush, comb your hair) or whole body commands (stand like a boxer, swing a cricket bat). *Conceptual apraxia* is defined as the loss of knowledge about the idea of the movements. Impairment is more obvious if the task involves multiple steps. For example, the following set of commands could be used for testing: Folding a letter, placing it in an envelope, sealing it, addressing it and putting a stamp on it. Non-dominant parietal lobe involvement could cause dressing or constructional apraxia. In *dressing apraxia,* the patient is unable to dress properly and makes mistakes. Patients with *constructional apraxia* have difficulty in drawing geometric figures, drawings of common objects, etc.

Agnosia

It is defined as failure to recognise or identify objects despite intact sensory functions. Depending upon the sensory modality affected, agnosia could be classified into visual, auditory, olfactory and tactile subtypes. For example, an individual with tactile agnosia may have normal tactile sensations but is unable to identify objects placed in his hands (e.g., coins or keys).

Impaired Executive Functioning

Disturbances of executive functioning are a common manifestation of dementia. Executive functioning involves ability to think abstractly and to plan, initiate, sequence, monitor, and stop complex motor behaviours. Abstraction is tested by asking the patient the similarities and differences between words or objects. Executive function can be tested by asking the person to count, recite the alphabet, subtract serial 7s or name as many animals as possible in a specified time frame.

The deficits listed above should be severe enough to cause a significant impairment in social and occupational functioning. Impairment in working, dressing, eating, bathing, handling finances, and other activities of daily living are often severe and incapacitating.

Patients with dementia tend to deteriorate in the level of self-care. They may forget to take bath, clean themselves, and forget their meals and medications. This could lead to an increase in morbidity.

In addition to significant memory disturbance, apraxia, agnosia, aphasia and loss of executive function, people with dementia often have other symptoms. Poor judgement and insight are commonly seen. They may make unrealistic assessments of their ability (e.g., making plans to start a new venture) and underestimate the risks involved in activities (e.g., driving). Occasionally, patients who develop paranoid delusions (e.g., delusions of persecution, of things being stolen) may turn violent. The initial stages of the disease may be associated with depression and can result in suicidal attempts. Inappropriate jokes, overfamiliarity with strangers, and disinhibited sexual behaviour may be seen.

Issues Related to Region, Culture and Education

The decline in the level of functioning is measured against the background of the individual's capacity prior to the onset of the disease. The local culture and educational background has to be specifically taken into consideration. Education plays a major role in determining the level of functioning and has to be kept in mind. Paper and pencil tests for people who have not routinely used such material can pose problems in diagnosis. Similarly people of certain cultural and educational backgrounds may not be familiar with certain types of information (e.g., national political leaders, geographical information), memory (e.g., date of birth in cultures that do not routinely celebrate birthdays), orientation (e.g., dates in cultures that do not routinely employ calendars). Regional differences in the causes of dementia (e.g., infections, nutritional deficiencies, etc.) can vary across regions and have to be also kept in mind.

CLINICAL DIFFERENTIAL DIAGNOSIS

The syndrome of dementia must be differentiated from other clinical presentations (APA, 1994; First et al., 1996). Common differential diagnoses include the following:

Delirium
Delirium is characterised by disturbance of consciousness. The major deficit is an impairment of attention and concentration. The onset is often acute, the course fluctuating and is usually of short duration.

Dementia should not be diagnosed if cognitive deficits are exclusively present during an episode of delirium. However, periods of delirium can occur in patients with a history of long standing dementia.

Amnestic Disorder

Amnestic disorder is characterised by severe memory impairment without significant impairment in cognitive functioning. There is no evidence of aphasia, agnosia, apraxia or a loss of executive function.

Substance Intoxication-or Withdrawal

The dementia syndrome can occur in patients in the context of substance abuse and withdrawal. It can also occur with exposure to toxins and to medication. It remits when the acute effects of intoxication or withdrawal settle. Substance-induced persistent dementia is diagnosed if the dementia persists long after the period of intoxication or withdrawal.

Mental Retardation

Mental retardation is characterised by markedly below average intellectual function and impairment in adaptive functioning. The onset is before the age of 18 years. Cognitive deficits are usually non-progressive in patients with mental retardation.

Schizophrenia

Cognitive impairment and deterioration in the functioning are commonly seen in schizophrenia. However, the age of onset in schizophrenia is generally earlier, the cognitive impairment is much less severe and the characteristic symptoms of psychosis are present.

Major Depression

Subjective memory problems, difficulty in concentrating and a general reduction in intellectual function can be seen in depressive disorders. However, they are usually abrupt in onset, associated with other characteristic depressive symptoms with a past or family history of the disorder. The cognitive symptoms improve with the remission of depression.

Malingering and Factitious Disorder
These conditions do not have the classic symptom profile and they are
not consistent over time.

Age Related Cognitive Decline
This is characterised by cognitive impairment that is in keeping with
what would be expected for the individual's age. Deficits such as
aphasia, agnosia, apraxia, and loss of executive function are not present
and the impairment in social and occupational function is much less
severe.

Associated Medical Conditions

The syndrome of dementia will be associated with different physical
findings depending on the nature of the underlying pathology, its location
and the stage of progression. The most common cause of dementia is
Alzheimer's disease followed by vascular disease and then by many
different causes. The other causes include Pick's disease, normal-
pressure hydrocephalus, Parkinson's disease, Huntington's disease,
traumatic brain injury, brain tumours, anoxia, infectious disease (e.g.,
human immunodeficiency virus, syphilis), Prion diseases (e.g.,
Creutzfeldt-Jakob disease), endocrine medical conditions,
(hypothyroidism, hypocalcaemia, hypoglycaemia), vitamin deficiencies
(e.g., deficiencies of thiamine, niacin, vitamin B_{12}), immune disorders
(e.g., polymyalgia rheumatica, systemic lupus erythematosus), hepatic
diseases, metabolic conditions (e.g., Kufs' disease,
adrenoleukodystrophy, metachromatic leukodystrophy) and other
neurological diseases (e.g., multiple sclerosis).

The cognitive and memory functions are assessed using the mental
status examination and neuropsychological testing. Neuroimaging (e.g.,
CT Scan, MRI) may reveal cerebral atrophy, focal brain disease (e.g.,
cortical strokes, tumours, subdural haematomas), hydrocephalus, or
periventricular ischaemic brain injury.

SPECIFIC DEMENTIAS AND THEIR CLINICAL FEATURES

This section focuses on the broad clinical types of dementias encountered in the practice and their clinical presentations.

The common clinical syndromes of dementia are: (i) Alzheimer's disease, (ii) Vascular (multi-infarct) dementia, (iii) Dementia with Lewy bodies, (iv) Frontotemporal dementia (Pick's disease), (v) Alcohol-related dementia (including Korsakoff's syndrome), (vi) AIDS-related dementia, (vii) Subcortical dementia, (viii) Depressive pseudo-dementia, (ix) Prion disease. These are briefly discussed.

ALZHEIMER'S DISEASE

Alzheimer disease (AD) is the most common cause of dementia, which is an acquired cognitive and behavioural impairment of sufficient severity to interfere significantly with social and occupational functioning. Prevalence of this disorder is expected to increase substantially in this century, since the disorder preferentially affects the elderly, who constitute the fastest growing age bracket in many countries, especially in industrialized nations.

Alzheimer's disease has onset in the middle or late life, rarely before 45 years of age.

The onset of dementia of Alzheimer's disease is gradual and involves continuing cognitive decline. Between 2% and 4% of individuals of the population over the age of 65 years are estimated to have Alzheimer's disease. The prevalence increases with increasing age, particularly after 75 years of age.

Clinical Features

Memory impairment: In the early stage, the memory impairment may go unrecognised and may be attributed to benign forgetfulness. The common pattern is an insidious onset, with an early deficit in recent memory followed by that of immediate recall and new learning ability. Remote memory is usually preserved.

Other cognitive deficits: Aphasia, apraxia and agnosia develop subsequently over several years after the onset of illness.

Other than cognitive impairment, the disease is characterised by neuropsychiatric and behaviour disturbances. Several types of neuropsychiatric and neurobehavioral disorders and symptoms occur in Alzheimer's disease (Chung, 2000). Hallucinations and delusions are common in AD. These are usually concrete and not too complex or bizarre. They may be present in isolation or with other symptoms of psychosis or depression. Sleep-wake patterns may be disturbed, and night time wandering may be very disruptive to the household.

Loss of inhibitions and belligerence may alternate with social withdrawal and passivity. These symptoms fluctuate and tend to recur and are associated with more rapid cognitive decline. They affect the functioning of the individual, and might be associated with earlier institutionalisation.

Often the patient is unaware of these problems (anosognosia) while their family member and others have considerable insight resulting in frustration and anxiety. Rarely, the AD patient may have a form of cortical blindness in which they deny their problem (Anton's syndrome). The sleep-wake pattern may be disturbed and this may lead to troublesome wandering in the nights. Neurologically there can be pyramidal signs, myoclonic jerks and seizures.

Diagnostic criteria for various sub-categories of Alzheimer's disease have been proposed (McKhann et al., 1984).

Unlikely AD
- Sudden onset
- Focal neurological signs
- Seizures or gait disturbance early in the course of the illness

Possible AD
- Atypical onset, presentation, or progression of a dementia syndrome without a known aetiology.
- A systemic or other brain disease capable of producing dementia but not thought to be the cause of the dementia is present.
- There is a gradually progressive decline in a single intellectual function in the absence of any other identifiable cause.

Probable AD

- Dementia established by clinical examination and documented by mental status questionnaire
- Dementia confirmed by neuropsychological testing
- Deficits in two or more of the following areas of cognition:
  - Memory
  - Language
  - Perceptual skills
  - Attention
  - Praxis
  - Orientation
  - Problem-solving
  - Functional abilities
- Progressive worsening of memory and other cognitive functions
- No disturbance of consciousness
- Onset between ages 40 and 90
- Absence of systemic or other brain diseases capable of producing a dementia syndrome

Definite Alzheimer's Disease

- Clinical criteria for probable Alzheimer's disease
- Histopathologic evidence of Alzheimer's disease (autopsy or biopsy)

A Diagnosis of Probable Alzheimer's Disease is Supported By:

- Progressive deterioration of specific cognitive functions: language (aphasia), motor skills (apraxia), and perception (agnosia).
- Impaired activities of daily living and altered patterns of behaviour.
- A family history of similar problems, particularly if confirmed by neurological testing.
- The following laboratory results:
  - Normal cerebrospinal fluid (lumbar puncture test).
  - Normal electroencephalogram (EEG) test of brain activity.
  - Evidence of cerebral atrophy in a series of CT scans.

Other Features Consistent with Alzheimer's Disease

- Plateaus in the course of illness progression.

- CT findings normal for the person's age.
- Associated symptoms, including: depression, insomnia, incontinence, delusions, hallucinations, weight loss, sex problems, and significant verbal, emotional, and physical outbursts.
- Other neurological abnormalities, especially in advanced disease, including: increased muscle tone and a shuffling gait.

Course and Prognosis

The course of the dementia tends to be slowly progressive, with a loss of 3–4 points per year on a standard instrument for assessment, e.g., Mini-Mental State Examination. Cognitive deficits start with memory impairment in the earlier phases and go through language impairment and involvement of other cognitive domains in the late phases. The typical duration of illness is 8 to 10 years but can range from 1 to 25 years. Death usually results from malnutrition, secondary infections or heart disease.

VASCULAR (MULTI-INFARCT) DEMENTIA

The vascular dementia is the second most common cause of dementia. The varied manifestations of this syndrome reflect complex interaction of the vascular aetiologies (cerebrovascular disease and vascular risk factors), changes in the brain (infarcts, white matter lesions, cerebral atrophy) and host factors such as age, education, and cognitive maturity. The subtypes of vascular dementia include the multiinfarct dementia (cortical dementia), the small vessels dementia (subcortical deep lesions) and strategic infarct dementia (Cummings, 1994).

Clinical Features

The cardinal features of vascular dementia are included in the Hachinski Ischaemic Score items: abrupt onset, step wise deterioration, fluctuating course, nocturnal confusion, relative preservation of personality, depression, somatic complaints, emotional incontinence, history of hypertension, history of strokes, evidence of associated atherosclerosis, focal neurological symptoms, and focal neurological signs (Hachinski, 1975). Step wise deterioration, fluctuating course, history of hypertension, history of stroke, and focal neurological symptoms differentiate definite vascular dementia from definite

Alzheimer's disease. The syndrome of vascular dementia is charac-terised by memory deficits, loss of executive function syndrome, slowed information processing, and mood and personality changes. Also, the memory deficits of vascular dementia are less severe than that found in Alzheimer's disease and are characterised by impaired recall, relatively intact recognition that benefits from cues (Desmond, 1999).

The dysexecutive syndrome in vascular dementia includes impairment in goal formulation, initiation, planning, organisation, sequencing, executing, set shifting and set maintenance, as well as abstracting. The executive functions are more involved if the vascular injury involves prefrontal subcortical circuits and thalamocortical circuits (Cummings, 1993). Personality and insight are relatively preserved in mild and moderate cases of vascular dementia.

NINDS-AIREN Criteria for the Diagnosis of Vascular Dementia (Roman et al., 1993)

I. The criteria for the clinical diagnosis of *probable* vascular demen-tia include *all* of the following:

Dementia defined by cognitive decline from a previously higher level of functioning and manifested by impairment of memory and of two or more cognitive domains (orientation, attention, language, visuospatial functions, executive functions, motor control, and praxis), preferably established by clinical examination and documented by neuropsychological testing; deficits should be severe enough to interfere with activities of daily living, not due to physical effects of stroke alone.

Exclusion criteria: Cases with disturbance of consciousness, delirium, psychosis, severe aphasia, or major sensorimotor impairment precluding neuropsychological testing; patients with systemic disorders or other brain diseases (such as AD), which could account for deficits in memory and cognition.

Cerebrovascular disease (CVD) defined by the presence of focal signs on neurologic examination, such as hemiparesis, lower facial weakness, Babinski sign, sensory deficit, hemianopia, and dysarthria consistent with stroke (with or without history of stroke), and evidence of relevant CVD by brain imaging (CT or MRI) including *multiple large vessel infarcts* or a *single strategically placed infarct* (angular gyrus, thalamus, basal forebrain, or posterior cerebral artery (PCA) or anterior cerebral artery (ACA) territories), as well as *multiple basal ganglia* and *white matter lacunes*, or *extensive periventricular white matter lesions*, or combinations thereof. ·

A relationship between the above two disorders, manifested or inferred by the presence of one or more of the following: (a) onset of dementia within 3 months following a recognized stroke; (b) abrupt deterioration in cognitive functions; or fluctuating, stepwise progression of cognitive deficits.

II. Clinical features consistent with the diagnosis of *probable* vascular dementia include the following:
(a) Early presence of gait disturbance (small-step gait or marche a petits pas, or magnetic, apraxic-ataxic or parkinsonian gait); (b) history of unsteadiness and frequent, unprovoked falls; (c) early urinary frequency, urgency, and other urinary symptoms not explained by urologic disease; (d) pseudobulbar palsy; and (e) personality and mood changes, abulia, depression, emotional incontinence, or other subcortical deficits including psychomotor retardation and abnormal executive function.

III. Features that make the diagnosis of vascular dementia *uncertain or unlikely* include:
(a) Early onset of memory deficit and progressive worsening of memory and other cognitive functions such as language (transcortical sensory aphasia), motor skills (apraxia), and perception (agnosia), in the absence of corresponding focal lesions on brain imaging; (b) absence of focal neurological signs, other than cognitive disturbance; and (c) absence of cerebrovascular lesions on brain CT or MRI.

IV. Clinical diagnosis of *possible* vascular dementia may be made in the presence of dementia with focal neurological signs in patients in whom brain imaging studies to confirm definite CVD are missing; or in the absence of clear temporal relationship between dementia and stroke; or in patients with subtle onset and variable course (plateau or improvement) of cognitive deficits and evidence of relevant CVD.

V. Criteria for diagnosis of *definite* vascular dementia are (a) clinical criteria for *probable* vascular dementia; (b) histopathologic evidence of CVD obtained from biopsy or autopsy; (c) absence of neurofibrillary tangles and neuritic plaques exceeding those expected for age; and (d) absence of other clinical or pathological disorder capable of producing dementia.

There is evidence from the history, clinical examination, or test of significant cerebrovascular disease, which may be reasonably judged to be aetiologically related to the dementia (history of stroke, evidence of cerebral infarction). However, recent pathological studies have suggested that isolated cerebrovascular disease (i.e., with no Alzheimer lesions) is rarely found in association with dementia (Hulette et al, 1997). With the development of more sensitive instruments, and clinicians who are more aware about the clinical syndrome of dementia, the boundary between the vascular and degenerative dementia may vanish as more subtle cases may be diagnosed.

Cortical vascular dementia is caused mainly due to large vessel disease, cardiac embolic events and subsequent hypoperfusion affecting the cortical and subcortical arterial territories and their distal fields (watershed infarcts). The typical clinical features are lateralised sensorimotor changes, sudden onset cognitive impairment and aphasia. Different clinical syndromes have been seen to occur in this type of dementia, due to specific vascular territory and lobar involvement, e.g., Anton's syndrome, Balint's syndrome etc. (Mahler et al, 1991). Subcortical vascular dementia or small vessel dementia includes the 'Binswanger's disease' and 'lacunar states'. Clinically, they are characterised by pure motor hemiparesis, bulbar signs, dysarthria, depression, emotional lability, and deficits in executive functioning (Babikian, 1987).

Current research undermines the usefulness of vascular dementia as a diagnostic category as it involves a high degree of subjective judgement, subsumes a large number of potentially heterogeneous conditions and overlaps considerably with Alzheimer's disease. The current system of classifying dementia into mutually exclusive subtypes poorly reflects mixed disease in older age groups and has become an important issue since these 'diagnoses' now determine eligibility for pharmacological intervention. Risk factors for cerebrovascular disease are also risk factors for dementia. However, the course of dementia, once it has developed, appears to be frequently determined by Alzheimer's disease (Stewart, 2002).

DEMENTIA WITH LEWY BODIES (DLB)

Lewy body dementia is the second most common cause of degenerative dementia in the old age. DLB shows a similar age range and insidious onset of dementia as AD and the terminal severity of cognitive impairment is comparable. Survival in published series is shorter than for AD, and DLB patients are especially vulnerable to neuroleptic medication, which further accelerates mortality. The features, which have been most consistently described as differentiating this group from Alzheimer's disease, are extrapyramidal signs, and psychiatric/behavioural symptoms.

Psychiatric and Behavioural Symptoms

Two prominent features in DLB are visual hallucinations and fluctuation in cognitive performance. The visual hallucinations are characteristically recurrent, well formed and detailed and in the earlier stages may be associated with insight into their nature. Data from several groups suggest that hallucinations involving other sensory modalities are considerably less frequent, and may be no more frequent than encountered in AD patients. To give an example, one of the authors of the current chapter had an elderly lady with Lewy Body dementia, who regularly discussed about the presence of a shark in her bath. She knew that it might be to do with her disease and never seemed to be afraid of the animal. There is a dedicated chapter on the neuropsychiatric symptoms of dementia in this book and thus we spare the reader from the details of the neuropsychiatric manifestations.

Another major feature of DLB in the elderly is fluctuation in the cognitive state and/or consciousness, which occur over periods ranging from a few hours to weeks or longer. They are sometimes associated with intercurrent illness, but can also be quite spontaneous. They are independent of normal diurnal variation in performance. However, this symptomatology remains controversial, not least because of difficulties in defining fluctuation, and in its quantification.

Consensus Criteria for the Clinical Diagnosis of Probable and Possible Dementia with Lewy Body (McKeith et al., 1996)

1. The central feature required for a diagnosis of DLB is progressive cognitive decline of sufficient magnitude to interfere with normal social or occupational function. Prominent or persistent memory impairment may not necessarily occur in the early stages but is usually evident with progression. Deficits on tests of attention and of frontal-subcortical skills and visuospatial ability may be especially prominent.

2. Two of the following core features are essential for a diagnosis of probable DLB, and one is essential for possible DLB:
   a. Fluctuating cognition with pronounced variations in attention and alertness.
   b. Recurrent visual hallucinations that are typically well formed and detailed.
   c. Spontaneous motor features of Parkinsonism.

3. Features supportive of the diagnosis are:
   a. Repeated falls
   b. Syncope
   c. Transient loss of consciousness
   d. Neuroleptic sensitivity
   e. Systematized delusions
   f. Hallucinations in other modalities.

4. A diagnosis of DLB is less likely in the presence of:
   a. Stroke disease, evident as focal neurological signs or on brain imaging.
   b. Evidence on physical examination and investigation of any physical illness or other brain disorder sufficient to account for the clinical picture.

FRONTOTEMPORAL DEMENTIAS (PICK'S DISEASE)

The clinical features of frontotemporal dementia (FTD) reflect its pathological anatomy regardless of the nature of the underlying lesions. The prefrontal cortex and the anterior temporal lobes carry the brunt of the involvement. Pick's disease is the prototype of the frontotemporal dementia. FTD has an earlier age of onset (50 to 60 years) than is typical for Alzheimer's disease and is often familial. The common symptoms of frontotemporal dementia include disinhibition, impulsivity, impaired judgement, and amotivational states. These changes result in inappropriate and disturbed social behaviour. The features, which help in assessing patients with such conditions, are listed in Table 2.1.

Table 2.1 Lund-Manchester consensus on clinical criteria of frontotemporal dementia

---

Core features

Behavioural disorder
    Insidious onset and slow progression
    Early loss of insight
    Early loss of personal and social awareness
    Early signs of disinhibition and lack of judgement
    Stereotyped, repetitive, and imitating behaviour
    Hyperorality, dietary changes
    Utilisation behaviour
    Distractibility, impulsivity, and impersistence

Affective symptoms
    Depression, anxiety, excessive sentimentality
    Hypochondriasis, bizarre somatic complaints
    Emotional bluntness, apathy, and lack of empathy
    Amnesia

---

contd.

Speech
Progressive reduction of speech output
Stereotypy of speech and perseveration
Echolalia
Late mutism

Spatial orientation, receptive speech and praxis comparatively spared

Physical signs
Early primitive reflexes
Early incontinence
Late akinesia, rigidity and tremor
Low and labile blood pressure

Investigations
Normal EEG in spite of clinically evident dementia
Brain imaging (structural and/or functional): Predominant frontal and/or anterior temporal abnormality
Neuropsychology: Profound failure on 'frontal-lobe' tests in the absence of severe amnesia or perceptual spatial disorder

Supportive diagnostic feature
Onset before 65 years of age
Positive family history or similar disorder in a first-degree relative
Bulbar palsy, muscular weakness and wasting, fasciculation (motor neuron disease)

CORTICAL BASAL GANGLIONIC DEGENERATION

Cortical basal ganglionic degeneration is a slowly progressive dementing illness. It is associated with severe gliosis and neuronal loss in both the neocortex and basal ganglia. The onset is often unilateral. Characteristic features include rigidity, dystonia, and apraxia of one arm and hand ("alien hand" syndrome). With time, the condition becomes bilateral. Patients develop dysarthria, slow gait, action tremor, and dementia (Bird, 2001). Autonomic nervous system dysfunctions may be found in this type of dementia.

ALCOHOL-RELATED DEMENTIA

About 9–23% of elderly patients receiving treatment for alcohol dependence syndrome have dementia. Chronic excessive alcohol intake can cause impairment of short and long term memory, learning, visuoperceptual abstraction, visuospatial organisation, maintenance of cognitive set and impulse control (Penington, 1998). The neuropsychological performances improve with abstinence, but are still detectable after 5 years (Brandt et al, 1983).

Diagnostic Criteria

1. Impairment in short- and long-term memory
2. At least 1 of the following:
   - Impairment in abstract thinking
   - Impaired judgement
   - Other disturbances of higher cortical function
   - Personality change
   - Memory impairment and intellectual impairment causing significant social and occupational impairments
3. Absence of occurrence exclusively during the course of delirium
4. Memory loss following prolonged, heavy ingestion of alcohol
5. Exclusion of all causes of memory loss other than alcoholism

Associated Features

- Learning problem
- Dysarthria/involuntary movement
- Hypoactivity
- Psychotic
- Depressed mood
- Somatic/sexual dysfunction
- Addiction
- Sexually deviant behaviour
- Odd/eccentric/suspicious personality
- Anxious/fearful/dependent personality
- Dramatic/erratic/antisocial personality

Wernicke-Korsakoff Syndrome

Chronic alcohol consumption can also lead to Wernicke-Korsakoff syndrome (WKS). The disease is characterized by mental confusion, amnesia (a permanent gap in memory) and impaired short-term memory. An estimated 80% of persons with WKS continue to have a chronic memory disorder. Individuals often appear apathetic and inattentive and some may experience agitation. In addition, WKS tends to impair the person's ability to learn new information or tasks. Individuals with WKS are known to "confabulate" (make up or invent information to compensate for poor memory). Other symptoms include ataxia (weakness in limbs or lack of muscle coordination, unsteady gait); slow walking; rapid, tremor-like eye movements or paralysis of eye muscles. Fine motor function (e.g., hand or finger movements) may be diminished and sense of smell may also be affected. In the advanced stages, coma can occur.

SUBCORTICAL DEMENTIAS

The term subcortical dementia was first used to describe a distinct clinical syndrome in association with progressive supranuclear palsy (PSP). Albert et al (1974) described subcortical dementia as a clinical syndrome characterised by forgetfulness, slowed thinking process (bradyphrenia), psychiatric changes (especially apathy, depression and irritability), and impaired ability to manipulate acquired knowledge. The differentiating features of subcortical dementias from those, which predominantly affect the cerebral cortex, are listed in Table 2.2. The various commonly encountered subcortical dementias have other clinical features, which may assist in the differential diagnosis (Table 2.3). The cognitive features of the three common subcortical dementia syndromes of Parkinson's disease, Huntington's disease, and progressive supranuclear palsy are briefly described.

Table 2.2 The distinguishing features of cortical and subcortical dementias

Characteristic	Subcortical dementia	Cortical dementia
Severity	Mild to moderate	More severe
Speed of cognition	Slow	Normal
Memory deficit	Initially failure of retrieval (forgetfulness amenable to cues)	Primarily a storage and recall deficit (occurs early)
Language	Less affected initially	Early aphasia
Gnostic-practic abilities	Less affected initially	Affected early
Personality	Apathetic, inert	Indifferent
Mood	Depressed	Euthymic
Abnormal movements	Chorea, trembling, tics	Rare (myoclonus)
Motor abnormalities	Extrapyramidal	Uncommon, gegenhalten
Posture	Stooped	Normal
Coordination	Affected	Normal
Pathology	Prominent changes in striatum and thalamus	Prominent changes in cortical association areas
Reversibility	Possible	Unlikely

Table 2.3 Supporting clinical features of diseases associated with subcortical dementias

Disease	Supporting clinical features
Parkinson's disease	Signs of frontal lobe involvement, memory deficits generally improving on cues, tremor, rigidity, bradykinesia
Huntington's disease	Behaviour changes, psychosis, slowing of mentation, choreiform movements
Wilson's disease	Predominantly a frontal-subcortical dysfunction, behavioural change, depression, psychosis, chorea, Kayser-Fleischer ring
Spinocerebellar degenerations	Memory and frontal dysfunction, cerebellar signs, sensory loss, signs of corticospinal tract disease
Corticoid basal ganglionic degeneration	Frontoparietal dysfunction predominates - apraxias, alien hand phenomenon, stimulus sensitive myoclonus
Normal-pressure hydrocephalus	Chronic increased pressure: predominantly gait disturbances, mild cognitive deficits, and urinary incontinence
Vascular dementias	Lacunar states, Binswanger's disease: risk factors for stroke present, focal neurological signs and symptoms

Parkinson's Disease

Dementia occurs in 20% to 60% of individuals with Parkinson's disease (PD), especially for those who are in the older age group and who have a more severe disease. The most consistent areas of cognitive impairment in PD are in the domains of visuospatial ability, memory, and executive function. The PD patients show a number of deficits of visuospatial functioning even in the early stages. There is impaired immediate and delayed free recall in the presence of normal or near normal retention, delayed cued recall, and delayed recognition.

The PD patients with dementia had significantly more impairment on motoric speech functions, that is on measures of dysarthria, phrase length, speech melody, and writing mechanics, as compared to Alzheimer's disease dementia (Freedman, 1990). The disturbances of the executive functions (planning, selecting, initiating, sequencing, implementing strategic actions, monitor and flexibly shift behaviour) are probably the earliest and most significant cognitive manifestations of PD (Ebersbach, 1994).

It has been proposed that the disturbances in the executive function represent the central feature of cognitive dysfunction in PD, and the visuospatial deficits are secondary to that. As a result of that there is difficulty in planning, selecting, sequencing complex motor programs (Marsden, 1984).

Huntington's Disease

Huntington's disease is an inherited progressive neurological disease characterised by choreiform and athetotic movements, psychiatric symptoms such as psychosis, depression and dementia. In the early and the mid stages, the dementia conforms to the general subcortical type, while in the late stages it becomes more of a generalised dementia.

Memory is probably the best characterised domain of cognitive dysfunction in patients with Huntington's disease. Visual memory is more affected than verbal memory. There is also defect in the executive function, the major problems being in the domains of planning and sequencing organisational strategies, cognitive flexibility and set shifting. The full scale IQ as measured by Wechsler Adult Intelligence Test drops modestly during the first years of illness, performance scale accounting for most of the decline (Josaissen, 1982). Studies have shown that the above cognitive changes can be identified in asymptomatic 'at risk' prior to the onset of the clinical syndrome (Lundervold, 1995).

Progressive Supranuclear Palsy

The patients of progressive supranuclear palsy (PSP) present with a number of cognitive problems involving visuospatial processing, auditory and visual inattention, impaired memory and slowed cognitive speed. Executive function derangement in PSP is more severe than Parkinson's disease and Huntington's disease. Patients with PSP are impaired on a number of executive functions measures requiring abilities such as abstraction, verbal fluency, and flexibility, shifting and sequencing. Problems on intelligence tests such as WAIS-R, are more pronounced especially for the arithmetic, similarities and picture arrangement subtests, which have requirements for the working memory, abstraction and sequencing respectively. As with other disorders of the basal ganglia, the investigators propose that the executive function deficits are primary and lead to the secondary problems in areas such as spatial ability and memory (Maher, 1985).

Interestingly, current clinical, neuropsychological and neuropathological findings do not allow the strict separation of the dementias into subcortical and cortical subgroups. Consequently, less emphasis should be placed on the issue of whether or not clinical and neuropsychological findings fit typical cortical or subcortical pictures. Assessments should be directed towards identifying the precise cause of a dementia and appraising functional deficits that have implications for management (Turner et al, 2002).

AIDS-RELATED DEMENTIA

The first report of a dementia syndrome associated with HIV infection was by Navia et al, in 1986. They named the syndrome of cognitive, motor and behavioural disturbances of patients infected with HIV as 'AIDS Dementia Complex'.

The onset of HIV associated dementia is generally insidious. Early cognitive symptoms include forgetfulness, loss of concentration, mental slowing, and reduced performance in sequential mental activities. Early behavioural changes are characterised by apathy, reduced expression of emotions and social withdrawal. Depression, emotional lability, agitation and psychosis may also occur.

Early motor symptoms include incoordination, difficulty with tasks involving motoric precision as writing and eating etc., leg weakness and frequent falls. Neurological examination may reveal tremor, hyperreflexia, ataxia, slowing of rapid alternating movements, frontal lobe release signs. Tests of ocular motility may show interruption of smooth pursuits and slowing of saccades.

In the late stage of the disease there is usually global deterioration of cognitive functions and a severe psychomotor retardation, which may progress to the stage of mutism. Patient becomes bed-bound and indifferent to the surroundings. The level of consciousness is preserved except for occasional hypersomnolence (Maj, 2001).

DEMENTIA ASSOCIATED WITH OTHER CHRONIC CNS INFECTIONS

Other infective causes of dementia include neurosyphilis, tuberculosis, progressive multifocal leukoencephalopathy, fungal and protozoal infections, sarcoidosis and Whipple's disease, to mention a few. Appropriate history of exposure, cerebrospinal fluid (CSF) and serum VDRL tests, MHA-TP tests may confirm the diagnosis of neurosyphilis. The dementia in neurosyphilis is thought to be caused by cerebral endarteritis. Whipple's disease is characterised by diarrhoea, weight loss, arthralgia, fever, oculomasticatory myoclonus and ophthalmoplegia. The diagnosis of Whipples's disease is confirmed by positive CSF polymerase chain-reaction for *T. whippelii,* and brain and meningeal biopsy in rare cases (Koroshetz, 2001).

Prion Diseases

Prion disease as Creutzfeldt-Jakob Disease (CJD) has been the area of extensive research in the past decade. The disease is relatively rare. The syndrome is characterised by rapidly progressive dementia associated with myoclonus, cortical blindness, pyramidal, cerebellar or extrapyramidal signs. Initially, patients experience problems with muscular coordination; personality changes, including impaired memory, judgement, and thinking. They may also have visual impairment. Patients commonly experience insomnia, depression, or unusual sensations. With time, the patients' mental impairment becomes severe. In the terminal stage, the patients develop myoclonus. They eventually lose the ability to move and speak and gradually become comatose. Pneumonia and other infections often occur in these patients and can lead to death.

There are several known variants of CJD. These variants differ somewhat in the symptoms and course of the disease. For example, a variant form of the disease—called new variant or variant (nv-CJD, v-CJD), described in Great Britain and France—begins primarily with psychiatric symptoms, affects younger patients than other types of CJD, and has a longer than usual duration from onset of symptoms to death. Another variant, called the panencephalopathic form, occurs primarily in Japan and has a relatively long course, with symptoms often progressing for several years. It tends to cause more rapid deterioration of a person's abilities than Alzheimer's disease or most other types of dementia.

DEMENTIA CAUSED DUE TO TOXINS AND HEAVY METALS

The various agents that have been attributed for causing dementia are lead, mercury, manganese, arsenic, aluminium, perchlorethylene, toluene, carbon tetrachloride, ethylene glycol, methyl alcohol, organophosphates, formaldehyde, and carbon monoxide. History of possibility of prolonged or intense exposure to the above agents should be ruled out when evaluating a patient with dementia.

DEMENTIA ASSOCIATED WITH BRAIN TUMOURS

Certain slow growing brain tumours may simulate the clinical picture of a primary dementia. Detailed neurological examination may or may not elicit any focal neurological signs. There is a gradual change in personality. For example, a person may become withdrawn, moody, and, often, inefficient at work. A person may feel drowsy, confused, and unable to think. Such symptoms are often more apparent to family members and co-workers than to the person. Absence of localising signs in these patients emphasises the need for routine structural imaging of brain, in the evaluation of patients with dementia.

DEMENTIA DUE TO METABOLIC DISTURBANCES

Electrolyte imbalances, hypoglycaemia, renal failure, liver failure or pancreatic disorders can provoke a confusional state simulating a syndrome of dementia. Prolonged organ failures by themselves can cause significant cognitive deficits, changes in sleep, appetite or emotions.

Deficiencies of folate, niacin, riboflavin and thiamine have been reported in the literature to produce cognitive impairment. Hypothyroidism, hyperthyroidism, parathyroid disturbances or adrenal abnormalities can cause delirium, mimicking dementia. Hypothyroidism can produce a retarded state, which can have dramatic response to treatment with thyroid supplementation.

DEMENTIA DUE TO HEAD TRAUMA AND DIFFUSE BRAIN DAMAGE

The common causes of dementia classified under this category include dementia pugilistica, dementia following chronic subdural haematoma, postanoxia, postencephalitis and cerebral irradiation. Generally the association of the offending agent and onset of symptoms are well demonstrated. There is no characteristic or unique presentation of these groups of dementias. Careful history taking and clinical examination is important as in all other types of dementia.

DEPRESSIVE PSEUDODEMENTIA

Depression is a complex condition that reflects the dynamic interaction of the subcortical and higher cortical structures. Elderly patients with depression often have cognitive deficits suggestive of dementia and people with dementia often have depressive symptoms. The cognitive deficits in both conditions are often similar and difficult to separate clinically. The clinical features, which distinguish the two conditions, are listed in Table 2.4.

Table 2.4 Differentiating features of dementia and pseudodementia

Characteristics	Pseudodementia	Dementia
Clinical course and history	Onset fairly well demarcated	Onset indistinct
	History short	Long history
	Rapidly progressive	Early deficits often go unnoticed
	Previous psychiatric history common	Uncommon
Clinical behaviour	More complaints of cognitive dysfunction	Little complaint of cognitive loss
	Little effort expended on examination items	Struggles with cognitive tasks
	Affective change often present	Usually apathetic, with shallow emotions
	Behaviour does not reflect cognitive loss	Behaviour compatible with cognitive loss
	Nocturnal exacerbation rare	Nocturnal accentuation common
Examination findings	Frequently answers "I don't know" even before trying	Usually tries items
	Inconsistent memory loss for both recent and remote items	Memory loss worse for recent than remote items
	Inconsistent performance	Rather consistent
	May have particular memory gaps	No specific memory gaps present

CONCLUSION

Dementia is a clinical syndrome that is seen in the elderly. It has many causes. While there are differences in clinical presentation, the identification of specific aetiology is often dependent on a comprehensive history, clinical evaluation and necessary laboratory investigations including brain imaging. The treatment includes treating the cause and also symptomatic treatment.

There will be, hopefully, newer insights into the presentation and treatment modalities for this complex group of disorders. The so-called bad news of being diagnosed to have dementia may have a silver lining. As per some of the newer reports, some of the patients with dementia had been seen to develop exceptional artistic talents, which were earlier suppressed. Loss of semantic knowledge, but preservation or even enhancement of visual and musical abilities often accompanies selective degeneration of the left anterior temporal lobe. Visual and musical abilities should be encouraged in the setting of left anterior temporal injury or dysfunction. Thus for a subgroup of patients with dementia, at least temporarily, the diagnosis of dementia may not be invariably associated with relentless loss of all intellectual abilities (Miller et al, 2000).

REFERENCES

- Albert ML, Feldman RG. (1974) The "subcortical dementia" of progressive supranuclear palsy. *Journal of Neurology, Neurosurgery and Psychiatry,* 37, 121–130.
- American Psychiatric Association (1994) *Diagnostic and Statistical Manual of Mental Disorders.* 4th Edition: 133–156. Washington DC: American Psychiatric Press.
- Babikian V and Ropper AH. (1987) Binswanger's disease: a review. *Stroke,* 18, 2–12.
- Bird TV. (2001) Alzheimer's disease and other primary dementias. In *Harrison's Principles of Internal Medicine CD* 15th Edition (Eds: Braunwald E, Fauci AS, Kaspe DL, et al) New York: McGraw-Hill.
- Brandt J, Butters N, Ryan C et al (1983) Cognitive loss and recovery in long term alcohol abusers. *Archives of General Psychiatry,* 40, 435–442.

- Chung JA, Cummings J. (2000) Neurobehavioral and neuropsychiatric symptoms in Alzheimer's disease: Characteristics and treatment. Dementia, *Neurological Clinical of North America,* 18, 829–846.
- Cummings JL. (1993) Fronto-subcortical circuits and human behaviour. *Archives of Neurology,* 50, 873–880.
- Cummings JL. (1994) Vascular subcortical dementias: Clinical aspects. *Dementia,* 5, 177–180.
- Desmond DW, Erkinjuntti, T, Sano, M, et al. (1999) The cognitive syndrome of vascular dementia: implications for clinical trials. *Alzheimer's Disease and Associated Disorders,* 13, Supp 3, S21–9.
- Ebersbach G, Hattig H, Schelosky L, et al (1994) Persevarative motor behaviour in Parkinson's disease. *Neuropsychologia,* 32, 799–804.
- Erkinjuntti T. (2001) Vascular dementia. In *New Oxford Textbook of Psychiatry* 1st Edition (Eds: Gelder MG, Lopez-Ibor JJ, Andreason N.), 428–436. New York: Oxford University Press.
- First MB, Frances A, Pincus HL. (1996) *DSM IV Handbook of Differential Diagnosis* 1st Edition:142–143. Washington DC: American Psychiatric Press.
- Freedman M. (1990) Parkinson's disease. In *Subcortical Dementia,* 1st Edition (Eds Cummings J.) p 108–122. New York: Oxford University Press.
- Hachinski VC, Iliff LD, Zilhka E, et al. (1975) Cerebral blood flow in dementia. *Archives of Neurology,* 32, 632–637.
- Hulette C, Nochlin D, McKeel D, et al (1997) Clinical neuropathological findings in multi-infarct dementia: a report of six autopsied cases. *Neurology,* 48, 668–672.
- Josaissen RC. (1982) Patterns of intellectual deficit in Huntington's disease. *Journal of Clinical and Experimental Neuropsychology,* 4: 173–183.
- Koroshetz WJ and Swartz MN. (2001) Chronic and recurrent meningitis (Chapter 374) In *Harrison's Principles of Internal Medicine CD,* 15th Edition (Eds Braunwald E, Fauci AS, Kaspe DL, et al) New York: McGraw-Hill.
- Lundervolt AJ and Reinvang I. (1995) Variability in Cognitive function among persons at high genetic risk of Huntington's disease. *Acta Neurologica Scandanavia,* 91, 462–469.
- Maher ER, Smith EM, Lees AJ. (1985) Cognitive deficits in the Steele-Richardson-Olszewski syndrome (progressive supranuclear palsy). *Journal of Neurology, Neurosurgery and Psychiatry,* 48, 1234–1239.

- Mahler ME and Cummings JL. (1991) The behavioural neurology of multi-infarct dementia. *Alzheimer's Disease and Associated Disorders,* 5, 122–130.
- Maj M. (2001) Dementia due to HIV disease. In *New Oxford Textbook of Psychiatry* 1st Edition (Eds Gelder MG, Lopez-Ibor JJ, Andreason N) p 436–439. New York: Oxford University Press.
- Marsden CD. (1984) Which motor disorder in Parkinson's disease indicates the true motor functions of the Basal Ganglia? In *Functions of Basal Ganglia* (Ed O'Connor) p 225–241. London: Pitman.
- McKeith IG, Galasko D, Kosaka K, et al. (1996) Consensus guidelines for the clinical and pathological diagnosis of dementia with Lewy bodies (DLB): report of the consortium on DLB International Workshop. *Neurology,* 47, 1113–24.
- McKhann G, Drachman D, Folstein M, Katzman R, Price D, Stadlan EM. (1984) Clinical diagnosis of Alzheimer's disease: Report of the NINCDS-ADRDA work group under the auspices of the Department of Health and Human Services task force on Alzheimer's disease. *Neurology,* 34, 939–944.
- Miller E, Morris R. (1993) *The psychology of dementia.* New York: John Wiley & Sons,
- Miller B, L, Boone K, Cummings JL, Read SL, Mishkin F. (2000) Functional correlates of musical and visual ability in frontotemporal dementia. *British Journal of Psychiatry,* 176, 458–463.
- Penington M. (1998) Welcome to Alzheimer's Outreach (Online) Available from: http://www.zarcrom.com/users/alzheimers/odem/al-d.html (Accessed on 21.06.2004).
- Roman GC, Tatemichi TK, Erkinjuntti T, et al (1993) Vascular dementia: diagnostic criteria for research studies. Report of the NINDS-AIREN International Workshop. *Neurology,* 43(2), 250–60.
- Stewart R. (2002) Vascular dementia: a diagnosis running out of time. *British Journal of Psychiatry,* 180, 152–156.
- Turner AM, Moran NF, Kopelman MD. (2002) Subcortical dementia. *British Journal of Psychiatry,* 180, 148–151.

3

Diagnostic Criteria of Dementia

Jisu Nath, Somnath Sengupta

INTRODUCTION

Dementia is a syndrome comprising cognitive deficits and certain behavioural disturbances, which most commonly affect the elderly population. It has to be differentiated from other causes of forgetfulness and intellectual impairments. Some of these are: age-related memory decline, mental retardation persisting into old age, delirium and other cognitive disorders such as amnestic disorders, mild cognitive impairment and depressive disorders in the elderly (pseudodementia). There is difficulty in distinguishing depression and dementia in late life as depressive states occur in early dementia and certain symptoms (lack of energy, lack of interest, poor concentration) actually overlap. Furthermore, late onset depression with pseudodementia has a higher risk of developing frank dementia (Alexopoulos et al., 1993). Several diagnostic criteria exist for different types of dementia syndromes. While some are used as routine screening instruments, some are specifically designed for research purposes. Moreover, as newer information and scientific data are gathered, diagnostic guidelines are reviewed and refined periodically.

MILD COGNITIVE IMPAIRMENT

Before coming to the area of dementia, the controversial area of mild cognitive impairment, which may herald onset of dementia proper needs some discussion. The concept has been variously defined leading to two broad groups of subjects, one with benign memory disturbances and the other that leads to eventual development of dementia. Thus a host of synonyms and related terminologies evolved over time, like: benign senescent forgetfulness, age-associated memory impairment (AAMI) , ageing-associated cognitive decline, age-related cognitive decline (ARCD), mild cognitive disorder, mild cognitive decline, questionable dementia, minimal dementia, limited cognitive disturbance, cognitively impaired not demented (CIND) and the mild cognitive impairment (MCI). When different constructs are assessed epidemiologically, the prevalence of such entities differs across studies (Bischkopf et al, 2002). One would assume that in future some of these subjects be included in dementia, given the rapid progress in the fields of neuroimaging, genetic and biological markers.

DIAGNOSTIC GUIDELINES OF DEMENTIA

According to ICD-10 (International Classification of Diseases, 10th edition) (World Health Organization, 1992), the primary requirements for diagnosis of dementia are evidence of a decline in both memory and thinking, which is sufficient to impair personal activities of daily living. The impairment of memory typically affects the registration, storage, and retrieval of new information, but previously learned and familiar material may also be lost, particularly in the later stages. Dementia is more than dysmensia: there is also impairment of thinking and of reasoning capacity, and a reduction in the flow of ideas. The processing of incoming information is impaired, in that the individual finds it increasingly difficult to attend to more than one stimulus at a time, such as taking part in a conversation with several persons, and to shift the focus of attention from one topic to another. If dementia is the sole diagnosis, evidence of clear consciousness is required. However, a double diagnosis of delirium superimposed upon dementia is common. The above symptoms and impairments should have been evident for at least 6 months for a confident clinical diagnosis of dementia to be made.

DEMENTIA OF ALZHEIMER'S DISEASE

Alzheimer's disease (AD) is the most common type of dementia worldwide. It is also the prototype of dementia that affects over 10.3% of the populations above the age of sixty-five (Evans et al, 1989). The aetiology of this degenerative brain disease is still unknown, but current understanding points towards immunologic and genetic hypothesis.

ICD-10 Criteria

The following features are essential for a definite diagnosis:
a) Presence of a dementia as described above.
b) Insidious onset with slow deterioration. While the onset usually seems difficult to pinpoint in time, realization by others that the defects exist may come suddenly. An apparent plateau may occur in the progression.
c) Absence of clinical evidence or findings from special investigations, to suggest that mental state may be due to other systemic or brain disease, which can induce a dementia (e.g., hypothyroidism, hypercalcaemia, vitamin B_{12} deficiency, niacin deficiency, neurosyphilis, normal pressure hydrocephalus, or subdural haematoma).
d) Absence of a sudden, apoplectic onset, or of neurological signs of focal damage such as hemiparesis, sensory loss, visual field defects, and in-coordination occurring early in the illness (although these phenomena may be superimposed later).

There can be subtypes such as early onset, late onset, atypical/mixed and unspecified.

DSM-IV Criteria

The DSM-IV (Diagnostic and Statistical Manual of Mental Disorders, 4th Edition) (American Psychiatric Association, 1994) requires the following criteria:

A) The development of multiple cognitive deficits manifested by both
  1. Memory impairment (impaired ability to learn new information and to recall previously learned information)
  2. One (or more) of the following cognitive disturbances
    ▪ Aphasia (language disturbance)
    ▪ Apraxia (impaired ability to carry out motor activities despite intact motor function)

- Agnosia (failure to recognize or identify objects despite intact sensory functions)
- Disturbance in executive functioning (i.e., planning, organizing, sequencing and abstracting)

B) The cognitive deficits in criteria A1 and A2 each cause significant impairment in social or occupational functioning and represent a significant decline from a pervious level of functioning.

C) The course is characterized by gradual onset and continuing cognitive decline.

D) The cognitive deficits in criteria A1 and A2 are not due to any of the following:
  1. Other CNS conditions that cause progressive deficits in memory and cognition (e.g., cerebrovascular disease, Parkinson's disease, Huntington's disease, subdural haematoma, normal pressure hydrocephalus, tumour)
  2. Systemic conditions that are known to cause dementia (e.g., hypothyroidism, vitamin B_{12} or folic acid deficiency, niacin deficiency, hypercalcaemia, neurosyphilis and HIV infection)
  3. Substance-induced conditions.

E) The deficits do not occur exclusively during the course of a delirium.

F) The disturbance is not better accounted for by another Axis I disorder (e.g., major depressive disorder and schizophrenia)

According to DSM-IV, dementia of Alzheimer type can be sub typed on the basis of age at onset (early or late) and presence or absence of behavioural disturbances. The central or defining principle of a dementia syndrome as given in ICD-10 and DSM–IV is actually based on cognitive deficits and decline from the previous level of functioning. While such criteria may be suitable for AD it may not be so for frontotemporal and subcortical dementias in which the cognitive deficits appear much after the onset of behavioural and personality changes.

NINCDS-ADRDA Criteria

This is one of the most commonly used clinical criteria for diagnosis of AD. A working group composed of the National Institute of Neurological and Communicative Disorders, and Stroke and Alzheimer's Disease and Related Disorders Association (NINCDS-ADRDA) has developed these criteria for the research diagnosis of definite, probable and possible AD to bring uniformity to the diagnosis of AD (McKhann et al, 1984). The criteria have proved valid for clinical and research purpose. The diagnosis of patients diagnosed with probable AD according to these criteria, is confirmed at autopsy in more than 85% cases.

a) Criteria for the clinical diagnosis of probable AD:
1. Dementia established by clinical examination and documented by the MMSE (Mini Mental State Examination), BDS (Blessed Dementia Scale) or other similar examination and confirmed by neuropsychological tests.
2. Deficit in two or more areas of cognition.
3. Progressive worsening of memory and other cognitive functions.
4. No disturbance of consciousness.
5. Onset between age 40 and 90, most often after age 65.
6. Absence of systemic disorders or other brain diseases that could account for the progressive deficits in memory and cognition.

b) The diagnosis of probable AD is supported by:
1. Progressive deterioration of specific cognitive functions such as language (aphasia), motor skills (apraxia) and perception (agnosia).
2. Impaired activities of daily living and altered pattern of behaviour.
3. Family history of similar disorders, particularly if neuropathologically confirmed.

c) Laboratory results of:
1. Normal lumbar puncture as evaluated by standard techniques.
2. Normal pattern or non-specific EEG (electroencephalogram) changes, such as increased slow-wave activity.
3. Evidence of cerebral atrophy on CT (computed tomography) with progression documented by serial observation.

d) Other clinical features consistent with probable AD, after exclusion of other causes of dementia:
   1. Plateaus in the course of progression of the illness.
   2. Associated symptoms of depression; insomnia; incontinence; delusions; illusions; hallucinations; catastrophic verbal, emotional, or physical outburst; sexual disorders and weight loss.
   3. Other neurological abnormalities in some patients, especially those with more advanced disease, including motor signs, such as increased muscle tone, myoclonus or gait disorder.
   4. Seizures in advanced disease.
   5. CT normal for age.

e) Features that make the diagnosis of probable AD uncertain or unlikely:
   1. Sudden apoplectic onset.
   2. Focal neurological findings such as hemiparesis, sensory loss, visual field deficits and incoordination early in the course of illness.
   3. Seizures or gait disturbances .t the onset of symptoms or very early in the course of the illness.

f) Diagnosis of possible AD:
   1. May be made on the basis of the dementia syndrome; in the absence of other neurologic, psychiatric, or systemic disorders sufficient to cause dementia; and in the presence of variations in the onset, presentation, or clinical course.
   2. May be made in the presence of a second systemic or brain disorder sufficient to produce dementia but not considered to be the cause of the dementia.
   3. Should be used in research studies when a single, gradually progressive, severe cognitive deficit is identified in the absence of another identifiable cause.

g) Criteria for diagnosis of definite AD:
   1. Clinical criteria for probable AD.
   2. Histopathologic evidence for probable AD

h) Subtype classification for research purpose:
1. Familial occurrence
2. Onset before age 65
3. Presence of trisomy 21
4. Coexistence of other relevant conditions, such as Parkinson's disease

VASCULAR DEMENTIA

Vascular dementia (VaD) is one of the poorly defined and agreed upon concepts. Besides problem occurring with the definition of dementia itself, the term vascular is vague and ill defined. Added to this the confusion of interpreting findings of white matter lesion, also seen in otherwise normal adult brains. Overemphasis of such findings in MRI (Magnetic Resonance Imaging) scan of the brain may falsely increase the prevalence of vascular dementia in a community as probably has happened in Japan (Meguro et al, 2002).

ICD-10 Criteria

The diagnosis presupposes the presence of a dementia as described above. Impairment of cognitive function is commonly uneven, so that there may be memory loss, intellectual impairment, and focal neurological signs. Insight and judgement may be relatively well preserved. An abrupt onset or a stepwise deterioration, as well as the presence of focal neurological signs and symptoms, increase the probability of the diagnosis: in some cases, confirmation can be provided only by computerized axial tomography or, ultimately, neuropathological examination.

Associated features are: hypertension, carotid bruit, emotional lability with transient depressive mood, weeping or explosive laughter, and transient episodes of clouded consciousness or delirium, often provoked by further infarction. Personality is believed to be relatively well preserved, but personality changes may be evident in a proportion of cases with apathy, disinhibition, or accentuation of previous traits such as egocentricity, paranoid attitudes, or irritability.

ICD-10 further divides vascular dementia into six subtypes: vascular dementia of acute onset, multi-infarct dementia, subcortical dementia, mixed cortical and subcortical, other and unspecified.

DSM-IV Criteria

Besides presence of dementia as described above (criteria A and B), there should be focal neurological signs and symptoms (like exaggeration of deep tendon reflexes, extensor plantar, pseudobulbar palsy, gait abnormalities or weakness of a limb) and laboratory evidence of cerebrovascular disease (e.g., multiple infarctions involving cortex and underlying white matter) that are judged to be aetiologically related to the disturbance.

Hachinski Ischaemic Score

The Hachinski ischaemic score (HIS) (Hachinski et al, 1975) is used to separate patients with VaD from those with primary degenerative dementia, like AD. The Ischaemic Score can be used to identify patients with vascular dementia by assessing the following clinical findings mentioned in Table 3.1. The HIS has been modified later by two groups of authors. Loeb and Gandolfo from Italy added CT findings to the original scale—the "Modified Ischaemic Score of Loeb and Gandolfo" (Loeb and Gandolfo, 1983). Small revised the scale with further standardization and descriptions—the "Revised Ischaemic Score of Small" (Small, 1985).

Table 3.1 Hachinski Ischaemic Score

Clinical findings	Points
Abrupt onset	2
Stepwise deterioration	1
Fluctuating course	2
Nocturnal confusion	1
Relative preservation of personality	1
Depression	1
Somatic complaints	1
Emotional incontinence	1
History of hypertension	1
History of strokes	2
Evidence of associated atherosclerosis	1
Focal neurological symptoms	2
Focal neurological signs	2

Interpretation: Minimum score: 0; maximum score: 18. More than 7: VaD; 4–7: Borderline mixed; Less than 4: Primary degenerative dementia.

NINDS-AIREN Criteria

The National Institute of Neurological Disorders and Stroke and the Association Internationale pour la Recherche et l'Enseignementen Neurosciences criteria was developed in 1993 in an international workshop (Roman et al, 1993). The criteria are:

a) Dementia
1. Impairment of memory
2. Impairment of memory and two or more cognitive domains
   - Orientation
   - Attention
   - Language
   - Visuospatial functions
   - Executive functions, motor control and praxis

b) Cerebrovascular disease
1. Focal signs on neurological examination (hemiparesis, lower facial weakness, Babinski's sign, sensory deficit, hemianopia, and dysarthria)
2. Evidence of relevant cerebrovascular disease by brain imaging (CT)
   - Large vessel infarcts
   - Single strategically placed infarct
   - Multiple basal ganglia and white matter lacunas
   - Extensive periventricular white matter lesions
   - Combination thereof

c) A relationship between the above disorders manifested or inferred by the presence of one or more of the following:
1. Onset of dementia within 3 months after a recognized stroke
2. Abrupt deterioration in cognitive functions
3. Fluctuating, stepwise progression of cognitive deficits

d) Clinical features consistent with the diagnosis of probable VaD
1. Early presence of a gait disturbance
2. History of unsteadiness or frequent, unprovoked falls
3. Early urinary incontinence

4. Pseudobulbar palsy
5. Personality and mood changes

e) Features that make the diagnosis of VaD uncertain
Early onset of memory deficit and progressive worsening of memory and other cognitive functions in the absence of focal neurological signs and cerebrovascular lesions on CT and MRI.

ADDTC (Alzheimer's Disease Diagnostic and Treatment Centres) Criteria

The ADDTC criteria (also known as "California Criteria") (Chui et al., 1992) and the NINDS-AIREN criteria were developed to overcome the problem of overinclusion of MRI findings of insignificant white matter hyperintensities resulting in possible overdiagnosis of VaD. The California criteria require presence of:

a) 1. Dementia
    2. Evidence of two or more ischaemic strokes by:
        ■ History, neurological signs, and/or
        ■ Neuroimaging studies (CT or T1-weighted MRI) or
        ■ Occurrence of a single stroke with a clearly documented temporal relationship to the onset of dementia
    3. Evidence of one or more infarct outside the cerebellum by CT or T1-weighted MRI

b) Diagnosis of probable ischaemic VaD is supported by:
    1. Evidence of multiple infarcts in brain regions known to affect cognition (as defined by NINDS-AIREN criteria)
    2. History of multiple transient ischaemic attacks
    3. History of vascular risk factors (e.g., hypertension, heart disease, diabetes mellitus)
    4. Elevated Hachinski ischaemic scale score (7 or more)

c) Clinical features that are thought to be associated with ischaemic VaD but await further research:
    1. Relatively early appearance of gait disturbance and urinary incontinence

2. Periventricular and deep white matter changes on T2-weighted MRI, those that are excessive for age.
3. Focal changes in electroencephalographic studies.

d) Other clinical features that do not constitute strong evidence either for or against a diagnosis of probable ischaemic VaD
   1. Periods of slowly progressive symptoms
   2. Illusions, psychosis, hallucinations, delusions
   3. Seizures

e) Clinical features that cast on a diagnosis of probable ischaemic VaD
   1. Transcortical sensory aphasia in the absence of corresponding focal lesions on neuroimaging studies.
   2. Absence of central neurological symptoms/signs other than cognitive disturbance.

FRONTOTEMPORAL DEMENTIA

Diagnosing the various non-Alzheimer dementias can be a difficult process as a result of overlap in cognitive and behavioural symptoms. This is undoubtedly true for frontotemporal dementia (FTD). It is to be remembered that FTD is a clinical syndrome rather than a single disease with a unitary pathology. These patients have dysfunction of the brain's prefrontal regions, temporal lobes, or both. In many cases, there may be significant atrophy visible with magnetic resonance imaging specific to the affected regions; in other instances, the abnormalities may be functional rather than structural. Although some of these patients have Pick bodies, most do not. When predominantly temporal lobes are involved they can present with aphasia (semantic dementia).

ICD-10 Criteria

ICD-10 does not give separate diagnostic criteria for FTD. However, it provides diagnostic guidelines for dementia in Pick's disease. It is recognized to be a progressive dementia, commencing in middle life (usually between 50 and 60 years), characterized by slowly progressive changes of character and social deterioration, followed by impairment of intellect, memory, and language functions, with apathy, euphoria, and (occasionally) extrapyramidal phenomenon. The neuro-pathological picture is one of selective atrophy of the frontal and temporal lobes, but without the occurrence of neuritic plaques and neurofibrillary tangles in excess of that seen in normal aging. Cases with early onset tend to exhibit a more malignant course. The social and behavioural manifestation often precedes frank memory impairment.

The following features are required for a definite diagnosis:
a) A progressive dementia
b) A predominance of frontal lobe features with euphoria, emotional blunting, and   coarsening of social behaviour, disinhibition, and either apathy or restlessness.
c) Behavioural manifestations, which commonly precede frank memory impairment.

Frontal lobe features are more marked than temporal and parietal, unlike Alzheimer's disease. The DSM-IV also gives diagnostic guidelines for dementia due to Pick's disease.

Lund-Manchester Criteria

The Lund-Manchester criteria (The Lund and Manchester Groups, 1994) require the presence of at least two of the following features: loss of personal awareness, strange eating habits, perseveration, and mood change. In addition, patients had to have one or more of the following: frontal executive dysfunction, reduced speech, and preserved visuospatial ability. Other important supporting features are: onset before age 65, a family history of FTD, early urinary incontinence, motor neuron disease, and (in the late stages) akinesia, rigidity, and tremor.

Consensus Diagnostic Criteria

The Work Group on Frontotemporal Dementia and Pick's Disease recommended the following clinical criteria for FTD (Neary et al, 1998):
a) The development of behavioural or cognitive deficits manifested by either (1) early or progressive change in personality, characterized by difficulty in modulating behaviour, often resulting

in inappropriate responses or activities, or (2) early and progressive change in language, characterized by problems with expression of language or severe naming difficulty and problems with word meaning.

b) The deficits outlined in a1 or b1 cause significant impairment in social or occupational functioning and represent a significant decline from a previous level of functioning.

c) The course is characterized by a gradual onset and continuing decline in function.

d) The deficits outlined in a1 or b1 are not due to other nervous system conditions (e.g., cerebrovascular disease), systemic conditions (e.g., hypothyroidism), or substance-induced conditions.

e) The deficits do not occur exclusively during a delirium.

f) The disturbance is not better accounted for by a psychiatric diagnosis (e.g., depression).

DEMENTIA WITH LEWY BODIES

Since the late 1980s, research has revealed that beyond dementia of the Alzheimer's type and vascular dementia, a common cause of progressive dementia may be related to the presence of Lewy bodies in the brainstem and cerebral cortex. Lewy bodies are intracytoplasmic, spherical, eosinophilic neuronal inclusion bodies, scattered through the brainstem, subcortical nuclei, limbic cortex and neocortex (temporal > frontal/parietal). Parkinson's disease, in contrast, manifests Lewy bodies in the subcortical nuclei, in addition to degeneration of dopaminergic neurones in substantia nigra.

Consensus Criteria for the Clinical Diagnosis of Probable and Possible Dementia With Lewy Bodies (CDLB) (McKeith et al, 1996)

a) The central feature required for a diagnosis of dementia with Lewy bodies (DLB) is progressive cognitive decline of sufficient magnitude to interfere with normal social or occupational function.

Prominent or persistent memory impairment may not necessarily occur in the early stages but is usually evident with progression. Deficits on tests of attention and of frontal-subcortical skills and visuospatial ability may be especially prominent.

b) Two of the following core features are essential for a diagnosis of probable dementia with Lewy bodies, and one is essential for possible dementia with Lewy bodies:
   1. Fluctuating cognition with profound variations in attention and alertness
   2. Recurrent visual hallucinations that are typically well formed and detailed
   3. Spontaneous motor features of parkinsonism

c) Features supportive of the diagnosis are:
   1. Repeated fall
   2. Syncope
   3. Transient loss of consciousness
   4. Neuroleptic sensitivity
   5. Systematized delusions
   6. Hallucinations in other modalities

d) A diagnosis of dementia with Lewy bodies is less likely in the presence of:
   1. Stroke disease, evident as focal neurological signs or on brain imaging
   2. Evidence on physical examination and investigation of any physical illness or other brain disorder sufficient to account for the clinical picture.

EVALUATION AND CRITICISM OF VARIOUS DIAGNOSTIC CRITERIA

Many of the commonly used diagnostic criteria for dementia (particularly AD and VaD, the two most common types), have been evaluated for their sensitivity and specificity. Construct validity is well studied with supporting data from neuropsychology, MRI scan and autopsy studies. Though, the discriminative validity from healthy individuals is well known, the discriminative validity from the pre–AD syndromes and depression is still not clear. For example, strictly defined MCI, amnesic type, is better recognized as part of early AD (Morris et al., 2001). In a study, comparison of NINCDS-ADRDA criteria with CERAD (Consortium to Establish a Registry for Alzheimer's Disease) histopathological criteria for AD showed that combining "possible" and "probable AD" categories of NINCDS-ADRDA resulted in a high sensitivity and accuracy in diagnosing AD, but with a low specificity. The authors recommended that the "probable AD" category should alone be used to increase specificity (Hogervorst et al., 2000). The inter-rater reliability of AD, FTD and DLB has been measured in a study using the NINCDS-ADRDA, Lund-Manchester and the CDLB criteria respectively. The mean sensitivity of AD, FTD and DLB were 95%, 97% and 34% respectively, but the mean specificity were 79%, 97% and 94% respectively, indicating a low sensitivity for CDLB to diagnose DLB (Lopez et al, 1999). In a community-based postmortem study, it was found that current clinical diagnostic criteria (NINCDS-ADRDA, NINDS-AIREN and CDLB) may be good at detecting pathology, but not at detecting pure pathology. Thus, a large proportion from the general population fulfilling probable NINCDS-ADRDA, probable NINDS-AIREN and probable CDLB will have mixed pathology (up to 33.8%) (Holmes et al, 1999). In a comparative study of different diagnostic criteria of VaD, it was found that different diagnostic guidelines of VaD pickup different groups of patients (Wetterling et al, 1996). The following reasons were given for the discrepancy:

1. Different criteria of "dementia" used in various criteria
2. ADDTC criteria restricting to only ischaemic VaD
3. DSM-IV criteria not differentiating VaD subtype on the basis of CT or MRI finding, and
4. Multifactorial aetiopathology of VaD

The quality standards subcommittee of the American Academy of Neurology recommended some guidelines in this regard. The DSM-III-R (Diagnostic and Statistical Manual of Mental Disorders, third revised edition) (American Psychiatric Association, 1987) definition of "Dementia of Alzheimer Type" and the NINCDS-ADRDA definition of "probable AD" were found to be on average 81% sensitive. As far as VaD goes, the recent view is that rather than simply stating vascular dementia present or absent, judgement should be made about amount of vascular pathology present, ranging from "none" to "pure" and correlating it with cognitive symptoms (which may be difficult, requiring knowledge and experience). The HIS is probably more suitable for identifying majority of the patients with VaD, while the NINDS-AIREN and the ADDTC criteria have much lower sensitivity (Knopman et al, 2001). A recent prevalence study from Japan in geriatric population showed that the prevalence of VaD is less common than that of AD/mixed dementia, contrary to what was thought earlier (Meguro et al, 2002). It was probably because of over-inclusion of white matter lesions in MRI as evidence of "vascular pathology". Clinical dilemma associated with mixed pathology has also been reported in India. In a tertiary care hospital in south India, out of 39 patients admitted in psychiatry ward over 12 years, it was found that a differential diagnosis of other dementia was considered along with dementia due to AD in one-third of the cases. Most frequently associated category was vascular dementia, about one-third of all other dementia types (Kar et al, 2000).

At present, functional imaging studies of the brain are not recommended for routine diagnosis of dementia. Sensitivity of SPECT (Single Photon Emission Computed Tomography) scan has been found to be lower than that of clinical diagnosis. PET (Positron Emission Tomography) scanning may have a promise for use as an adjunct to clinical diagnosis. Biological markers such as CSF (cerebrospinal fluid) β (beta)-amyloid and tau for inclusion as adjunct to diagnosis require further study (Knopman et al, 2001).

CONCLUSION

The various diagnostic criteria used in detection of different dementia syndromes have different purposes for which they have been designed and, therefore, have different degrees of sensitivity and specificity. Future research should focus on clarifying the difficulties in defining "dementia" and differential diagnosis of various syndromes, particularly AD, VaD and DLB precisely. Clinicians should be able to predict development of AD on the basis of functional imaging or biological markers.

REFERENCES

- Alexopoulos GS, Meyers BS, Young RC et al. (1993) The course of geriatric depression with "reversible dementia": a controlled study. *Am J Psychiatry,* 150, 1693–1699.
- American Psychiatric Association (1987) *Diagnostic and Statistical Manual of Mental Disorders,* 3rd revised edition, Washington DC: American Psychiatric Association.
- American Psychiatric Association (1994) *Diagnostic and Statistical Manual of Mental Disorders,* 4th edition, Washington DC: American Psychiatric Association.
- Bischkopf J, Busse A, Angermeyer MC (2002) Mild cognitive impairment- a review of prevalence, incidence and outcome according to current approaches. *Acta Psychiatr Scand,* 106, 403–414.
- Chui HC, Victoroff JI, Margolin D et al. (1992) Criteria for the diagnosis of ischaemic vascular dementia proposed by the State of California Alzheimer's Disease Diagnostic and Treatment Centers. *Neurology,* 42, 473–480.
- Evans DA, Funkenstein HH, Albert MS, et al. (1989) Prevalence of Alzheimer's disease in a community population of older persons: Higher than previously reported. *JAMA,* 262, 2551–6.
- Hachinski VC, Iliff LD, Zilhka E et al. (1975) Cerebral blood flow in dementia. *Arch Neurol,* 32, 632–637.
- Hogervorst E, Barnetson L, Jobst KA et al. (2000) Diagnosing dementia: interrater reliability assessment and accuracy of the NINCDS/ADRDA criteria versus CERAD histopathological criteria for Alzheimer's disease. *Dement Geriatr Cogn Disord,* 11, 107–113.
- Holmes C, Cairns N, Lantos P et al. (1999) Validity of current clinical criteria for Alzheimer's disease, vascular dementia and dementia with Lewy bodies. *Br J Psychiatry,* 174, 45–50.
- Kar N, Sengupta S, Sharma PSVN (2000) Diagnosing dementia due to Alzheimer's disease. *Indian J Psychiatry,* 42, 267–270.
- Knopman DS, DeKosky ST, Cummings JL et al. (2001) Practice parameter: diagnosis of dementia (an evidence based review) - report of the quality standards subcommittee of the American Academy of Neurology. *Neurology,* 56, 1143–1153.
- Loeb C, Gandolfo C (1983) Diagnostic evaluation of degenerative and vascular dementia. *Stroke,* 14, 399–401.
- Lopez OL, Litvan I, Catt KE et al. (1999) Accuracy of four clinical diagnostic criteria for the diagnosis of neurodegenerative dementias. *Neurology,* 53, 1292–1299.

- Mckeith IG, Galasko D, Kosaka K et al. (1996) Consensus guidelines for the clinical and pathologic diagnosis of dementia with Lewy bodies (DLB): report of the consortium on DLB international workshop. *Neurology*, 47, 1113–1124.
- Mckhann G, Drachman D, Folstein M et al. (1984) Clinical diagnosis of Alzheimer's disease: report of the NINCDS-ADRDA Work Group under the auspices of Department of Health and Human Services Task Force on Alzheimer's disease. *Neurology*, 12, 939–944.
- Meguro K, Ishi H, Yamaguchi S et al. (2002) Prevalence of dementia and dementing diseases in Japan - the Tajiri Project. *Arch Neurol*, 59, 1109–1114.
- Morris JC, Storandt M, Miller JP et al. (2001) Mild cognitive impairment represents early-stage Alzheimer disease. *Arch Neurol*, 58, 1705–1706.
- Neary D, Snowden JS, Gustafson I et al. (1998) Frontotemporal lobar degeneration: a consensus on clinical diagnostic criteria. *Neurology*, 51, 1546–1554.
- Roman GC, Tatemichi TK, Erkinjuntti T et al. (1993) Vascular dementia: diagnostic criteria for research studies. Report of the NINDS-AIREN international workshop. *Neurology*, 43, 250–260.
- Small GW (1985). Revised Ischemic Score for diagnosing multi-infarct dementia. *J Clin Psychiatry*, 46, 514–517.
- The Lund and Manchester Groups (1994) Clinical and neuropathological criteria for frontotemporal dementia. *J Neurol Neurosurg Psychiatry*, 57, 416–418.
- Wetterling T, Kanitz RD, Borgis KJ (1996) Comparison of different diagnostic criteria for vascular dementia (ADDTC, DSM-IV, ICD-10, NINDS-AIREN). *Stroke*, 27, 30–36.
- World Health Organization (1992) *The ICD-10 Classification of Mental and Behavioural Disorders. Clinical Descriptions and Diagnostic Guidelines.* Geneva: World Health Organization.

4

Behavioural & Psychological Symptoms of Dementia

Nilamadhab Kar

INTRODUCTION

For decades, the cognitive paradigm has prevented the adequate mapping of the non-cognitive symptoms of dementia and hindered research (Berrios, 1989), even though, behaviour changes, paranoid delusions, hallucinations and long periods of screaming were described by Alzheimer in 1907 in his original case description of the disease (Deutsch and Rovner, 1991).

International Classification of Mental and Behavioural Disorders Diagnostic Criteria for Research (ICD-10-DCR) (WHO, 1992) requires decline in emotional control or motivation, or a change in social behaviour manifesting as emotional lability, irritability, apathy and coarsening of social behaviour as one of the diagnostic criteria for dementia. This gives credence to behvaioural and psychological symptoms of dementia (BPSD) as an essential component of dementia syndrome. These often influence the diagnostic process for dementia, especially their subtyping (Kar et al, 2000).

BPSDs are often the reasons for which the consultation is sought (Deutsch and Rovner, 1991), and often the reason for the first contact of a dementia patient with the health care professionals. They are a cause of concern to the caregivers and are often more difficult to cope with than cognitive changes (Rabins et al, 1982). They are often the cause of institutionalization of dementia patients (Steele et al., 1990). Inappropriate behaviour (constant restlessness, crying, screaming, fearfulness etc.) is not a normal state of being for dementia patients; it is an altered state of being and is sometimes the only way a dementia patient can convey distress (Cheong, 2004).

It may be stressed that most of these noncognitive abnormalities, which increase the morbidity of patients and burden of caregivers (Morgan et al., 1997; Cohen-Mansfield, 2004), are treatable. These symptoms are a major cause of diminished quality of life for both patients and caregivers (Wynn and Cummings, 2004; and Kar et al., 2001). Periodic assessment of these symptoms can measure the effectiveness of pharmacological and environmental interventions in dementia (Deutsch and Rovner, 1991; Kluger and Ferris, 1991).

PREVALENCE

Though all dementia patients have noncognitive symptoms, one of the reasons for different prevalence figures in different studies is the methodology and definitions used. In one study, caregivers reported an average of 10 problems for each patient out of a 48-item behavioural problem checklist (Stern et al, 1991). Almost all patients with Alzheimer's disease (AD) develop 'noncognitive neuropsychiatric symptoms (NPS) at some point during the course of their illness (Lyketsos and Lee, 2004). Lifetime risk of neuropsychiatric disturbances is nearly 100% (Lyketsos et al, 2000). Depression is most common, affecting up to 50% of patients (Lyketsos and Lee, 2004). On a cross sectional evaluation, 60% had at least one symptom (Lyketsos et al, 2000). Tariot et al (1994) reported that up to 90% of patients develop behavioural problems. However, if the whole range of BPSD are studied, all patients with dementia exhibit those during the course of their illness.

Behavioural and psychological symptoms of dementia, also known as 'neuropsychiatric symptoms', 'behavioural disturbances', and 'noncognitive mental disturbances' affect over 80% of patients with AD, a prevalence that is 3–4 times higher than that seen in comparably aged persons without dementia (Lyketsos et al, 2002). These neuropsychiatric symptoms appear to cluster into at least two syndromes: a psychotic syndrome and an affective syndrome (Lyketsos et al., 2001). The psychotic syndrome may affect as many as 15–20% of patients in any given month, and the 'affective syndrome' may affect as many as 25–30% of patients (Lytetsos and Lee, 2004). Other studies report 41% of AD patients having delusions, 33% having persecutory types and 33% having misidentification syndromes (Deutsch and Rovner, 1991).

Prevalence of a major depressive episode in AD is 20–25%, with other depressive syndromes, including minor depression affecting an additional 20–30% of patients. Consortium to establish a registry for AD (CERAD) suggested that the clinical features as reported by informants are personality change in 47.5%, depressive manifestation in 23.0% and impaired ADL in 77% besides the cognitive deficits.

TYPES OF BPSD

Major BPSDs are listed below for comprehension. This is not an exhaustive list.

Table 4.1 A list of behavioural and psychological symptoms of dementia

Motor behaviour
- Agitation
- Hypermetamorphosis
- Hyperorality
- Hyperphagia
- Passivity, inactivity
- Physical aggression
- Restlessness
- Violence
- Wandering

Social interactions
- Decreased interaction
- Disinhibited behaviour
- Insensitive behaviour
- Lack of restraint
- Socially inappropriate behaviour
- Verbal aggression

contd.

- Withdrawn
- Sexual misadventure

Speech
- Decreased talk
- Increased talk
- Almost mute
- Muttering
- Screaming

Mood and anxiety disturbances
- Anger
- Anxiety
- Apathy
- Catastrophic reaction
- Decreased interest
- Emotional lability
- Euphoria
- Fear
- Frequent crying
- Irritability
- Phobias
- Reduced initiative
- Sadness

Thought disturbances
- Death wishes
- Delusions of persecution
- Delusions of misidentification
- Depressive cognitions
- Marked suspiciousness
- Misinterpretation
- Paranoid ideas
- Suicidal ideas

Perceptual disturbances
- Auditory hallucinations
- Visual hallucinations

Personality changes
- Increasingly passive

contd.

- Less responsive, active and cheerful
- Self-centered behaviour
- Individual characteristics blunted
- Obsessional traits exaggerated
- Personality: it appears 'there is not any'

Biological functions
- Disturbed sleep
- Decreased appetite
- Incontinence of urine
- Incontinence of stool
- Urination at inappropriate places –
- Defecation at inappropriate places
- Excessive dependency for needs

Physical infirmity
- Complaining of pain
- Generalized weakness
- Remaining bedridden
- Dependency for hygiene maintenance

There are a few attempts to subtype certain groups of BPSDs. Inappropriate behaviours have been divided into four main subtypes: physically aggressive behaviour, such as hitting, kicking or biting; physically non-aggressive behaviour, such as pacing or inappropriately handling objects; verbally non-aggressive agitation, such as constant repetition of sentences or requests; and verbal aggression such as cursing or screaming (Cohen-Mansfield, 2004).

Motor Behaviour

Agitation
Cohen-Mansfield and Billig (1986) defined agitation as 'inappropriate verbal, vocal, or motor activity unexplained by apparent needs or confusion'. The term 'inappropriate' may refer to abusive or aggressive behaviour, to the frequency of behaviour, or to its relation to social standards. Commonly observed agitated behaviours are general restlessness, pacing, complaining, repetitive sentences, negativism, requests

for attention, cursing and verbal aggression. Agitation is common in dementias and has a marked impact on caregivers (Senanarong et al., 2004). The frequency of agitation in patients with Alzheimer's disease has been reported as 24% and 48% (Deutsch and Rovner, 1991; Reisberg et al., 1987).

Physical violence and hitting occurs in approximately 30% (Reisberg et al., 1987) of patients with dementia of Alzheimer's type. Premorbid history of aggression, troubled premorbid relationship between caregiver and patient, and a greater number of patient problems are predictors of aggressive behaviour.

Screaming: Behavioural oddities like screaming (Deutsch and Rovner, 1991) are seen in almost 25% of nursing home residents. It is often associated with toileting and bathing, severe cognitive impairment and high degree of dependency.

Wandering
Wandering is reported in 3 to 26% of outpatients of Alzheimer's disease. Four types of wandering patterns have been described: exit-seekers, self-stimulators, akathesiacs and modelers. Exit-seekers attempt to leave; self-stimulators may manipulate the door as an activity rather than for the purpose of leaving; akathesiacs show restlessness, pacing and fidgeting; and modelers follow other people around and may leave the building only to follow another person. It has been found that elderly wanderers have language impairment, disorientation and hyperactivity compared to non-wanderers; on the other hand, wanderers exhibit better social skills, are less withdrawn (Deutsch and Rovner, 1991).

Other symptoms include: Hyperorality (tendency to touch and examine objects with mouth), hypermetamorphosis (tendency to contact and touch every object in sight) and hyperphagia.

Extreme Dependency
High degree of dependency for activities of daily living is marked (Deutsch and Rovner, 1991). Dependency for excretory functions

and hygiene maintenance come as a burden to caregivers. Besides physical infirmity, various cognitive disabilities contribute to this dependency.

Mood Disturbances

Depression

Depression is commonly overlooked in dementia patients as it does not have a typical presentation – often there is a lack of sad or depressed affect or mood. The aphasic patient is often unable to articulate the subjective experience of being depressed (Cheong, 2004).

Other predominant mood disturbances are anxiety and fear. Emotional lability, explosive emotional outbursts, weeping or laughing are also seen (Lishman, 1987). Fatuous euphoria or apathy, elevated mood, inappropriate laughter have also been described.

Apathy

Apathy, a syndrome of decreased initiation and motivation, decreased social engagement, emotional indifference and diminished reactivity, and lack of persistence, affects over 70% of individuals with Alzheimer's disease in the mild to moderate stages and over 90% of patients in the later stages; and is the most common neuropsychiatric symptom reported in AD patients (Boyle and Malloy, 2004). The diagnosis of apathy in AD requires the differentiation between loss of initiation versus the loss of ability and emotional indifference versus a primary mood disturbance (e.g., depression). Apathy is underdiagnosed in AD, but is distinct from depression and can be reliably identified in AD patients (Landes et al, 2001). Distinction of the syndrome of apathy as mentioned above from depression is to be made considering dysphoria, hopelessness, guilt, self-criticism, suicidal ideation, sleep problems and appetite disturbances associated with the latter (Boyle and Malloy, 2004). However, overlapping symptoms like lack of interest in events and activities, anergia, psychomotor retardation and fatigue may make the differentiation difficult. Apathy can be assessed by Neuropsychiatric Inventory (NPI) (Cummings et al, 1994 and Cummings, 1997), the Frontal Systems Behaviour Inventory (FrSBe) (Grace and Malloy, 2001), the Apathy Evaluation Scale (AES) (Marin et al, 1991) and the Apathy Inventory (AI) (Robert et al, 2002).

Changes in Personality

Passivity, coarsening of affect and decreased spontaneity, inactivity, feelings of insecurity, less cheerfulness and responsiveness are common. Loss of socialization, companionship, and irritability are also seen.

Psychotic Features

Examples of common psychotic features are given in Table 4.2. Paranoid delusions, especially persecutory type, are commonly seen. Often these are the cause for violent behaviour, agitation and combativeness.

Table 4.2 Common psychotic features in patients with dementia

Delusions
- Persecutory (someone is stealing things, someone is present in the room, someone is living inappropriately in the home (phantom boarder), someone is mishandling personal finances, someone is planning to harm physically)
- Infidelity
- Hypochondriacal delusion
- Delusional zoopathy (worm infestation)
- Dead relatives are still alive
- Erotomania
- Ongoing daily work (different from previous occupation)

Misidentification symptoms
- Capgras syndrome (e.g., spouse is an imposter, caregivers are different persons)
- Strangers are family members or vice versa
- Television images are real
- Personal image in a mirror is a different person
- Misidentifying home (not recognizing own home, demanding to go home when already at home)

Hallucinations
- Auditory
- Visual

(Lishman, 1987; Sultzer, 2004; Kar et al., 1998 and 2001)

Social Behaviour

Changes of social behaviour, reduced initiative and drive, grossly insensitive behaviour, lack of restraint, sexual misadventure, indolence, foolish jokes and pranks (Lishman, 1987) have been described.

Sleep Problems

Nighttime and early morning awakenings are common. Sleep disturbance and daytime behavioural problems are related whereas it is not related to score of language or visuospatial performance, activities of daily living or MMSE. Subjects with AD are more likely to have sleep apnoea compared to normal or depressed elders (Deutsch and Rovner, 1991).

TYPES OF DEMENTIA AND BPSD

Alzheimer's Dementia

In early stages of dementia of Alzheimer's type passivity, aspontaneity and reduced initiative have been described (Deutsch and Rovner, 1991), which may get interpreted as depression. Wandering, abusiveness, harming self due to clumsiness or accident, restlessness, agitation, repetitive futile behaviour, psychotic features, sleep disturbance, loss of control, personality change have been reported in senile dementia of Alzheimer's type (Lishman, 1987; Deutsch and Rovner, 1991).

In 178 Alzheimer's patients, Burns and Levy (1992) found hallucinations (17%) at some time, visual being slightly more common than auditory. Misidentification (30%), failing to recognize others (12%), believing events in television to be real (6%), failing to recognize self in the mirror (4%) and belief that others are there in the house (17%) were also observed. Delusions at some point were noticed in 16%, usually with simple delusions of suspicion or theft; paranoid ideations were noticed in 20%. At least one symptom of depression was there in two-thirds. Only 4% had elevated mood. Those who complained of depression were less cognitively impaired than those who did not.

Behavioural symptoms occurred more frequently as the severity of dementia increased (Teri et al., 1988). Aggression (20%), wandering (19%), incontinence (48%), and at least one symptom of Kluver-Bucy syntrome was found in 72%, namely misrecognition (44%), apathy (41%), rage (36%), hypermetamorphosis (31%), binge eating (10%), sexual disinhibition (7%) or hyperorality (6%).

Inability to recognize relatives or self in mirror, strong tendencies to examine and touch objects with mouth (hyperorality) and tendencies to be stimulus bound to contact and touch every object in sight (hyper-metamorphosis), indiscriminate eating of any material available and excessive eating (hyperphagia) have been described (Sourander and Sjogren, 1970; Lishman, 1987).

Patients of dementia of Alzheimer's disease may have a different profile of BPSD than that of patients with other dementia. Table 4.3 presents the difference in a sample of inpatients (Kar et al., 1998).

Table 4.3 Prevalence of behavioural and psychiatric symptoms in dementia inpatients in an Indian population

	Alzheimer's dementia (n=24)	Other dementias (n=15)
Motor behaviour		
■ Physical aggression*	12.5	40.0
■ Restlessness	33.3	26.7
■ Wandering	25.0	20.0
■ Passivity, inactivity	33.3	46.7
Social interactions		
■ Verbal aggression	33.3	33.3
■ Decreased interaction	33.3	33.3
■ Withdrawn	20.8	26.6
■ Socially inappropriate behaviour*	8.3	33.3
■ Disinhibited behaviour	12.5	13.3
Speech		
■ Decreased talk	54.2	26.6
■ Increased talk	8.3	13.3
■ Almost mute	8.3	13.3
■ Muttering	37.5	20.0

contd.

	Alzheimer's dementia (n=24)	Other dementias (n=15)
Mood disturbances		
▪ Irritability	33.3	40.0
▪ Sadness	29.2	33.3
▪ Decreased interest	25.0	26.6
▪ Anxiety	20.8	13.3
▪ Frequent crying	12.5	13.3
▪ Fear	16.7	6.7
Thought disturbances		
▪ Persecution	25.0	13.3
▪ Death wishes	12.5	13.3
▪ Suicidal ideas	20.8	13.3
▪ Depressive cognitions	12.5	6.7
Biological functions		
▪ Disturbed sleep**	70.8	26.6
▪ Decreased appetite	58.3	26.6
▪ Incontinence of urine	25.0	46.7
▪ Incontinence of stool	12.5	13.3
▪ Urination at inappropriate places	12.5	20.0
▪ Defecation at inappropriate places	8.3	20.0
Physical infirmity		
▪ Complaining of pain	8.3	20.0
▪ Generalized weakness	16.7	13.3
▪ Remaining bedridden	4.2	13.3
▪ Needs supervision for hygiene maintenance	29.2	26.6
▪ Needs complete care for hygiene maintenance	25.0	33.3

*The study sample was inpatients at psychiatric ward, Kasturba Hospital, Manipal, India. Figures are in percentages; *p<0.05, ** p<0.01.*

In this study, lesser frequency of physical violence and socially inappropriate behaviour in patients of AD in comparison to those of other dementias assumes significance. The duration of illness in both groups being comparable, the findings that the patients of AD were significantly older, have later age of onset and have more gradual onset may explain the above, allowing time for adjustment to the deteriorating cognitive functions. However, the differences may result from loss of ability to modulate affect and behaviour and may be directly related to the disease process.

Lewy Body Dementia

Visual hallucinations are more commonly found in Lewy body dementia than Alzheimer's and are more complex, vivid and rapidly moving. Auditory hallucinations, persecutory delusions are also present. These fluctuate in their severity and become more at night. Depression is significantly more common in these patients (Lishman, 1987).

Vascular Dementia

It is well known that intracerebral vascular events result in not only cognitive deficits, but also other psychiatric symptoms, mostly anxiety and depression (Kar and John, 2003). Common early features of vascular dementia include many somatic symptoms such as headache, dizziness, tinnitus, and syncope (Lishman, 1987). As in vascular dementia, capacity for judgement and a remarkable degree of insight is sometimes maintained for a long time; patient often reacts to the awareness of decline by extreme anxiety and depression, which are seldom present in AD. Lability and explosive emotional outbursts are also present. Episodes of noisy weeping or laughing may occur on minor provocation, often without accompanying subjective distress or elation (Lishman, 1987).

Pick's Dementia

The distinctive early features include changes of character and social behaviour rather than impairment of memory and intellect. Diminished drive, grossly insensitive behaviour, lack of restraint leading to stealing, odd manner, sexual misadventure, indulgence in foolish jokes and pranks, alcoholism, and other social misconduct are seen. Mood remains as a fatuous euphoria or apathetic may be interspersed with brief periods of restless overactivity. Delusions and hallucinations are relatively rare. Oral tendencies, overeating, tendencies to touch and seize objects within the field of vision appear early in contrast to AD where these appear late.

Dementia due to Huntington's Disease

Emotional disturbance is more prominent as a premonitory feature (Lishman, 1987). Change of disposition and paranoia are also seen. Often psychiatric changes are present for some considerable time before chorea or intellectual impairment develops. A change in personality, patient becoming morose and quarrelsome, or slowed, apathetic, and neglectful of home and person is often observed. These are well-recognized premonitory symptoms. Paranoid developments may be earliest change, with marked sensitivity and ideas of reference. Sometimes a florid schizophrenic or paraphrenic illness may be present for years before the Huntington's disease becomes clearly apparent. Delusions of persecution, religiosity, reference and grandiosity are common. Depression, sometimes recurrent depressive psychosis, and anxiety may be marked from the outset. There are reports of severe personality change (Lishman, 1987).

Creutzfeldt-Jakob Disease

A prodromal stage is described, which lasts for weeks or months characterized by neurasthenic symptoms. Fatigue, insomnia, anxiety, depression, mental slowness and unpredictability of behaviour are the usual complaints. Occasionally, mood is mildly elevated with loquacity and inappropriate laughter. Bouts of uncontrollable laughing and crying may be seen due to brain stem involvement. Episodes of delirium are common. Auditory hallucinations and delusions may be marked (Lishman, 1987).

Alcoholic Dementia

Profound social disorganization, deterioration of personality have been described (Lishman, 1987).

AETIOLOGY OF BPSD

Three theoretical models help in understanding the behavioural disturbances of the dementia patients and guide the non-pharmacological intervention. They are: 'unmet needs' model; a behavioural/learning model; and an environmental vulnerability/reduced stress-threshold model (Cohen-Mansfield, 2004).

Often the needs are not apparent to the observer or the caregiver, or the caregivers do not feel able to fulfill these needs. Most dementia patients suffer from sensory deprivation, boredom and loneliness. Therefore, providing sensory stimulation, activities, and social contacts are among the most commonly described interventions. For example, provision of hearing aids, an easily accessible outdoor area can improve sensory stimulation and activity. Reduced level of restraint, sufficient level of light, good toileting procedures, better communication, prompt and proper treatment of pain are other needs (Cohen-Mansfield, 2004). Unmet biological, social and psychological needs lead to discomfort and distress, and in a background of impaired cognitive state and ineffective communication, these often manifest as behavioural and psychological symptoms.

Many problem behaviours are learned through reinforcement by caregivers or staff members, who provide attention when problem behaviour is displayed. A modification of reinforcement contingencies is needed to change the behaviour.

It is known that these noncognitive abnormalities frequently arise possibly from the intensive approach to care where patients are stressed beyond their cognitive capabilities. Severity of cognitive impairment is associated with increased frequency and number of behavioural problems, whereas age, gender and duration of illness are not (Deutsch and Rovner, 1991). Agitation has been clearly linked to dementia severity (Senanarong et al., 2004). They may also be due to brain-damaged state or specific psychiatric syndromes or symptoms (Deutsch and Rovner, 1991). Agitation has been proved to be related to specific types of associated psychopathology implicating frontal lobe dysfunction (Senanarong et al., 2004).

It is assumed that dementia process results in greater vulnerability to the environment, and a lower threshold at which stimuli affect behaviour. Therefore, a stimulus that may be appropriate for a cognitively intact person may result in overreaction in the cognitively impaired person. Persons with dementia progressively lose their coping abilities and therefore perceive their environment as more and more stressful (Hall, 1994). This results in anxiety and inappropriate behaviour.

BPSD has also been linked to premorbid personality adjustment. Dementia accompanied by florid paranoid or affective symptoms is associated with abnormal personality earlier in life; persons with simple downward course were found to have been more stable (Post, 1944; Lishman, 1988).

Apathy is one of the primary manifestations of frontal lobe dysfunction and AD-related apathy is thought to reflect the interaction between cholinergic deficiency and neuropathological changes in frontal brain regions (Boyle and Malloy, 2004).

Cultural Variation

Most of the patients in India are taken care of by their own family members at home, not in a dementia care set up or old age home. In a typical Indian family, elders are loved, respected and are taken care of. The caregivers are often unaware of the nature of the illness.

Comparing to Western reports, Kar et al (2001) found similar noncognitive problems in dementia patients in India. The frequency of restlessness and wandering were comparable. While physical violence was more commonly reported than verbal aggression by Reisberg et al (1987), Kar et al (2001) found it reversed in their sample. Screaming was reported in almost 25% of nursing home residents (Deutsch and Rovner, 1991), but was not observed in Indian patients; similarly, compared to reported figures (Deutsch and Rovner, 1991) passivity was observed in fewer persons in the latter.

Though one in five persons in the study by Kar et al (2001) felt persecuted, the frequency was less than that (33%) reported by Deutsch and Rovner (1991). However, it remained the most common theme as observed by Wragg et al (1991). This can often be a risk factor for violent aggressive behaviour. Hallucinations were not common in the sample compared to around 25% as reported by Deutsch and Rovner (1991).

Death wishes and suicidal ideas are common in dementia patients. A considerable proportion of Indian patients expressing these thoughts is possibly reflective of death accepting attitude of the Indian culture

(Kar et al, 2001). There remains a considerable risk for suicide attempt by the demented persons everywhere, at least in earlier stages.

ASSESSMENT

Assessment of the noncognitive problems is important as they may be associated with rapid rate of disease progression (Mortimer et al., 1992) or signify severity of morbidity. The stress of the caregiver is increased by the behavioural disturbances and these are often the cause for which demented patients come in contact of psychiatric services. These disturbances may predict the institutional placement (Steele et al, 1990; Rubin et al, 1989). Assessment of the status of noncognitive abnormalities in dementia presents particular difficulty since both cognitive deficits and lack of insight may make the history from patients unreliable. Most scales in use for the assessment of noncognitive features depend upon interviews with caregivers (Allen et al, 1996).

Some Scales that can Help in Assessing BPSD

- Apathy Evaluation Scale (AES) (Marin et al, 1991)
- Beck Depression Inventory (BDI) (Beck et al, 1961)
- Behavioural Rating Scale for Geriatric Patients (van der Kam, et al, 1971)
- Behaviour Pathology in Alzheimer's Disease Rating Scale (BEHAVE-AD) (Reisberg et al, 1987)
- Behavioural Rating Scales for Dementia of the Consortium to Establish a Registry for Alzheimer's Disease behaviour (Tarriot et al, 1995)
- Brief Psychiatric Rating Scale (BPRS) (Overall and Gorham, 1962)
- Clinical Global Impression of Severity (CGI-S) and of Change (CGI-C) (Guy, 1976)
- Cohen-Mansfield Agitation Inventory (CMAI): a 29-item questionnaire rated by caregivers (Cohen-Mansfield et al, 1989).
- Cornell Scale for Depression in Dementia (CSDD) (Alexopoulos et al, 1988)
- Frontal Systems Behaviour Inventory (FrSBe) (Grace and Malloy, 2001)
- Geriatric Depression Scale (GDS) (Yesavage, 1988)
- Hamilton Depression Rating Scale (HAM-D) (Hamilton, 1960)

- Montgomery-Asberg Depression Rating Scale (Montgomery and Asberg, 1979)
- Neuropsychiatric Inventory (NPI) (Cummings et al, 1994; Cummings, 1997)
- Neuropsychiatric Inventory – Nursing Home version (NPI-NH) (Wood et al, 2000)
- The Apathy Inventory (AI) (Robert et al, 2002).
- A new scale for the assessment of depressed mood in demented patients (Sunderland et al, 1988)

CONCLUSION

Noncognitive abnormalities in many areas are commonly present in patients with dementia and are useful in differential diagnostic process. They affect quality of life of patient and caregivers. Presence of these should be systematically probed as management of these is expected to improve the biopsychosocial function of these patients and decrease the burden of caregivers. These have immense relevance for home-based service of the demented patients. Details of their management are given in a different chapter of this book.

REFERENCES

- Alexopoulos GS, Abrams RC, Young RC, Shamoian CA (1988) Cornell scale for depression in dementia. *Biol Psychiatry,* 23, 271–284.
- Allen NHP, Gordon S, Hope T, Burns A. (1996) Manchester and Oxford Universities Scale for the Psychopathological Assessment of Dementia (MOUSEPAD). *British Journal of Psychiatry,* 169, 293–307.
- Beck T, Ward CH, Mendelson M, et al (1961) An inventory for measuring depression. *Arch Gen Psychiatry,* 4, 561–585.
- Berrios GE. (1989) Noncognitive symptoms and diagnosis of dementia. historical and clinical aspects. *British Journal of Psychiatry,* 154 (Suppl. 4), 11–16.
- Boyle PA and Malloy PF (2004) Treating apathy in Alzheimer's disease. *Dementia and Geriatric Cognitive Disorders,* 17, 91–99.
- Burns A and Levy R (1992) Clinical diversity in Late Onset Alzheimer's Disease, *Maudsley Monograph No 34.* Oxford: Oxford University Press.

- Cheong JA (2004) An evidence-based approach to the management of agitation in the geriatric patient. *Focus: The Lifelong Learning in Psychiatry,* 2, 197–205.
- Cohen-Mansfield J (2004) Nonpharmacologic interventions for inappropriate behaviours in dementia: A review, summary, and critique. *Focus: The Journal of Lifelong Learning in Psychiatry,* 2, 288–308.
- Cohen-Mansfield J and Billig N (1986) Agitated behaviour in the elderly. 1. A conceptual review. *J Am Geriatr Soc,* 34, 711–721.
- Cohen-Mansfield J, Marx MS, Rosenthal AS. (1989) A description of agitation in nursing home. *J Gerontology,* 44 (3), M77–84.
- Cummings JL (1997) The Neuropsychiatric Inventory: Assessing psychopathology in dementia patients. *Neurology,* 48(5 suppl 6), S10–S16.
- Cummings JL, Mega M, Gray K, et al (1994) The Neuropsychiatric Inventory: Comprehensive assessment of psychopathology in dementia patients. *Neurology,* 44, 2308–2314.
- Deutsch LH, Rovner BW. (1991) Agitation and other noncognitive abnormalities in Alzheimer's disease. *The Psychiatric Clinics of North America,* 14 (2), 341–351.
- Gauthier S, Fedman H, Hecker J, et al. (2002) Efficacy of donepezil on behavioural symptoms in patients with moderate to severe Alzheimer's disease. *Int Psychogeriatr,* 14, 389–404.
- Grace J and Malloy PF. (2001) *Frontal System Behaviour Scale (FrSBe): Professional Manual.* Lutz: Psychological Assessment Resources.
- Guy W (ed) (1976) *ECDEU Assessment Manual for Psychopharmacology, Revised.* Rockville: National Institute of Mental Health.
- Hall GR (1994) Caring for people with Alzheimer's disease using the conceptual model of progressively lowered stress threshold in the clinical setting. *Nurs Clin North Am,* 29, 129–141.
- Hamilton MA. (1960) A rating scale for depression. *J Neurol Neurosurg Psychiatry,* 23, 56–62.
- Kar N and John SP (2003) Site of stroke: Correlation with cognitive deficits, symptoms of anxiety and depression, amd quality of life. *Indian Journal of Psychiatry,* 45 (4), 218–220.
- Kar N, Sengupta S, Sharma PSVN. (2000) Diagnosing dementia due to Alzheimer's disease: Clinical perspective. *Indian Journal of Psychiatry,* 42, 267–270.
- Kar N, Sengupta S, Sharma PSVN. (1998) Noncognitive abnormalities in dementia. Paper presented at 14th International Conference of Alzheimer's Disease International, September 24–27, at Cochin.

- Kar N, Sharma PSVN, Sengupta S. (2001) Behavioural and psychological symptoms in dementia – clinical features in an Indian population. *Int J Geriatr Psychiatry,* 16, 540–541.
- Kluger A, Ferris SH. (1991) Scales for the assessment of Alzheimer's disease. *Psychiatric Clinics of North America,* 14, 309–326.
- Landes AM, Sperry SD, Strauss ME, Geldmacher DS. (2001) Apathy in Alzheimer's disease. *J Am Geriatr Soc,* 49, 1700–1707.
- Lishman WA. (1987) *Organic Psychiatry, The Psychological Consequences of Cerebral Disorder.* Oxford: Blackwell Scientific Publication.
- Lyketsos CG, Olin J. (2002) Depression in Alzheimer's disease: Overview and Treatment. *Biological Psychiatry,* 52, 243–252.
- Lyketsos CG, Sheppard JM, Steinberg M, et al. (2001) Neuropsychiatric disturbance in Alzheimer's disease cluster into three groups: The Cache County Study. *International Journal of Geriatric Psychiatry,* 16, 1043–1053.
- Lyketsos CG, Steinberg M, Tschanz JT, Norton MC, Steffens DC, Breitner JC (2000) Mmental and behavioral disturbances in dementia: Findings from the Cache County Study on Memory in Aging. *American Journal of Psychiatry,* 157, 708–714.
- Lytetsos CG, Lee HB. (2004) Diagnosis and treatment of depression in Alzheimer's disease: A practical update for the clinician. *Dementia and Geriatric Cognitive Disorders,* 17, 55–64.
- Marin RS, Beiedrzycki RC, Firinciogullari S. (1991) Reliability and validity of the Apathy Evaluation Scale. *Psychiatry Res,* 38, 143–162.
- Montgomery SA and Asberg M (1979) New depression scale designed to be sensitive to change. *British Journal of Psychiatry,* 134, 382–389.
- Morgan CD, Baade LE. (1997) Neuropsychological testing and assessment scales for dementia of the Alzheimer's type. *Psychiatric Clinics of North America,* 20, 1, 25–43.
- Mortimer JA, Ebbitt B, Jun SP et al. (1992) Predictors of cognitive and functional progression in patients with probable Alzheimer's disease. *Neurology,* 42, 1689–1696.
- Overall JE Gorham DR. (1962) The brief psychiatric rating scale. *Psychol Rep,* 10, 799–812.
- Rabins PV, Mace NL, Lucas NJ. (1982) The impact of dementia on the family. *Journal of American Medical Association,* 248, 333–335.
- Reisberg B. (1986) Dementia: A systematic approach to identifying reversible causes. *Geriatrics,* 41, 30–46.

- Reisberg B, Borenstein J, Salob SP, et al. (1987) Behavioural symptoms in Alzheimer's disease: Phenomenology and treatment. *Journal of Clinical Psychiatry*, 48 (suppl), 9–15.
- Robert PH, Clarinet S, Benoit M, et al. (2002) The apathy inventory: Assessment of apathy and awareness in Alzheimer's disease, Parkinson's disease and mild cognitive impairment. *Int J Geriatr Psychiatry*, 17, 1099–1105.
- Rubin EH, Kinscherf DA. (1989) Psychopathology of very mild dementia of Alzheimer's type. *American Journal of Psychiatry*, 146, 1017–1021.
- Senanarong V, Cummings JL, Fairbanks L, et al. (2004) Agitation in Alzheimer's disease is a manifestation of frontal lobe dysfunction. *Dementia and Geriatric Cognitive Disorders*, 17, 14–20.
- Small GW, Donohue JA, Brooks RL (1998) An economic evaluation of donepezil in the treatment of Alzheimer's disease. *Clin Ther*, 20, 838–850.
- Sourander P and Sjogren H (1970) The concept of Alzheimer's disease and its clinical implications. In Alzheimer's disease. Ciba Foundation Symposium (eds WolstenHolme GEW and O'Connor M). London: Churchill.
- Steele C, Rovnor B, Chase A et al. (1990) Psychiatric symptoms and nursing home placement of patients with Alzheimer's disease. *American Journal of Psychiatry*, 147, 1049–1051.
- Stern RG, Duffelmeyer ME, Zemishlani Z, Davidson M. (1991) The use of benzodiazepines in the management of behavioral symptoms in demented patients. *The Psychiatric Clinics of North America*, 14 (2), 375.
- Sultzer DL (2004) Psychosis and antipsychotic medications in Alzheimer's Disease: Clinical management and research perspectives. *Dementia and Geriatric Cognitive Disorders*, 17, 78–90.
- Sunderland T, Alterman IS, Yount D, et al. (1988) A new scale for the assessement of depressed mood in demented patients, *Am J Psychiatry*, 145, 955–959.
- Tariot PN, Erb R Leibovici A et al. (1994) Carbamazepine treatment of agitation in nursing home patients with dementia: a preliminary study. *J Am Geriatr Soc*, 42, 1160–1166.
- Tariot PN, Mack JL, Patterson MB (1995) The behaviour rating scale for dementia of the Consortium to Establish a Registry for Alzheimer's disease. *Am J Psychiatry*, 152, 1349–1357.
- Teri L, Larson EB, and Reifler BV. (1988) Behavioural Disturbance in dementia of Alzheimer's type. *Journal of the American Geriatric Society*, 36, 1–6.

- van der Kam P, Mol F, Wimmers MFHC. (1971) Beoordelingsschaal voor oudere patienten (BOP). Deventer, Van Loghum Slaterus.
- Wood S, Cummings JL, Hsu MA, (2000) The use of the neuropsychiatric inventory in nursing home residents: Characterization and measurement. *Am J Geriatr Psychiatry,* 8, 75–83.
- World Health Organization (1992) *The ICD-10 Classification of Mental and Behavioural Disorders. Clinical descriptions and diagnostic guidelines.* Geneva: World Health Organization.
- Wynn ZJ and Cummmings JL. (2004) Cholinesterase inhibitors therapies and neuropsychiatric manifestations of Alzheimer's disease. *Dementia and Geriatric Cognitive Disorders,* 17, 100–108.
- Yesavage JA (1988) Geriatric depression scale. *Psychopharmacol Bull,* 24, 709–711.

5

Epidemiology of Dementia

The Demography of Ageing

Population ageing is a global phenomenon, which is no longer restricted to developed countries. From 1980 to 2025 there will be a threefold increase in the size of the world population aged over 60. However, the increase will be largest in the developing world, four fold compared with only two fold in developed world. In India according to 1981 census, out of the total population of 682.2 million, 44 million (6.4%) people were elderly (aged over 60 years). According to 1991 Census, 55.3 million people (6.6%) were over 60 years. Their number increased to 70 million (7%) by 2001 AD. It is the number of elderly that is formidable rather than the percentage. Along with this demographic transition that is occurring throughout the world there will be an increase in age-associated morbidity. Dementia being an important cause of age-associated morbidity, is expected to rise steadily.

Prevalence of Dementia

Prevalence is the proportion of existing cases of the disease in a defined population at a given point or over a brief period in time. It is estimated through cross-sectional study (survey) design, examining all persons (or a random sample of persons) in a community. Prevalence represents the disease burden of a population and is important when planning services and allocating resources. Prevalence itself depends on two other measurements: (1) incidence rate, or the proportion of new cases occurring in a defined population over a given period of time (e.g., 2 years). (2) Duration of disease is how long affected persons live with the disease. Thus, either high incidence or long duration can lead to high prevalence, whereas the reverse is true of low prevalence. Prevalence of dementia also depends on the age structure and life expectancy of the population (Ganguli and Pandav, 2002).

An important concept is "age specific prevalence rate," i.e., the prevalence examined separately in different age groups (60–64, 65–70, etc.) rather than in the entire over-65 population. It has been shown consistently across all studies in all populations that prevalence of dementia increases exponentially with age (Evans et al., 1989). Exact estimation of the prevalence of dementia depends on the definition and specific threshold used. The syndrome affects approximately 5–8% of individuals over age 65, 15–20 % of individuals over age 75 and 25–50% of individuals over age 85. Alzheimer's disease is the most common form of dementia, accounting for 50–70% of the total, with a greater proportion in the higher age ranges. Vascular dementia is probably next common, but its prevalence is unknown. The remaining type of dementia account for a much smaller fraction of the total, although in the last few years it has been suggested that Lewy body disease may be more prevalent than previously realized (Rabins et al., 2000). A worldwide average age specific prevalence curve can be approximated by a trajectory that begins at about 1% at age 60, then rises to 2% at 70, 4% at 75, 8% at 80, and 16% at age 85 years. These rates are for dementia of all causes and of at least moderate severity (White, 1992).

Studies of Dementia in India

Shankar et al. (1988) reported the first autopsy confirmed case of Alzheimer's disease in a man with disease onset at age 73 and no family history of dementia. Satishchandra et al. (1997) reported a histologically confirmed familial case of Alzheimer's disease in a woman, with onset at age 47. Barodawala and Ghadi (1992) noted that typical Alzheimer's disease pathology was present, but rare in an autopsy series of 100 patients aged 60 years and above from Bombay.

Wadia (1992) observed that in the Zorostrian Community (primarily in Bombay) where average survival had reached the eighth decade of life, Alzheimer's disease had become quite prevalent.

Prevalence of various dementing disorders has been well documented in developed countries. In India, a few epidemiological studies have been conducted during the last decade. Rajkumar et al (1996) conducted two studies in Tamilnadu, one in Madras city, and the other in a rural community. Using the multistage stratified random sampling technique, 1300 individuals aged 65 years and above were selected from the city of Madras. The selected elderly persons were assessed using the third edition of Geriatric Mental Status Schedule Test (GMS) by trained staff. The prevalence of dementia was found to be 2.7%. A study to estimate the prevalence of dementia in a rural population was conducted in Thiruporur, a community located in the outskirts of Madras city (Rajkumar et al, 1997). 750 elderly persons aged 60 years of age and above were selected using the cluster sampling technique and were interviewed using the Geriatric Mental Status Schedule. The prevalence of dementia was found to be 3.6% in this community.

Shaji et al. (1996) investigated the prevalence of various dementing disorders in a rural community in Kerala. A door-to-door survey was conducted to identify elderly persons aged 60 years and above. A total of 2067 elderly persons were screened with the vernacular adaptation of MMSE. All those scored at or below the cut off score of 23, had a detailed neuropsychological evaluation by Cambridge Mental Disorders of the Elderly Examination - Section B (CAMDEX-Section B), and the caregivers of the people with confirmed cognitive impairment were interviewed using CAMDEX - Section H to confirm the history of deterioration or impairment in social or personal functioning. In the third phase, the subjects with confirmed cognitive impairment were evaluated at their home, and diagnosis was made as per DSM-III R criteria. The prevalence rate was found to be 3.4%. 58% cases were diagnosed as vascular dementia and 41% satisfied the criteria for Alzheimer's disease. Shaji et al. (2001) conducted a study in the city of Cochin using similar methodology and the prevalence rate was found to be 3.4% in elderly persons aged 65 and above. Amongst them 53% of dementia cases were diagnosed as Alzheimer's disease, 40% satisfied the criteria for vascular dementia and 7% were due to causes like infection, tumour and trauma.

Chandra et al. (1998) performed a community survey of a cohort of 5126 individuals aged 55 years and older, 73.3% of whom were illiterates. Hindi cognitive and functional screening instruments developed for and validated in this population, were used to screen the cohort, a total of 536 subjects (10.5%) who met operational criteria for cognitive and functional impairment and a random sample of 270 unimpaired control subjects underwent standardized clinical assessment for dementia using DSM-IV diagnostic criteria, the Clinical Dementia Rating Scale and National Institute of Neurological and Communicative Disorders and Stroke-Alzheimer's Disease and Related Disease Association (NINCDS-ADRDA) criteria for probable and possible Alzheimer's disease. An overall prevalence of 0.84% was observed in the population aged 55 years and older and an overall prevalence rate of 1.36% in the population aged 65 years and older.

A prevalence study of major neurological disorders in the far northern Indian State of Kashmir found no subjects with Alzheimer's disease (Razdan et al, 1994). However, 42% of the population of that region was younger than 14 years, and the Kashmir survey included only 31 subjects aged 60 years and above. Vas et al (2001) reported an overall prevalence of 1.8% for those aged 65 years and above in an urban population in Mumbai.

Epidemiological studies made it clear that there are differences in prevalence rates of dementia across various regions. All three studies conducted in southern part of India reported higher total and age-specific prevalence rates than those of Ballabgarh study conducted in Haryana in Northern part.

Regional Differences

Most studies in "developed" countries have reported the overall prevalence of dementia to be between 5% and 10% of the elderly, usually defined as age 60 or 65 years and older. Most of these studies have been carried out in white populations in Europe, Britain, Australia, USA and Canada (Ganguli and Pandav, 2002). Prince (2002) reviewed seven published prevalence surveys from the developing world and reported that the prevalence of dementia ranged from 1.3% to 5.3% for all those aged 60 and over and 1.7% to 5.2% for all those aged 65 and over (Shaji et al., 1996; Shaji et al., 2001; Rajkumar and Kumar, 1996; Chandra et al, 1998; Li et al, 1989; Zhang et al, 1990; Phanthumchinda et al, 1991 and Hendrie et al, 1995). In general estimated rates from the Asian nations have been lower than from the US, England and Europe.

Alzheimer's disease is the most common form of dementia in Western countries. For most European and American populations, prevalence rates of Alzheimer's disease have been approximately half the total dementia figures, while the rates for vascular dementia have varied between 0 and 30% of the total dementia prevalence values. In most surveys from Japan, China and Taiwan, the relative frequencies are reversed, with the rates of vascular dementia being 30–60% of the values for total dementia and the rate of Alzheimer's disease being 20–40% of the total dementia prevalence rates. It appears that prevalence rate for AD in US and Europe are 2–3 times than in Japan while vascular dementia prevalence rate in Japan is 1.5–2 times than those for the US and Europe. This apparent difference in prevalence rates between the two populations indicates that the difference may be related to some biological factor, rather than to methods of case detection (White, 1992).

A lower incidence of Alzheimer's disease could be mediated by differences in environmental or lifestyle determinants or a lower prevalence of familial predisposition of Alzheimer's disease. The differences between Asian and European ancestry populations in the Alzheimer's disease: vascular dementia ratio is best documented for Japan. Similar findings have been reported from China, Taiwan and India (White, 1992). The relative proportion of Alzheimer's disease in studies reported from India ranged from 41–65% while the proportion of vascular dementia ranged from 22–58% (Shaji et al., 1996; Shaji et al, 2001; Rajkumar and Kumar, 1996; Vas et al, 2001).

Risk Factors

Epidemiological studies suggest that a variety of factors contribute to the occurrence of Alzheimer's disease (AD), particularly late onset AD. Age is clearly the most important risk factor for AD (Larson et al., 1963; Shang et al. 1990). Meticulous epidemiological studies have established that being a woman is an independent risk factor for Alzheimer's disease (Rocca et al., 1990; Gao et al., 1998). The higher prevalence of AD in older women has not yet been explained. Possible explanations include unrecognized environmental influences, unspecified hormonal effects, the presence of one or more predisposing genes on the X-chromosome, and the higher incidence of the apolipoprotein E4 allele in the women.

Family history of Alzheimer's disease is one of the most consistent risk factors, increasing disease risk by approximately four fold at any age. Established genetic risk factors are strongest for early onset, familial AD (three separate genes known as APP, PSI and PS_2) (St George-Hyslop et al., 1992; Schellenberg et al., 1993) but another gene called ApoE4 is a risk factor for late onset and non-familial cases as well (Lery-Lahad et al., 1995; Saunders et al., 1993).

Head trauma (Chandra et al., 1989; Geyde et al., 1989) has been reported as a risk factor for AD in several, but not all, studies considering its potential role in the disease. In dementia pugilistica, repeated head trauma leads to dementia with the accumulation of neuropathological abnormalities associated with AD, including many neurofibrillary tangles and diffuse Alzheimer amyloid. Epidemiological studies have not identified an environmental toxin that contributes to the development of AD, other than aluminium, and the data for this are contradictory (Doll et al., 993; Graves et al., 1990). Vascular disease appears to be a risk factor for Alzheimer's disease (Aroson et al., 1990; Sparks et al., 1990). Other risk factors reported include Down's syndrome (Wisniewski et al., 1985), major depression (Berger et al. 1999), diabetes (Ott et al., 1996), heart disease (Sparks et al., 1990; Aronson et al., 1990) and thyroid disease (Ganguly et al., 1996). Protective factors for Alzheimer's disease reported in the literature include higher education (Stern et al., 1994; White et al., 1994), the ApoE2 gene (Farrer et al., 1997), intake of antioxidant substances (e.g., vitamins E and C) (Jama et al, 1996, Perkins et al, 1999, Sano et al, 1997), use of oestrogen supplements in women (Henderson, 1997), use of some anti-inflammatory drugs (Stewart et al, 1997) and cigarette smoking (van Duijn et al, 1991).

Methodological Issues in Epidemiological Research

Age ascertainment of elderly population is an important issue especially in illiterate populations. Many elderly people do not know their exact ages and may give differing ages at different times. The identification and classification of cases of dementia in a community survey require the use of appropriate instruments, methods and criteria, and extremely rigorous attention to standardization and quality control at every step. It is possible that many cases of dementia may be missed if the screening instruments and diagnostic methods are not sufficiently sensitive. Use of cognitive screening tests not appropriate for poorly educated or illiterate elderly may overestimate cognitive impairment based on test scores. At times it is very difficult to estimate the functional impairment as the lifestyles of rural elderly persons do not require them to perform instrumental activities of daily living comparable to those in industrialized societies. It is possible that many signs and symptoms of mild dementia may be misattributed as a part of 'normal ageing'. In most of the published reports comparing autopsy findings with premorbid diagnosis of Alzheimer's disease or vascular dementia, there was agreement for 75–85% of cases, i.e., the diagnosis made during life were incorrect for 15–25% of cases.

REFERENCES

- Aronson MK, Ooi WL, et al. (1990) Women, myocardial infarction and dementia in the very old. *Neurology,* 40 (7), 1102–1106.
- Barodwala S and Ghadi P. (1992) A progress report on the prevalence of Alzheimer's lesion in a Bombay hospital population. *Curr Sci,* 4, 44–55.
- Chandra V, Kokmen E, Schoenberg BS, et al. (1989) Head trauma with loss of consciousness as a risk factor for Alzheimer's disease. *Neurology,* 39, 1576–1578
- Chandra C Ganguli M, Pandav R, et al. (1998) Prevalence of Alzheimer's disease and other dementia in rural India: the Indo-US study, *Neurology,* 51 (4), 1000–1008.

- Doll R (1993) Review: Alzheimer's disease and environmental aluminium. *Age and Aging,* 22 (2), 138–153.
- Evans DA, Funkenstein HH, Aibert MS, et al. (1989) Prevalence of Alzheimer's disease in a community population of older persons, higher than previously reported. *JAMA,* 262, 2551–2556.
- Farrer LA, Cupples LA, Haines JL, et al (1997) Effects of age, sex, and ethnicity on the association between apolipoprotein E genotype and Alzheimer's disease, Meta-analysis Consortium. *JAMA,* 278, 16:1349–1356.
- Ganguli M and Pandav R. (2002) Epidemiology of Alzheimer's disease: An overview. In *Alzheimer's Disease in India.* p: 27–42. New Delhi: Society for Gerontological Research.
- Gao S, Hendrie HC et al (1998) The relationships between age, sex and the incidence of dementia and Alzheimer's disease: a meta analysis. *Archives of General Psychiatry,* 155 (9), 809–815.
- Geyde A, Beattie BL, Tuokko H et al (1989) Severe head injury hastens age of onset of Alzheimer's disease. *Journal of American Geriatric Society,* 37, 970–973.
- Graves AB, White E, et al (1990) Genetic evidence for a novel familial Alzheimer's disease. *Journal of Clinical Epidemiology,* 43 (1), 35–44.
- Henderson VW. (1997). The epidemiology of estrogen replacement therapy and Alzheimer's disease. *Neurology,* 48, 27–35.
- Hendrie HC, Osuntokun BO, Hall KS, et al (1995) Prevalence of Alzheimer's disease and dementia in two communities: Nigerian Africans and African Americans. *American Journal of Psychiatry,* 152 (10), 1485–1492.
- Jama JW, Launer LJ, et al (1996) Dietary and cognitive function in a population-based sample of older persons. The Rotterdam study. *American Journal of Epidemiology,* 150, 275–280.
- Larson I, Syogren T, Jacobson G (1963) Senile dementia: a clinical, sociomedical, and genetic study. *Acta Psychiatrica Scandinavica,* (suppl 167), 1–259.
- Lery-Lahad E, Wijsman EM, et al (1995) A familial Alzheimer's disease locus on chromosome. *Science,* 269 (5226), 970–973.
- LiG, Shen YC, Chen CH, et al (1989) An epidemiological survey of age related dementia in an urban area of Beijing. *Acta Psychiatrica Scandinavica,* 79, 557–563.
- Ott A, Stalk RP et al (1996) Association of diabetes mellitus and dementia: The Rotterdam Study. *Diabetologia,* 39, 11, 1392–1397.
- Perkins AJ, Hendrie HC, et al (1999) Association of antioxidants with memory in a multicentric study sample using the third national health and nutrition examination survey. *American Journal of Epidemiology,* 150, 37–44.

- Phanthumchintha K, Jitapunkal S, Sitthi Amorn C, Bunnag SC et al. (1991) Prevalence of dementia in an urban slum population in Thailand: Validity of screening methods. *International Journal of Geriatric Psychiatry*, 6, 639–646.
- Prince M. (2000) Methodological issues for population based research into dementia of developing countries. *International Journal of geriatric psychiatry*, 15, 21–30.
- Rabins PV, Blacker D, Bland A, et al (1997) Practice guideline for the treatment of patients with Alzheimer's disease and other dementias of late life: American Psychiatric Association. *American Journal of Psychiatry*, 154, (suppl), 1–39.
- Rabins PV, Blacker D, Bland A, et al (2000) *Practice guideline for treatment of psychiatric disorders. Compendium 2000*, pp 73–125. Washington DC: American Psychiatric Association.
- Rajkumar S, Kumar S, Thara R. (1997) Prevalence of dementia in a rural setting, A report from India. *International Journal of Geriatric Psychiatry*, 12, 702–707.
- Rajkumar S, Kumar S (1996) Prevalence of dementia in the community: a rural-urban comparison from Madras, India. *Australian Journal of Ageing*, 15, 9–13.
- Razdan S, Kau RL, Motta A, Kau S, Bhatt RK (1994) Prevalence and pattern of major neurological disorders in rural Kashmir (India) 1986. *Neuroepidemiology*, 13 (3), 113–119.
- Rocca WA, Bonaiuto S, Lippi A, et al (1990) Prevalence of clinically diagnosed Alzheimer's disease and other dementing disorders: a door-to-door survey in Appignano, Maccrata province, Italy. *Neurology*, 40, 626–631.
- Sano M, Ernesto C, et al (1997) A controlled trial of selegiline, alpha-tocopherol, or both as treatment for Alzheimer's disease. The Alzheimer's disease cooperative study. *New England Journal of Medicine*, 336, 1216–1222.
- Satishchandra P, Yasha TC, Shankar L, et al (1997) Familial Alzheimer's disease: First report from India. *Alzheimer's Disease and Associated Disorders*, 11(2), 107–109.
- Saunders AM, Stictmatter WJ et al (1993) Association of apolipoprotein E allele epsilon 4 with late onset familial and sporadic Alzheimer's disease. *Neurology*, 43, (8), 1467–1472.
- Schellenberg GD, Payami H, et al (1993) Chromosome 14 and late onset familial Alzheimer disease. *American Journal of Human Genetics*, 53 (3), 619–628.
- Shaji S, and Roy KJ (2001) An epidemiological study of dementia in an Urban Community in Kerala, India. Book of Abstracts - 2001. Alzheimer's Disease International Conference. Christ Church, New Zealand.

- Shaji S, Pramodu K, Abraham R, Roy KJ & Varghese A. (1996) An epidemiological study of dementia in a rural community in Kerala, India. *British Journal of Psychiatry*, 168 (8), 745–749.
- Shang M, Katzman R, Salmon D et al (1990) The prevalence of dementia and Alzheimer's disease and other dementing disorders: a door-to-door survey in Appignano, Maccrata Province, Italy. *Neurology*, 40, 626–631.
- Shankar S, Chandra P, Rao T, et al (1988) Alzheimer's disease-histological, ultrastructural and immunochemical study of autopsy-proven case. *Indian Journal of Psychiatry*, 30, 219–298.
- Sparks DL, Hunsaker JC, et al (1990) Cortical senile plaques in coronary artery disease, aging and Alzheimer's disease. *Neurobiology of Aging*, 11 (6), 601–607.
- St. George Hyslop P, et al (1992) Genetic evidence for a novel familial Alzheimer's disease locus on chromosome 14. *Nature Germetics*, 2 (4), 330–334.
- Stern Y, Gurland B, Tatemichi TK, et al (1994) Influence of education and occupation on incidence of Alzheimer's disease, *JAMA*, 271, 13, 1004–1010.
- Stewart WF, Kawas C, et al (1997) Risk of Alzheimer's disease and duration of NSAID use. *Neurology*, 48, 626–632.
- Van Duijn CM, Stijnen T, Hofman A. (1991) Risk factors for Alzheimer's disease: overview of the EURODEM collaborative re-analysis of case-control studies. EURODEM Risk Factor Research Group. *International Journal of Epidemiology*, 20, Suppl: 4–12.
- Vas CJ, Pinto C, Panikker D et al (2001) Prevalence of dementia in an urban Indian population. International *Psychogeriatrics*, 13, 439–450.
- Wadia N. (1992) Experience with the differential diagnosis and prevalence of dementing illnesses in India. *Curr Science*, 63, 419–430.
- White LR. (1992) Towards a program of cross-cultural research on the epidemiology of Alzheimer's disease. *Current Science*, 63, 8, 456–469.
- White L, Katzman R, Losonczy K et al (1994) Association of education With Incidence of cognitive Impairment in three established populations for epidemiological studies of the elderly. *Journal of Clinical Epidemiology*. 1994, 47 (4), 363–374.
- Wisniewskike, Wisniewskike HM & Wen GY (1985) Occurrence of neuropathological changes and dementia of Alzheimer's disease in Down's syndrome. *Annals of Neurology*, 17, 278–282.
- Zhang MY, Katzman R, Salmon D et al (1990) The prevalence of dementia and Alzheimer's disease in Shanghai, China: Impact of age, gender and education. *Annals of Neurology*, 27, 428–437.

6

Aetiology of Dementia

Salman Karim, Alistair Burns

Introduction

The word dementia stems from "demens", a Latin term, which literally means without mind. The French Encyclopaedia of 1765 described it as a syndrome characterised by deterioration of memory and personality with multiple causes, some of which are reversible. By 1900s three main types of dementia were recognised as senile, arteriosclerotic and subcortical and were distinguished from cognitive deficits seen in other psychiatric illness like depression, mania and schizophrenia. Over the next half of the century, a number of specific disorders including epilepsy, alcoholism, myxoedema and lead poisoning were described, which can present with symptoms similar to dementia. Last 30 years have seen huge advances in the understanding of neuropathology and neurochemistry of dementia, which have provided useful insights into their aetiology. The common causes of dementia have been summarized in Table 6.1. This chapter aims at giving an overview of the current knowledge about the aetiology of the three most common types of dementia including Alzheimer's disease (AD), vascular dementia (VaD) and dementia with Lewy bodies (DLB).

Table 6.1 Causes of dementia

Endocrine
- Diabetes mellitus
- Thyroid disorder
- Parathyroid disorder
- Cushing's disease
- Addison's disease

Infections
- Syphilis
- Encephalitis
- HIV
- Creutzfeldt-Jakob disease

Toxic
- Alcohol
- Heavy metals (lead, mercury)
- Organic solvents
- Carbon monoxide

Metabolic
- Vitamin deficiency (B_{12}, B_6, folate)
- Liver disease
- Renal disease

Space occupying lesions
- Normal pressure hydrocephalus
- Tumours
- Subdural haematoma

Anoxic
- Chronic respiratory disease

Traumatic
- Head injury

Neurodegenerative
- Alzheimer's disease
- Dementia with Lewy bodies
- Vascular dementia
- Parkinson's disease
- Pick's disease
- Huntington's disease
- Multiple sclerosis
- Motor neurone disease

ALZHEIMER'S DISEASE

Alois Alzheimer in 1907 described an illness in a 51-year-old lady characterised by cognitive impairment and psychotic symptoms along with the postmortem neuropathological findings of senile plaques and neurofibrillary tangles in the brain. The eponym "Alzheimer's disease" was coined by Kraepelin and appeared for the first time in his textbook of psychiatry in 1910. Since then the clinical syndrome that commonly occurs later in life and is characterised by cognitive impairment along with the neuropathological findings of senile plaques, neurofibrillary tangles, granulovacular degeneration and nerve cell loss is referred as AD. The aetiology of AD can be described on the basis of risk factors (Table 6.2).

Table 6.2 Risk factors in Alzheimer's disease

Demographic factors
■ Age
■ Sex
■ Ethnicity
■ Intelligence
■ Education
Genetic factors
■ Family history
■ Apolipoprotein E polymorphisms
■ Down's syndrome
■ Autosomal dominant gene mutations
Systemic illness
■ Depression
■ Diabetes mellitus
■ Hypertension
■ Hypercholesterolaemia
■ Vitamin deficiency
■ Hyperhomocysteinaemia
Environmental factors
■ Head injury
■ Aluminium
■ Smoking
■ Increased fat intake
■ Obesity

RISK FACTORS

Age

Age is an established risk factor for Alzheimer's disease. The prevalence of AD rises sharply after the age of 60 years and doubles every 5 years. However, it is not clear whether it continues to rise indefinitely. There is some evidence that the prevalence of AD drops for the people who are in their 90s or older (Richie and Kildea, 1995). Incidence studies looking at age as a causal factor in AD have shown that the incidence of AD continues to rise until the age of 98 although it does slow down in the 90s (Gao et al, 1998).

Sex

AD is known to be more common in females but it is still not clear whether the female gender is an independent risk factor as women tend to live longer than men and have consequently a higher risk of developing AD. Studies looking at the incidence of AD have shown a higher incidence in females as compared to males (Gao et al, 1998). However, this higher rate of incidence appears to be significant in very old age. Andersen et al (1999) in a pooled analysis of prospective studies found that women above 90 years of age had a 3 times higher rate of AD as compared to men. These gender differences have been postulated to be linked with postmenopausal changes in oestrogens and sex interactions with apolipoprotein E geno type (Gao et al, 1998).

Ethnic Background

A higher incidence of AD disease has been reported in Europe and North America as compared to Asia and the developing countries. Jorm and Jolley (1998) in a meta-analysis of multiple studies found a higher incidence of AD in Europe as compared to East Asia. These findings however should be viewed under the light of the difficulties of not having uniform standardised methods of diagnosing AD. Most instruments used in the Western cultures to diagnose AD are not culturally sensitive and the differences in the prevalence and incidence between different populations based on ethnic backgrounds cannot be viewed with confidence (Prince et al, 2003).

Family History

Amongst known patients of AD, about 25 to 50% have a family history. People with a first-degree relative of AD have a 3.5 fold increased risk of developing the illness (Van Duijn et al., 1991). The early onset type of AD, where onset is before 65 years of age carries a stronger family risk although it is rare and comprises only 5% of all AD cases. The risk of the illness becomes smaller if the relatives develop AD in older age.

ApoE genotype

Apolipoprotein E (ApoE) is a plasma protein involved in lipid transport and probably in neuronal repair. It is located on chromosome 19 and has three common alleles, E2, E3 and E4. A number of studies have shown that about 30 to 50% of AD patients have the E4 allele. The E4 allele is known to increase the risk of AD in a dose dependent manner and the E2 allele decreases the risk. The E4 allele has also been shown to bring forward the time of onset of AD (Roses, 1996).

Down's Syndrome

Almost all people with Down's syndrome (trisomy 21) have neuropathological features of AD by the time they reach the age of 40 years. This pathology is due to having an extra copy of amyloid precursor protein gene on chromosome 21. However, the prevalence of dementia in people with Down's syndrome is much less than 100% even by the age of 50 years (Zigman et al., 1996). The reasons for this discrepancy are not clearly understood although a number of studies have indicated links between AD and Down's syndrome. Family history of Down's syndrome is associated with AD (Van Duijn et al., 1991). A higher frequency of ApoE 4 allele has been reported in younger mothers with children having Down's syndrome suggesting that ApoE 4 allele is a risk factor for Down's syndrome.

Autosomal Dominant Gene Mutations

A number of genetic mutations have been identified which can cause AD. These are mutations of beta amyloid precursor protein on chromosome 21 and the presenilin genes on chromosome 1 and 14. These mutations lead to an excessive production of the pathogenic long chain form of amyloid beta protein, accumulation of which results in AD. These mutations are associated with the early onset type of AD (before 65 years) but they do not seem to be present in the majority of early onset familial AD cases (Farrer et al, 1997).

Education

A number of studies have reported a higher incidence of AD in people belonging to less educated groups of populations (Farmer et al, 1995) although some studies have not shown this relationship. The reasons for the association of AD with educational levels can be explained on the hypothesis that people with higher levels of education are able to compensate for any cognitive decline in the early stages of illness thus leading to a delay in the diagnosis. Some imaging studies have supported this hypothesis as Stern et al (1992) reported that highly educated people had better regional blood flow to parietal and temporal lobes as compared to people with lower education levels.

Pre-morbid Intelligence

As education is correlated to intelligence it can be inferred that pre-morbid intelligence is a protective factor against AD. Schmand et al. (1997) in a longitudinal study showed that a reading vocabulary test was a better predictor of subsequent dementia as compared to education. Imaging studies have shown a higher rate of cerebral glucose metabolism in AD people of higher pre-morbid intelligence (Alexander et al, 1997). In an interesting epidemiological study, Snowden et al (1996) showed verbal ability's direct influence on AD pathology. The study involved assessments of verbal ability of a group of nuns, which was followed up for 58 years. A neuropathological examination of those who died was also carried out. The results showed that low scores on verbal abilities were associated with poorer cognitive functioning in old age. Verbal ability in early life was also found to be related to AD pathology after death. The postmortem findings of the nuns who died during the study showed AD type neuropathology in all those with low verbal ability. This evidence suggests that high intelligence may be an independent protective factor rather than being just a compensatory mechanism.

Cognitive Reserve

Brain imaging studies have revealed a relationship of brain size to the IQ and there is some evidence that brain reserve could be protective for AD (Jorm et al, 1997). Schofield (1999) reported that individuals with larger head size or a larger brain on a scan had reduced risk of AD and moreover non-demented individuals showing AD changes on autopsy tend to have larger brains as compared to demented individuals (Katzman et al, 1988).

Head Trauma

Head injury has been associated with AD in a number of studies. Mortimer et al (1991) in a meta-analysis of case controlled studies show that a history of head trauma with loss of consciousness was associated with an 80% increase in risk of AD and that head injuries occurring in the 10 years before the onset of the illness were more important as compared to ones in earlier years. Head injury has been shown to increase the deposition of beta amyloid protein, which is one of the pathological hallmarks of AD (Roberts et al, 1991). Beta amyloid protein is more likely to be deposited after brain injury in individuals carrying ApoE 4 allele (Nicoll et al., 1995) and head injury has been reported to be a risk factor for AD in only those people who were carrying ApoE 4 allele (Mayeux et al., 1995).

Depression

Depression is known to be prodromal feature of AD but whether it is a risk factor for developing the illness is not clear. Jorm et al (1991) in a meta-analysis of 4 case controlled studies reported depression as a risk factor but others (Henderson et al, 1997; Chen et al, 1999) have not found it to be a risk factor for cognitive decline or dementia. It has been postulated that depression could predispose to AD by activating the hypothalamic-pituitary-adrenal axis leading to excessive release of cortisone, which has been shown to lead to hippocampal atrophy (O'Brien, 1997).

Vascular Factors

A number of vascular risk factors like high blood pressure, raised cholesterol levels and diabetes mellitus are established risk factors for

AD. Skoog et al. (1996) in a prospective study reported that hypertension 10 to 15 years earlier increased the rate of AD disease and treatment studies have reported a reduction in AD with adequate treatment of systolic hypertension. Similarly, lowering of cholesterol levels and use of cholesterol lowering drugs have been widely reported to reduce the risk of AD. Diabetes mellitus, which is known to cause peripheral vascular disease, is also an established risk factor for AD. Considering all these vascular risks factors together it is evident that multiple factors leading to cerebral ischaemia may be involved in the pathogenesis of AD (Kalaria, 2000).

Homocystine

Homocystine is a plasma protein produced in the body in the process of metabolism of the amino acid methionine. Folic acid, vitamin B_6 and B_{12} are involved in its metabolism. Diet deficient of these vitamins or some systemic diseases can lead to elevated homocystine levels and some studies have reported high homocystine levels in AD patients (McCaddon et al, 1998). A more recent study (Sheshadri et al, 2002) showed raised plasma homocystine level as a strong and independent risk factor for the development of AD.

Inflammation

In recent years increasing evidence has accumulated on the role of inflammatory process in pathology of AD. The evidence of increased inflammatory process in the brain comes from studies that have shown increased activation of microglia in the brain, increased serum level of mediators of inflammation like interleukin-6 and C-reactive protein and the protective effect of anti-inflammatory drugs in AD (Casserly and Topol, 2004).

Summary

According to the current evidence it appears that AD is a progressive neurodegenerative process with a number of demographic, genetic, systemic and environmental risk factors. These factors converge as pathogenic events leading to the culmination and deposition of amyloid beta peptide inside or outside the neurones. This process initiates a chronic inflammatory reaction and a cascade of events leading to microglial and astrocyte activation, oxidative injury to the neurones, alteration in the neuronal ionic homeostasis resulting in neuronal dysfunction, neuronal death and dementia (Figure 6.1).

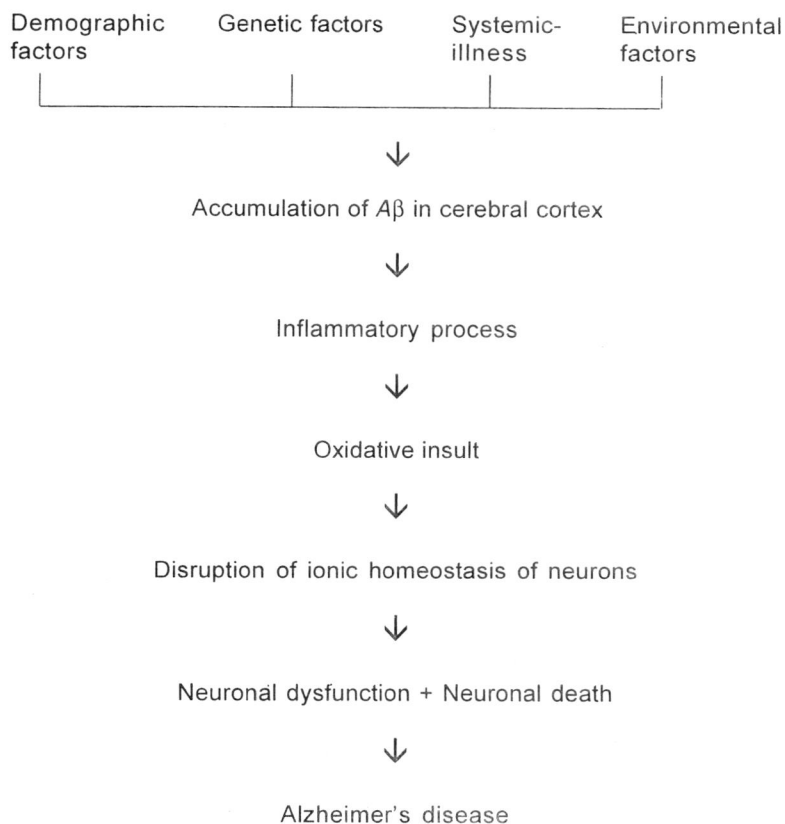

Demographic factors	Genetic factors	Systemic-illness	Environmental factors

↓

Accumulation of $A\beta$ in cerebral cortex

↓

Inflammatory process

↓

Oxidative insult

↓

Disruption of ionic homeostasis of neurons

↓

Neuronal dysfunction + Neuronal death

↓

Alzheimer's disease

Figure 6.1 Convergence of various factors responsible for AD

VASCULAR DEMENTIA

The term vascular dementia (VaD) when used as a diagnostic category refers to cases of dementia where vascular disease is believed to be the main cause. Historically it was recognised as early as 1896 when Kraepelin separated arterial sclerotic dementia from senile dementia. Since then up to the 1970s, disturbance to the blood supply of the brain was thought to be commonest cause of dementia until Tomlinson et al.

(1970) suggested that AD was a more frequent cause of dementia. Hachinski and colleagues in 1974 introduced the term "multi-infarct dementia" to describe dementia caused by small or large brain infarcts. More recently there has been a resurgence of interest in the vascular causes of dementia and there is growing evidence that VaD does not just include multi-infarct dementia but also a complex interaction between a host of cerebral vascular disorders, vascular risk factors and other factors like age and education. Thus, the concept of VaD describes a dementia syndrome due to vascular causes and its aetiology will be described under genetic disorders, cerebrovascular disorders and risk factors.

Table 6.3 Cerebrovascular disorders: aetiology of vascular dementia

Large artery disease ■ Artery to artery embolism ■ Occlusion
Small-vessel disease ■ Lacunar infarct ■ White matter ischaemia
Cardiac emboli **Haemorrhages** ■ Intracranial ■ Subarachnoid

Genetic Disorders

Amongst the genetic disorders that are known to cause VaD, "cerebral autosomal dominant arteriopathy with subcortical infarcts and leukoencephalopathy" (CADASIL) is the most well known. The disorder, caused by mutations on chromosome 19 (Joutel et al., 1997), is familial and usually presents as recurrent strokes in the absence of other vascular risk factors in the fourth to sixth decade of life. Clinically it commonly presents as a subcortical dementia combined with pseudobulbar palsy and smooth muscle abnormalities of cerebral arteries on histopathology.

Other genetic syndromes that can cause VaD dementia include Fabry's disease, familial British dementia with amyloid angiopathy, hereditary endotheliopathy with retinopathy, nephropathy and stroke (HERNS) and mitochondria myopathy, encephalopathy, lactic acidosis and stroke-like episodes (MELAS).

Cerebrovascular Disorders

A number of cerebrovascular disorders, summarised in Table 6.3, have been described as aetiological factors of VaD. In large artery disease, the blood supply to a certain part of the brain is compromised by embolisms arising from larger arteries like the internal carotids and travelling upwards and ultimately blocking off the smaller arteries. Occlusion of large size extra- or intracranial arteries can also lead to the disruption of blood supply to certain parts of the brain, ultimately leading to VaD. Emboli arising from heart can travel up through the carotids to the brain and block the small size blood vessels leading to VaD. Disease of the small vessels of the brain like the deep penetrating arteries can result in lacunar infarcts and ischaemic white matter lesions causing VaD. Similarly, haemorrhages, either intracranial or subarachnoidal, can also lead to VaD.

Table 6.4 Risk factors: aetiology of vascular dementia

Demographic
- Age
- Race
- Education

Vascular
- Hypertension
- Ischaemic heart disease
- Atrial fibrillation
- Hyperlipidaemia
- Transient ischaemic attacks
- Smoking

Others
- Diabetes mellitus
- Hyper-homocysteinemia
- Polycythaemia
- Alcohol abuse
- Obesity
- High fat intake

Risk Factors for Vascular Dementia

Risk factors for VaD have been usually described in relation to the risk factors for stroke (Table 6.4). In general, these risk factors can be divided into demographic, vascular and general risk factors. Most of these risk factors predispose to atherosclerotic process directly or indirectly, which can ultimately lead to VaD (Skoog, 1998; Gorelick, 1997).

CONVERGENCE OF RISK FACTORS FOR ALZHEIMER'S DISEASE AND VASCULAR DEMENTIA

Considering the risk factors described for AD and VaD, it is apparent that they share a number of common risk factors such as hypertension, hyperlipidaemia, hyper-homocystinaemia, diabetes mellitus, increased fat intake and obesity. Recent research in looking at ApoE4 polymorphisms and raised levels of inflammatory markers are also suggestive of a common theme in both AD and VaD dementia (Farrer et al, 1997, Schmidt et al, 2002). The evidence of decrease in the risk of developing both AD and VaD with the use of statins, anti-inflammatory drugs like nonsteroidal anti-inflammatory agents are also suggestive of common aetiology (Casserly and Topol, 2004).

DEMENTIA WITH LEWY BODIES

Lewy bodies are neuronal inclusion bodies that were first described by Frederick Lewy in 1923 in his landmark monograph on the neuropathology of Parkinson's disease (Gibb, 1986). The Lewy bodies were later on found to be associated with a number of neurodegenerative disorders like motor neurone disease, progressive supranuclear palsy, cortical basal degeneration. However, they are most frequently associated with Parkinson's disease (PD) and dementia with Lewy bodies (DLB), which have many other features in common (McKeith et al, 1994).

Aetiology

The aetiology and risk factors of DLB have been less extensively investigated as compared to AD, and PD. Its clinical and neuropathological similarity with these disorders, especially PD, suggests that it might share some of the aetiological risk factors with PD.

Genetic Factors

Abnormal processing and aggregation of alpha synculein proteins in to filamentous aggregation have been described as key events in the pathogenesis of both autosomal dominant and sporadic PD (Polymeropoulos, 1998; Spillantini et al., 1997).

Exposure to Toxins

Exposure to toxins like chemical pesticides has been postulated as a risk factor for the development of PD (Liou et al., 1997; Herishanu et al., 1998). The exact mechanism of exposure to toxins leading a culmination of Lewy bodies in the brain is not clear. Hubble et al. (1998) have proposed a possible gene-toxin interaction as risk factor for PD with dementia. They reported that subjects who were exposed to pesticides and had CYP2D629 B+ allele had a high probability of developing dementia in association with PD.

Oxidating Agents

Nitric oxide is produced in the nerve cells from the amino acid arginine with the help of an enzyme called nitric oxide synthetase. Excessive activity of this enzyme can lead to oxidative damage and cell death (Dawson et al., 1996). Nitric oxide synthetase inhibitors have been shown to prevent neuronal damage in animal studies. Nitric oxide mediated neuronal damage has been reported in PD and DLB (Tompkins et al., 1997; Molina et al., 1998). Protective effect of anti-oxidants, anti-inflammatory drugs and oestrogens have also been reported in PD (Cummings, 1995). These agents along with vitamin E could have a possible role in preventing DLB.

REFERENCES

- Alexander GE, Furey ML, Grady CL, et al. (1997) Association of premorbid intellectual function with cerebral metabolism in Alzheimer's disease: implications for the cognitive reserve hypothesis. *American Journal of Psychiatry,* 154, 165–72.
- Anderson K, Launer LJ, Dewwy ME, et al. (1999) Gender differences in the incidence of AD and vascular dementia: The EURODEM Studies. EURODEM Incidence Research Group. *Neurology,* 53, 1992–7.

- Casserly I & Topol E. (2004) Convergence of atherosclerosis and Alzheimer's disease: inflammation, cholesterol, and misfolded proteins. *The Lancet,* Vol 363, 1139–1146.
- Chen P, Ganguli M, Mulsant BH, & DeKosky ST. (1999) The temporal relationship between depressive symptoms and dementia: a community-cased prospective study. *Archives of General Psychiatry,* 56, 261–6.
- Cummings LJ. (1995) Lewy body diseases with dementia: pathophysiology and treatment. *Brain and Cognition,* 28, 266–80.
- Dawson VL, Kizushi VA, Huang PL, Synder SH & Dawson TM. (1996) Resistance to neurotoxicity in cortical cultures from neuronal nitric oxide synthase-deficient mice. *Journal of Neurosciences,* B16,B 2479–87.
- Farmer ME, Kittner SJ, Rae DS, Bartko JJ, & Regier DA. (1995) Education and change in cognitive function. The Epidemiologic Catchment Area Study. *Annals of Epidemiology,* 5, 1–7.
- Farrer LA, Cupples LA, Haines JL, et al. (1997) Effects of age, sex and ethnicity on the association between Apolipoprotein E genotype and Alzheimer's disease. A meta-analysis. APOE and Alzheimer Disease Meta Analysis Consortium. *Journal of the American Medical Association,* 278, 1349–56.
- Gao S, Hendrie HC, Hall KS, & Hui S. (1998) The relationships between age, sex and the incidence of dementia and Alzheimer disease: a meta-analysis. *Archives of General Psychiatry,* 55, 809–15.
- Gibb WRG. (1986) Idiopathic Parkinson's disease and the Lewy body disorders. *Neuropathology and Applied Neurobiology,* 12, 223–34.
- Gorelick PB, (1997) Status of risk factors for dementia associated with stroke. *Stroke,* 28, 459–63.
- Hachinski VC, Lassen NA & Marshall J. (1974) Multi-infarct dementia. A cause of mental deterioration in the elderly. *Lancet,* 2, 207–10.
- Henderson AS, Korten AE, Jacomb PA, et al (1997) The course of depression in the elderly: a longitudinal community-based study in Australia. *Psychological Medicine,* 27, 119–29.
- Herishanu YO, Kordysh E & Goldsmith JR. (1998) A case-referent study of extrapyramidal signs (pre-parkinsonism) in rural communities of Israel. *Canadian Journal of Neurological Sciences,* 25, 127–33.
- Hubble JP, Kurth JH, Glatt SL, et al (1998) Gene-toxin interaction as a putative risk factor for Parkinson's disease with dementia. *Neuroepidemiology,* 17, 96–104.
- Jorm AF, & Jolley D. (1998) The incidence of dementia: a meta-analysis. *Neurology,* 51, 728–33.

- Jorm AF, Creasey H, Broe GA, Sulway MR, Kos & Dent OF. (1997) The advantage of being broad-minded: brain diameter and neuropsychological test performance in elderly war veterans. *Personality and Individual Differences,* 23, 371–7.
- Jorm AF, Van Duijn CM, Chandra V, et al. (1991) Psychiatric history and related exposures as risk factors of Alzheimer's disease: a collaborative re-analysis of case-control studies. EURODEM Risk Factors Research Group. *International Journal of Epidemiology,* 20, S43–7.
- Joutel A, Vahedi K, Corpechot C, Troesch A, Chabriat H, Vayssiere C et al. (1997) Strong clustering and stereotyped nature of Notch3 mutations in CADASIL patients. *Lancet,* 350, 1511–15.
- Kalaria RN (2000) The role of cerebral ischaemia in Alzheimer's disease. *Neurobiology of Aging,* 21, 321–30.
- Katzman R, Terry R, DeTeresa R, et al. (1988) Clinical, pathological and neurochemical changes in dementia: a subgroup with preserved mental status and numerous neocortical plaques. *Annals of Neurology,* 23, 138–44.
- Kraepelin E. (1910) *Psychiatrie: Ein Lehrbuch Fur Studierende und Arzte,* Johann Ambrosius Barth, Leipzig.
- Liou HH, Tsai MC, Chen CJ, et al. (1997) Environmental risk factors and Parkinson's disease: a case-control study in Taiwan. *Neurology,* 48, 1583–8.
- Mayeux R, Ottman R, Maestre G, et al. (1995) Synergistic effects of traumatic head injury and Apolipoprotein E4 in patients with Alzheimer's disease. *Neurology,* 45, 555–7.
- McCaddon A, Davies G, Hudson P, Tandy S & Cattell H. (1998) Total serum homocysteine in senile dementia of Alzheimer type. *International Journal of Geriatric Psychiatry,* 13, 235–9.
- McKeith IG, Fairbairn AF, Perry RH & Thompson P. (1994) The clinical diagnosis and misdiagnosis of senile dementia of Lewy body type. *British Journal of Psychiatry,* 165, 324–32.
- Molina JA, Jiminez-Jiminez FJ, Orti-Pareja M & Navarino JA. (1998) The role of nitric oxide in neurodegeneration potential for pharmacological intervention. *Drugs and Aging,* 12, 251–9.
- Mortimer JA, van Duijn CM, Chandra V, et al. (1991) Head trauma as a risk factor for Alzheimer's disease: a collaborative re-analysis of case control studies. EURODEM Risk Factors Research Group. *International Journal of Epidemiology,* 20, S28–35.
- Nicoll JA, Roberts GW & Graham DI. (1995) Apolipoprotein E epsilon 4 allele is associated with deposition of amyloid beta-protein following head injury. *Nature Medicine,* 1, 135–7.
- O'Brien JT (1997) The 'Glucocorticoid cascade' hypothesis in man. Prolonged stress may cause permanent brain damage. *British Journal of Psychiatry,* 170, 199–201.

- Polymeropoulos MH. (1998) Autosominal dominant Parkinson's disease and alpha synculein. *Annals of Neurology,* 44 (suppl. 1), 563–4.
- Prince M, Acosta D, Chiu H, Scazufca M, Varghese M. (2003) Dementia diagnosis in developing countries: a cross-cultural validation study. *Lancet,* 361(9361), 909–17.
- Ritchie K & Kildea D. (1995) Is senile dementia 'age-related' or 'ageing-related'? – Evidence from meta-analysis of dementia prevalence in the oldest old. *Lancet,* 346, 931–4.
- Roberts GW, Gentleman SM, Lynch A, & Graham DI. (1991) Beta A4 amyloid protein deposition in brain after head trauma. *Lancet,* 338, 1422–3.
- Roses AD (1996) Apolipoprotein E alleles as risk factors in Alzheimer's disease. *Annual Review of Medicine,* 47, 387–400.
- Schmand B, Smit JH, Geerlings MI & Lindeboom J. (1997) The effects of intelligence and education on the development of dementia. A test of the brain reserve hypothesis. *Psychological Medicine,* 27, 1337–44.
- Schmidt R, Schmidt H, Curb JD, Masaki K, White LR, Launar LJ. (2002) Early inflammation and dementia: a 25 year follow-up of the Honolulu-Asia Aging Study. *Annals of Neurology,* 52, 168–74.
- Schofield P. (1999) Alzheimer's disease and brain reserve. *Australasian Journal on Ageing,* 18, 10–14.
- Seshadri S, Beiser A, Selhub J, et al. (2002) Plasma homocysteine as a risk factor for dementia and Alzheimer's disease. *New England Journal of Medicine,* 346 (7), 476–83.
- Skoog I. (1998) Status of risk factors for vascular dementia. *Neuroepidemiology,* 17, 209.
- Skoog I, Lernfelt B, Landahl S, et al. (1996) 15 year longitudinal study of blood pressure and dementia. *Lancet,* 347, 1141–5.
- Snowden DA, Kemper SJ, Mortimer JA, Greiner LH, Wekstein DR, & Markesbery WR. (1996) Linguistic ability in early life and cognitive function and Alzheimer's disease in late life. Findings from the Nun Study. *Journal of the American Medical Association,* 275, 528–32.
- Spillantini MG, Schmidt ML, Lee VM-Y, Trojanowski JQ, Jakes R & Goedert M. (1997) Alpha synculein in Lewy bodies. *Nature,* 388, 839–40.
- Stern Y, Alexander GE, Prohovnik I, and Mayeux R. (1992) Inverse relationship between education and parietotemporal perfusion deficit in Alzheimer's disease. *Annals of Neurology,* 32, 371–5.
- Tomlinson BE, Blessed G & Roth M. (1970) Observations on the brains of demented old people. *Journal of the Neurological Sciences,* 11, 205–42.

- Tompkins MM, Basgall EJ, Zamrini E & Hill WD. (1997) Apoptotic-like changes in Lewy body associated disorders and normal ageing in substantia nigral neurons. *American Journal of Pathology,* 150, 119–31.
- Van Duijn CM, Clayton D, Chandra V, et al (1991) Familial aggregation of Alzheimer's disease and related disorders: a collaborative re-analysis of case-control studies. EURODEM Risk Factors Research Group. *International Journal of Epidemiology,* 20, S13–20.
- Zigman WB, Schupf N, Sersen E, & Silverman W. (1996) Prevalence of dementia in adults with and without Down syndrome. *American Journal of Mental Retardation,* 100, 403–12.

7

Factors Influencing Risk of Dementia

Sandip Deshpande, Nilamadhab Kar

Introduction

A person's chance of being affected by a particular disease may be influenced by many different factors—known and unknown—which interact together in complex ways. While some factors may increase the risk, some may decrease it (protective factors). Risk factors may not be enough by themselves to cause the disease. For example, not everyone who smokes develops a heart disease and not everyone with a heart disease has been a smoker. However, smoking is still a strong risk factor for heart disease. One needs to study the risk factors because their influence can be reduced and some protective factors can be increased, leading to a decrease in the chance of developing the disease. In dementia, many risk factors have been identified. This chapter describes these factors that influence risk for dementia and analyse the evidence for them.

DETERMINANTS INFLUENCING RISK OF DEMENTIA

Table 7.1 summarises the risk factors in dementia that have been commonly cited and researched (there is no particular significance in the order in which the risk factors are presented here).

Table 7.1 Factors influencing risk of dementia

Demographic factors	Age, gender, educational level, marital status, occupational exposure (to neurotoxic substances)
Constitutional factors	Family history, genetic, carrier of apolipoprotein e4 allele

Physical factors

■ Cardiovascular illness	Atrial fibrillation, hypertension, inflammation, vascular diseases
■ Physical trauma	Head injury, repeated minor trauma to head
■ Infections	HIV, syphilis, chronic meningitis, viral encephalopathy, Creutzfeldt-Jakob disease
■ Other physical disorders	Down's syndrome, hypertension, diabetes, inflammatory diseases, normal pressure hydrocephalus, hepatic disturbances, renal failure
■ Toxins	Aluminium, mercury and carbon monoxide
■ Hormones	Oestrogen

Psychosocial factors

■ Lifestyle	Dietary factors, alcohol, caffeine, tobacco, exercise
■ Social environment	Early life environment, social ties and leisure
■ Psychiatric illness	Delirium, alcohol dependence, depression

DEMOGRAPHIC FACTORS

Age

Age is a risk factor for dementia (Cummings, 1995). Dementia may occur at any age but is rare below the age of 60 years. Jorm et al. (1998) in their meta-analysis from 23 studies have reported that the incidence of dementia rose exponentially till the age of 90 years. In a study by Strauss et al. (1999) the prevalence of dementia was found to be 13% in 77–84-year-old subjects and 48% in those 95 years or older (18% and 61% respectively when questionable cases were included). The odds ratio for subjects 90–94 years and 95 and above in comparison with 77–84 year olds was 3.7 and 6.5 for dementia; 4.8 and 8.0 for Alzheimer's disease (AD); 2.3 and 4.6 for vascular dementia respectively. This suggests dementia prevalence continues to increase even in the most advanced ages; this increase is more clear for AD. Age is also a known risk factor for vascular dementia (odds ratio [OR] 1.19) (Ross et al., 1999).

Ravaglia et al (1999) studied 92 centenarians in Italy and found an overall prevalence of dementia in 62%, with 70% of them having severe disability; however only 20% of the sample was cognitively normal. In a study by Thomassen et al. (1998) in a Dutch town, all nine persons above the age of 100 years had dementia with eight of them having moderate-severe grade. These findings suggest, although dementia does not appear to be an inevitable consequence of aging, it is possible that aging itself makes the brain more susceptible to multiple addictive damaging factors.

It is found that East Asian countries have a lower incidence of AD than Europe and United States, but the exponential rise with age tended to be steeper. In other words, the advantage of the East Asian countries diminished with increased age. This difference could be a methodologic artefact and needs to be confirmed. However, it is consistent with the lower prevalence of the ApoE-e4 allele in Japanese subjects and might also reflect environmental differences (Jorm and Jolley, 1998).

Gender

There is no sex difference in dementia incidence, but women tend to have a higher incidence of Alzheimer's disease in very old age and men tend to have a higher incidence of vascular dementia at younger ages (Jorm and Jolley, 1998). Higher incidence of vascular dementia in younger men could reflect the effects of smoking. Prevalence studies have noted a general tendency for a higher prevalence of AD in women and vascular dementia in men; but an age-specific sex difference did not emerge in meta-analyses (Jorm and Jolley, 1998). The reasons stated for the higher prevalence of dementia in women are hormonal and also the fact that women tend to live longer than men (Alzheimer's Disease International, 2002).

Education

Available evidence suggests low educational level as a risk factor for AD (Cummings, 1995). Most prevalence studies have reported a higher frequency of dementia in persons with low levels of education. To address the excess of dementia among poorly educated persons, Katzman (1993) has hypothesised that education may increase the brain reserve by increasing the synaptic density in the neurocortical association cortex (the cerebral reserve hypothesis). Thus, individuals with more brain reserve might have more synapses to lose before AD is expressed clinically. Some studies have suggested that a larger brain size might be protective against dementia (Stern et al., 1999).

Since patients with a higher educational and occupational attainment have more cognitive reserve, more pathology is required before memory begins to be affected. Having no education is associated with dementia independent of gender, occupation, life habits, and hypertension. This association is stronger among younger old persons, and decreased with increasing age. The first decade of life is a critical period for developing dementia in later life. The decrease in dementia risk may be due to schooling, according to the cerebral reserve hypothesis or to the factors associated with higher educational level during childhood (De Ronchi et al., 1998).

Other hypotheses related to education and dementia are: the educated elderly may get more brain stimulation ('use it or lose it'), higher brain reserve capacity of educated persons could postpone the onset of dementia; and factors related to education such as lifestyle, occupational exposure, morbidity and health care may be responsible for the association with dementia (Ott et al., 1999). The Rotterdam study (Ott et al., 1999) found that low education was associated with a higher risk of dementia in women but not in men, thereby suggesting that the association is modified by sex.

Marital Status

Living alone and never having married pose a higher risk for dementia. Helmer et al. (1999) found that the risk was twice more for dementia in general and thrice for AD in these as compared to married ones. The explanation given to this effect is that being unmarried leads to a lesser cognitive stimulation due to a narrow social network, fewer leisure activities and a greater exposure to other risk factors like undernutrition.

Occupational Exposure

Exposure to mercury, carbon monoxide and aluminium have been suggested to be related to dementia. Details are described below.

CONSTITUTIONAL FACTORS

Family History and Genetic Factors

Rarely, dementia may occur in people aged below 60 years. This is found to be due to an inherited cause. A proof to this is the fact that majority of patients with Downs' syndrome who survive into adulthood develop AD. So Down's syndrome is a known risk factor for AD (Cummings, 1995). First-degree relatives are three to four times more likely to develop this than those without a family history.

Early onset familial AD is inherited as an autosomal dominant disorder associated with mutations on chromosomes 14 or 21 but vast majority of cases are sporadic and of late onset (Cummings, 1995).

Apolipoprotein E (ApoE) genotype, has been found to affect risk of future Alzheimer's disease. ApoE gene is found on chromosome 19. The gene has got instructions that enable the body to make a protein called apolipoprotein E. It is synthesized in several organs in the body, with diverse functions. The most well known function is to transport cholesterol into the cells. In the nervous system it is synthesized by the astrocytes and it participates in nervous tissue repair following injury. During postmortem studies, accumulation of ApoE has been observed throughout senile plaques and neurofibrillary tangles. People with 'at risk' form of this gene are about 3–4 times more likely to develop Alzheimer's disease. Having this gene does not necessarily mean that a person will develop Alzheimer's disease in their lifetime. Not having it does not mean that they will not.

PHYSICAL FACTORS

Cardiovascular Risk Factors

Ravaglia et al (1999) found that risk factors for stroke were present in almost one-third of the AD cases. In a study by Pohjasvaara et al (1998) to examine the clinical determinants of post-stroke dementia in a group of 337 patients, found dementia in 1/3rd of patients who survive to 3 months after a stroke. Stroke features (dysphasia, major dominant stroke syndrome), host characteristics (education levels) and prior cerebrovascular disease, each independently contributed to the risk. The following mechanisms have been proposed for this association:

- Direct effect on the pathology: severe coronary artery disease leading to an increase in the senile plaque count. Vascular amyloid deposition was found to be associated with cerebral arteriosclerosis.
- Vascular disease unmasks subclinical AD.
- Role of ApoE: ApoE allele is known to be a risk factor for both cardiovascular disease and for AD.
- Adding further to the vascular risk factors are: atrial fibrillation, hypertension, inflammation and vascular diseases, including diabetes mellitus.

Atrial Fibrillation

Atrial fibrillation is a common finding in the elderly. Patients with atrial fibrillation frequently develop cerebral infarctions, which often remain clinically silent. In the Rotterdam study (Ott et al, 1997) involving 6584 patients, the conclusion was that both vascular and AD are related to atrial fibrillation even if no clinical stroke occurred. The mechanism proposed for the association is that atrial fibrillation leads to thromboemboli formation that act like multiple silent infarcts. This coupled with a decrease in cardiac output leads to underperfusion of cerebral hemispheres leading to cognitive decline.

Hypertension

Several longitudinal investigations have established an association between elevated blood pressure (BP) in middle aged and the observation of subsequent (range 12–30 years later) decreased neurobehavioural functioning in old age. This appears to be independent of antihypertensive medication status, age, education, and incidence of cardiovascular disease. Elevated BP, especially systolic BP and hypertension are both known to be associated cross sectionally with the presence and amount of white matter hyperintensities (WMHIs) and cerebral atrophy. Larger WMHIs are associated with lower levels of cognitive function (Swan et al., 1998). So, midlife elevated systolic BP is a significant predictor of decline in cognitive function. Studies by Tzourio et al (1999) showed that high BP and chronicity of it were associated with a higher risk of cognitive decline, the highest risk being in untreated hypertensives.

Further studies that strengthen the association are the ones like Guo et al (1999) who have found that use of antihypertensives is protective against dementia. It was found that persons taking antihypertensives had a reduced incidence of dementia (adjusted relative risk, 0.7; 95% confidence interval 0.6–1.0; p=0.03). Persons taking diuretics had further lower risk. Further, patients with dementia who were not taking diuretics had a 2-fold faster rate of decline in score on mini-mental status examination (MMSE), than those taking diuretics.

The mechanism by which hypertension plays a role is by a disturbance in cerebral perfusion or metabolism leading on to a white matter disease secondary to ischaemia, demyelination and cerebral atrophy. Hypertension is also associated with increased plaque and tangle density.

Vascular Diseases
Vascular risk factors are important not only in the aetiology of vascular dementia but also in the aetiology of AD (Stewart et al., 1998). Coronary heart disease (OR 2.50) is a known risk factor for vascular dementia (Ross et al, 1999). Clinical predictors of dementia among individuals with ischaemic stroke include increasing age, low level of education, non-white race and diabetes mellitus (Ross et al, 1999).

Inflammation

Increased evidence indicates that inflammation is involved in the pathogenesis of AD. Neuritic plaques, a cardinal neuropathologic marker of AD, are composed of amyloid peptides and numerous other proteins indicative of an inflammatory response. It has been found that relative risk (RR) for AD decreased with increasing duration of non-steroidal anti-inflammatory drugs (NSAID) use (Stewart et al., 1997). In those with 2 or more years of reported NSAID use, the RR is 0.40, compared with 0.65 for those with less than 2 years of NSAID use. No association was found between AD risk and use of acetaminophen (a pain-relief medication with little or no anti-inflammatory activity) (Stewart et al, 1997).

Although the precise role of inflammation in AD pathogenesis is not known, the association of immune system proteins and immune competent microglial cells with senile plaques (SP) suggests that inflammation may play a role in the development of SP. Alternatively, pre-established SP may attract microglia and stimulate them to produce various pro-inflammatory mediators, thus helping to sustain and propagate the inflammatory process. In either case, activated microglial cells are capable of secreting a variety of potentially neurotoxic substances that could contribute to neurodegeneration in AD. NSAID may be more beneficial than steroids in preventing AD by virtue of their superior ability to suppress the specific type of inflammation that occurs in AD brain tissue. A possible role of NSAID for treatment of AD is also suggested (Mackenzie, 2000).

An alternate mechanism explained by Sevush et al (1998) involved the activation of platelets in AD. Platelets of patients with AD exhibit greater unstimulated activation than those of controls. Potential causes of such activation include possible stimulation of platelets by damaged cerebral endothelial cells or platelet activation induced by membrane abnormalities reported to be present in platelets of patients with AD. Evidence has suggested that platelets are the principal source of both amyloid precursor proteins and beta-amyloid peptide in human blood. It is possible that AD platelet activation may reflect or even contribute to the pathogenesis of the disease (Sevush et al, 1998).

Early observations of a low dementia prevalence rates among cases of rheumatoid arthritis have been supported by case-control studies reporting an inverse association between arthritic conditions and AD. In a study by Prince et al (1998) a significant, although modest, association between change in the paired associate learning test score over time and NSAID use was found, which was modified by age. NSAID users showed less decline, with younger subjects seeming to benefit more than the older. This suggests more studies and randomised control trials of NSAID are required to delineate their role more clearly.

Head Injury

Head injury is a risk factor for AD (Cummings, 1995). People who take part in boxing are at risk for developing a particular type of dementia, which is believed to be caused by repeated blows to the head. Some studies have also found that head injuries have occurred about two times more commonly than expected in people with AD. Head injury in this context means any blow to the head resulting in a loss of consciousness for at least 15 minutes. There have been studies that did not find any association between head injury and dementia; however, the hypotheses proposed (Mayeux et al., 1995) for this association are that:

■ There is a possible association of trauma and ApoE epsilon 4 allele. The presence of ApoE increases the risk of developing dementia even with a minor head trauma.

■ Trauma is seen to cause overexpression of beta-amyloid precursor proteins causing an increase in the deposition of beta-amyloid proteins in the brain, similar to that in patients of AD.

Infections

Human Immunodeficiency Virus

Human Immunodeficiency virus (HIV) associated dementia complex (HIV dementia) has been estimated to affect 60% of all individuals in the late stages of HIV disease typically presenting as a subcortical disease. McArthur et al (1993) have studied the risk factors and have found that low pre-AIDS haemoglobin and body mass index, more constitutional symptoms 7–12 months before AIDS and older age at AIDS onset were the most significant predictors of dementia, pre-AIDS haemoglobin being the most significant predictor of dementia. There were no significant risks from demographic characteristics, specific AIDS defining illnesses, zidovudine use before AIDS or CD4+ lymphocyte count before AIDS. McArthur et al. (1993) projected that 12 months after the first AIDS diagnosis, 7.1% of survivors will have dementia. The observed association between anaemia, low weight, constitutional symptoms, and dementia suggests a role for cytokines inducing both systemic and neurologic disease.

Other Infections
Other infections like syphilis, Creutzfeldt-Jakob disease, chronic meningitis have been implicated in the aetiology of dementia (Cummings, 1995).

Other Physical Illnesses

Medical disorders like Parkinson's disease, Huntington's disease, deficiencies of certain vitamins (thiamine, vitamin B_{12}, folic acid), renal failure and hepatic disturbances (Cummings, 1995), severe chronic bronchitis and advanced malignancies have all been reported to be associated with predisposition to development of dementia (Alzheimer's Disease International, 2002).

Diabetes Mellitus
Diabetes mellitus has been well studied in dementia. There is interplay between Stroke-Diabetes Mellitus (especially type II) and dementia. Curb et al. (1999) found no association between AD and diabetes mellitus present either 25 or 15 years previously, after adjustment for age and education. A significant association was reported however between impaired glucose tolerance at baseline and vascular dementia (Curb et al., 1999). One-hour postprandial glucose (OR: 1.41) is significantly predictive of vascular dementia (Ross et al., 1999).

The question that arises is whether brain is another site of end organ damage in diabetes mellitus. The following mechanisms have been proposed for the association: (a) it is not diabetes mellitus per-se but the vascular complications of diabetes that result in neurodegeneration; and, (b) glycoprotein and glycosylation may be associated with the development of neuritic plaques in AD.

Toxins

Role of Aluminium
Aluminium has been a matter of much debate in the causation of AD. The 'aluminium hypothesis' originated in 1965 with the discovery that injections of aluminium salts into the brain or cerebrospinal fluid of rabbits induces a progressive encephalopathy that is associated with the development of lesions reminiscent of neurofibrillary tangles. This

logic was further extended to aluminium in drinking water (McLachlan et al., 1996), in dialysis and in antacids. This issue has caused an 'aluminium phobia' with families throwing away their aluminium cooking ware and utensils.

However, dialysis encephalopathy has been found to bear no similarity to AD. In addition, the examinations of brain specimens reveal a total absence of neuritic senile plaques and tangles, thereby refuting the argument for aluminium as a causative agent in AD (Munoz, 1998). Several large controlled studies have documented the lack of association between aluminium in drinking water and dementia. In addition, patients who consume antacids that contain aluminium do not demonstrate an increased incidence of dementia (Munoz, 1998). Using autopsy verified cases of AD, control subjects and an aluminium concentration cut off level of 100 microgram per litre, McLachlan et al. (1996) have determined the odds ratio for developing AD was 2.6 (95% confidence interval 1.2–5.7); and the relative risk of developing AD increased with higher aluminium concentration cut off levels (Forbes and Hill, 1998). However, these studies have methodological limitations. Available evidence answers the question of link between aluminium exposure and risk of Alzheimer with a tentative yes and resounding no (Hachinski, 1998).

Other Toxins
Other toxins that have been implicated as potential risk factors in AD are mercury and carbon monoxide. The final word about their involvement is awaited.

Oestrogen

Since women have a higher prevalence of dementia than men, it is thought that hormone depletion in postmenopausal women is the cause. In addition, evidence from many case control and cohort studies suggest that a woman's use of oestrogen after menopause is associated with a reduced risk of developing AD, and in women with AD, oestrogen therapy is linked to better performance on a variety of cognitive measures (Waring et al., 1999; Henderson et al., 1996). Small intervention studies have shown that oestrogen treatment might improve AD symptoms. However, two randomized double blind placebo controlled studies by Henderson et al. (2000) and Mulnard et al. (2000) have not shown any improvement in short term, by oestrogen, in symptoms of most women with AD.

PSYCHOSOCIAL FACTORS

Life Style

As prevalence of dementia varies in different cultures, researchers have tried to find variations in life style considering factors like diet, substance use, and exercise. There have been some interesting observations.

Dietary Factors

The role of both micro- and macronutrients has been studied with regards to cognitive decline. Of the micronutrients, deficiencies of vitamin B_1, B_2, B_6, B_{12}, C, and folate are significantly associated with cognitive impairment.

Elevated plasma homocysteine levels were associated with AD (Clarke et al., 1998). Reduced dietary intake of folate and vitamin B_{12} leading to elevation in plasma homocysteine levels is a possibility but cause or consequence, abnormalities in levels may be still relevant to the clinical course of the AD (Clarke et al., 1998).

The association of low folate and vitamin B_{12} levels with AD may be related to their effects on methylation reactions in the brain or may be mediated by their effects on plasma homocysteine levels. Homocysteine may have a neurotoxic effect by activating N-methyl-D-aspartate receptors, leading to cell death. In addition, elevated homocysteine levels are a strong risk factor for the development of vascular diseases (Clarke et al., 1998).

On the other hand, a few data are available on the role of micronutrient intake in AD. In a study by Solfrizzi et al. (1999), it was found in an elderly population of Italy with a typical Mediterranean diet, that, high monounsaturated fatty acids (MUFA) intake appeared to be protective against age related cognitive decline. It was hypothesised that the effect could be related to the role of fatty acids in maintaining the structural integrity of neuronal membranes. With advancing age, the neuronal membranes demonstrate an increase in MUFA content.

In an interesting study, Lim et al. (2001) have noted that curcumin, a yellow curry spice derived from turmeric, is a potent antioxidant and is several times more potent a free radical scavenger than vitamin E. It is also found to reduce oxidative damage and amyloid pathology in an AD transgenic mouse. It is now thought that factors like these could be implicated in the 4.4 fold lower rate of AD in prevalence in 70–79 year olds in India compared to the United States.

The antioxidant vitamin E and presently unknown factors related to a Western diet as opposed to Oriental diet may be protective against developing vascular dementia. So, supplemental vitamin E may be beneficial (Ross et al., 1999).

Caffeine

Caffeine is the most widely consumed behaviourally active substance in the world. Neuroprotective effects of caffeine in low doses, chronically administered, have been shown in different experimental models. Case control studies have shown that caffeine intake was associated with a significantly lower risk of AD. These results if confirmed with future prospective studies may have a major impact on the prevention of AD.

Alcohol

People who drink excessive amounts of alcohol over a prolonged period of time may develop dementia. Saunders et al. (1991) found that men with a history of heavy drinking (>17.5 units of alcohol per week) for greater than 5 years were found to have a greater than a 5 fold risk of suffering from dementia. Alcohol by virtue of its direct damage on the brain and also the malnourishment commonly associated with its chronic use becomes a risk factor. Though some reports claim that a small amount of alcohol is beneficial, this protective effect needs to be well researched.

The risk of dementia related to alcohol drinking is modified by the presence of apolipoprotein e4 allele. In a study of risk of dementia associated with alcohol drinking in middle age, Anttila et al. (2004) reported that compared to persons who never drank and did not carry the apolipoprotein e4 allele, e4 carriers who drank infrequently (less than once a month) were 2.3 times more likely to develop dementia, and carriers who drank frequently (several times a month) were 3.6 times more likely. However, the risk of dementia for e4 carriers who never drank was not different from that of non-carriers who never drank. Among the non-carriers, there was no association between alcohol drinking and the risk of dementia.

Tobacco Use

Early researchers suggested that an inverse association exists between smoking and AD, meaning thereby that smoking was protective in AD. It was proposed that smoking augments cholinergic metabolism by up-regulation of cholinergic nicotinic receptors in the brain. Many of the manifestations of AD are attributed to alterations in acetylcholine metabolism and as a result, smoking was thought to decrease the risk or at least retard the onset of symptoms associated with AD through this mechanism.

However, the Rotterdam study (Ott et al, 1998) and a study by Merchant et al (1999) and others have proven that on the contrary, smoking increases the risk of AD. The observations in the previous studies were found to be due to methodological limitations of case-control study designs. It is now believed that smoking leads to a reduction in cerebral perfusion and adversely alters the capacity of cells to repair DNA, which is already low in the aged. The RR of AD among former smoker was 0.7, for current smoker 1.9; smokers without an ApoE-e4 allele had the highest risk with RR 2.1, compared to those with an ApoE-e4 allele (RR=1.4). There may be slight reduction in the risk of AD in smokers who quit smoking (Merchant et al, 1999).

Exercise

Regular physical exercise is an important and a potent *protective* factor for cognitive decline and dementia in the elderly. This has been proven in a prospective study by Laurin et al. (2001) in Canada, where exercise data of 9008 men and women were collected when subjects were non-demented. High levels of physical activity were associated with reduced risks of cognitive impairment. The possible mechanisms suggested for the protective effect of exercise are that: exercise improves cerebral blood flow and thereby improves cerebral nutrient supply; it decreases blood lipid levels; and it inhibits platelet aggregation.

Social Environment

Early Life Environment
The early life environment and its effect on growth and maturation of children and adolescents are linked to many adult chronic diseases (heart diseases, stroke, hypertension, and diabetes mellitus). AD may also have an early life link. The areas of the brain that show the earliest signs of AD are the same areas of the brain that take the longest to mature during childhood and adolescence (hippocampal formation, reticular formation, intracortical association areas). A poor quality childhood and adolescent environment could prevent the brain from reaching complete levels of maturation. Lower levels of brain maturation may put people at a higher risk for AD. Moceri et al. (2000) in a systematic study found that the area of residence (urban) before the age of 18 years and a higher number of siblings are associated with subsequent development of AD. For each additional child in the family, the risk of AD increases by 8% (odds ratio: 1.08). Both these factors reflect the socioeconomic level and therefore the quality of life enjoyed. Moceri et al. (2000) did not find any association between mother's age at patient's birth and subsequent onset of AD.

Social Ties and Leisure
Recent findings suggest that a rich social network may decrease the risk of developing dementia. It is hypothesised that such a protective effect may be due to social interaction and intellectual stimulation. Wang et al. (2002) did a longitudinal study in Sweden and suggested that stimulating activity, either mentally or socially oriented. may protect against dementia. This indicates that both social interaction and intellectual stimulation may be relevant to preserving mental functioning in the elderly.

Psychiatric Illness

Delirium when it becomes too frequent or lasts longer then there is risk of dementia due to the underlying pathology. Alcohol dependence can also lead to dementia.

Depression

People with depressed mood have a higher risk of developing dementia. With a late onset first episode of depression, dementia was seen to develop within 3–8 years after onset of depression (Berger et al., 1999). Another feature associating depression and dementia is that depressive symptoms are found in 15–50% of patients with AD compared to 1–10% in non-demented elderly (Berger et al., 1999).

The following hypotheses have been proposed to explain the association: (i) depression may be an early prodrome of an impending dementia (Mowry et al., 1998); (ii) depression may bring forward the clinical manifestations of dementing diseases like cognitive deficits that are also seen in depression; and (iii) depression leads to a damage to the hippocampus (through a glucocorticoid cascade) which plays an important role in memory functions.

CONCLUSION

Doing AD research is like doing a jigsaw puzzle with a thousand pieces. One would not know if a risk factor in question would be in the centre or at the periphery of the picture in the puzzle. While substantial progress has been made in identifying the possible risk factors, research in this area is only a few decades old and there is still a long way to go. Having learnt more about the underpinnings and the risk factors for dementia, one can hope for many more promising therapies and cautions for its prevention and treatment.

REFERENCES

- Alzheimer's Disease International (2002) Risk factors for dementia. http://www.alz.co.uk/adi/pdf/9riskfactors.pdf (accessed January, 2004).
- Anttila T, Eeva-Liisa H, Viitanen M, et al. (2004) Alcohol drinking in middle age and subsequent risk of mild cognitive impairment and

dementia in old age: a prospective population based study. *British Medical Journal,* 329, 539–542.

■ Berger AK, Fratiglioni L, Forsell Y, Winblad B, Backman L. (1999) The occurrence of depressive symptoms in the preclinical phase of AD: a population-based study. *Neurology.* 53(9), 1998–2002.

■ Clarke R, Smith AD, Jobst KA, Refsum H, Sutton L, Ueland PM. (1998) Folate, vitamin B_{12}, and serum total homocysteine levels in confirmed Alzheimer disease. *Arch Neurol.* 55(11), 1449–55.

■ Cumings JL (1995) Dementia: the failing brain. *Lancet,* 345:1481–1484.

■ Curb JD, Rodriguez BL, Abott RD, et al. (1999) Longitudinal association of vascular and Alzheimer's dementias, diabetes and glucose tolerance. *Neurology,* 52, 971–975.

■ De Ronchi D, Fratiglioni L, Rucci P, Paternico A, Graziani S, Dalmonte E. (1998) The effect of education on dementia occurrence in an Italian population with middle to high socioeconomic status. *Neurology.* 50(5), 1231–8.

■ Forbes WF, Hill GB. (1998) Is exposure to aluminium a risk factor for the development of Alzheimer disease? - Yes. *Arch Neurol.* 55(5), 740–741.

■ Guo Z, Fratiglioni L, Zhu L, Fastbom J, Winblad B, Viitanen M. (1999) Occurrence and progression of dementia in a community population aged 75 years and older: relationship of antihypertensive medication use. *Arch Neurol.* 56(8), 991–6.

■ Hachinski, V. (1998) Aluminium exposure and risk of Alzheimer's disease. *Arch Neurol,* 55, 742.

■ Helmer C, Damon D, Letenneur L, et al. (1999) Marital status and risk of Alzheimer's disease: a French population-based cohort study. *Neurology.* 53(9), 1953–8.

■ Henderson VW, Paganini-Hill A, Miller BL, et al. (2000) Estrogen for Alzheimer's disease in women: randomized, double-blind, placebo-controlled trial. *Neurology.* 54(2), 295–301.

■ Henderson W, Watt L, Buckwalter JG (1996) Cognitive skills associated with estrogen replacement in women with Alzheimer's disease. *Psychoneuroendocrinology,* 21, 421–430.

■ Jorm AF, Jolley D. (1998) The incidence of dementia: a meta-analysis. *Neurology.* 51(3), 728–33.

■ Katzman R. (1993) Education and the prevalence of dementia and Alzheimer's disease. *Neurology.* 43(1), 13–20.

- Laurin D, Verreault R, Lindsay J, MacPherson K, Rockwood K. (2001) Physical activity and risk of cognitive impairment and dementia in elderly persons. *Arch Neurol,* 58(3), 498–504.
- Lim GP, Chu T, Yang F, Beech W, Frautschy SA, Cole GM. (2001) The curry spice curcumin reduces oxidative damage and amyloid pathology in an Alzheimer transgenic mouse. *J Neurosci.* 21(21), 8370–7.
- Mackenzie IR. (2000) Anti-inflammatory drugs and Alzheimer-type pathology in aging. *Neurology,* 8, 54(3), 732–4.
- Mayeux R, Ottman R, Maestre G, et al. (1995) Synergistic effects of traumatic head injury and apolipoprotein-epsilon 4 in patients with Alzheimer's disease. *Neurology,* 45(3 Pt 1), 555–7.
- McArthur JC, Hoover DR, Bacellar H, et al. (1993) Dementia in AIDS patients: incidence and risk factors. Multicenter AIDS Cohort Study. Neurology. 43(11), 2245-52.
- McLachlan DR, Bergeron C, Smith JE, Boomer D, Rifat SL. (1996) Risk for neuropathologically confirmed Alzheimer's disease and residual aluminium in municipal drinking water employing weighted residential histories. *Neurology.* 46(2), 401–5.
- Merchant C, Tang MX, Albert S, Manly J, Stern Y, Mayeux R. (1999) The influence of smoking on the risk of Alzheimer's disease. *Neurology.* 52(7), 1408–12.
- Moceri VM, Kukull WA, Emanuel I, van Belle G, Larson EB. (2000) Early-life risk factors and the development of Alzheimer's disease. *Neurology.* 54(2), 415–20.
- Mowry BJ, Burvill PW. (1988) A study of mild dementia in the community using a wide range of diagnostic criteria. *Br J Psychiatry.* 153, 328–34.
- Mulnard RA, Cotman CW, Kawas C, et al. (2000) Estrogen replacement therapy for treatment of mild to moderate Alzheimer disease: a randomized controlled trial. Alzheimer's Disease Cooperative Study. *JAMA.* 283(8), 1007–15.
- Munoz DG. (1998) Is exposure to aluminium a risk factor for the development of Alzheimer disease?-No. *Arch Neurol.* 55(5), 737–9.
- Ott A, Breteler MM, de Bruyne MC, van Harskamp F, Grobbee DE, Hofman A. (1997) Atrial fibrillation and dementia in a population-based study. The Rotterdam Study. *Stroke.* 28(2), 316–21.

- Ott A, Slooter AJ, Hofman A, et al. (1998) Smoking and risk of dementia and Alzheimer's disease in a population-based cohort study: the Rotterdam Study. *Lancet.* 351(9119), 1840–3.
- Ott A, Stolk RP, van Harskamp F, Pols HA, Hofman A, Breteler MM. (1999) Diabetes mellitus and the risk of dementia: The Rotterdam Study. *Neurology.* 53(9), 1937–42.
- Ott A, vanRossum CTM, vanHarskampF, vande Mheen H, Hofman A, Breteler MMB (1999) Education and the incidence of dementia in a large population based study: The Rotterdam Study. *Neurology,* 52, 663–666.
- Pohjasvaara T, Leppavuori A, Siira I, Vataja R, Kaste M, Erkinjuntti T. (1998) Frequency and clinical determinants of post-stroke depression. *Stroke.* 29(11), 2311–7.
- Prince M, Rabe-Hesketh S, Brennan P. (1998) Do antiarthritic drugs decrease the risk for cognitive decline? An analysis based on data from the MRC treatment trial of hypertension in older adults. *Neurology.* 50(2), 374–9.
- Ravaglia G, Forti P, De Ronchi D, et al. (1999) Prevalence and severity of dementia among northern Italian centenarians. *Neurology.* 53(2), 416–8.
- Ross GW, Petrovitch H, White LR, et al. (1999) Characterisation of risk factors for vascular dementia: The Honolulu-Asia Aging Study. *Neurology,* 53, 337–343.
- Saunders PA, Copeland JR, Dewey ME, et al. (1991) Heavy drinking as a risk factor for depression and dementia in elderly men. Findings from the Liverpool longitudinal community study. *British Journal of Psychiatry,* 159, 213–6.
- Sevush S, Jy W, Horstman LL, Mao WW, Kolodny L, Ahn YS. (1998) Platelet activation in Alzheimer disease. *Arch Neurol.* 55(4), 530–6.
- Solfrizzi V, Panza F, Torres F, et al. (1999) High monounsaturated fatty acids intake protects against age-related cognitive decline. *Neurology.* 52(8): 1563–9.
- Stern Y, Albert S, Tang MX, Tsai WY. (1999) Rate of memory decline in AD is related to education and occupation: cognitive reserve? *Neurology.* 53(9), 1942–7.
- Stewart R. (1998) Cardiovascular factors in Alzheimer's disease. *J Neurol Neurosurg Psychiatry.* 65(2), 143–7.

- Stewart WF, Kawas C, Corrada M, Metter EJ. (1997) Risk of Alzheimer's disease and duration of NSAID use. *Neurology.* 48(3), 626–32.
- Strauss EV, Viitanen M, DeRonchi D, Winblad B, Fratiglioni L. (1999) Aging and the occurrence of dementia. *Arch Neurol,* 56, 587–592.
- Swan GE, DeCarli C, Miller BL, et al. (1998) Association of midlife blood pressure to late-life cognitive decline and brain morphology. *Neurology.* 51(4), 986–93.
- Thomassen R, van Schaick HW, Blansjaar BA. (1998) Prevalence of dementia over age 100. *Neurology.* 50 (1), 283–6.
- Tzourio C, Dufouil C, Ducimetiere P, Alperovitch A. (1999) Cognitive decline in individuals with high blood pressure: a longitudinal study in the elderly. EVA Study Group. Epidemiology of Vascular Aging. *Neurology.* 53(9), 1948–52.
- Wang HX, Karp A, Winblad B, Fratiglioni L. (2002) Late-life engagement in social and leisure activities is associated with a decreased risk of dementia: a longitudinal study from the Kungsholmen project. *Am J Epidemiol.* 155(12), 1081–7.
- Waring SC, Rocca WA, Peterson RC, O'Brien PC, Tangalos EG, Kokmen E. (1999) Postmenopausal oestrogen replacement therapy and risk of AD: A population based study. *Neurology,* 52, 965–970.

8

Neuropathology of Dementia

P Ravikala V Rao

Introduction

Since dementia is a common component of diffuse diseases of the brain of varied aetiology, histopathological study is imperative in the accurate diagnosis of these disorders. This chapter deals with neuropathology of Alzheimer disease and primary dementias.

Dementias of varying aetiology involve selected areas of the brain (Table 8.1). Important regions of brain that are involved in dementia are: subthalamus (12), hippocampus cornu ammonis (18, a – CA1, b – CA2, c – CA3, d – CA4), dentate gyrus (19), subiculum (20), entorhinal region (21), collateral sulci (22), tail of caudate nucleus (25), putamen (31), globus (32), internal capsule (33), caudate nucleus (36) (Duvernoy, 1991).

HISTOLOGICAL HALLMARKS OF DEMENTIA

Senile plaque (SP): Haematoxylin and Eosin (H & E) stain: Spherical 5–100 micron central dense congophilic core is surrounded by radiating argyrophilic structures measuring 5 micron. Plaque core is surrounded by debris of degenerating neuron, microglia and argyrophilic macrophages (Hirano, 1988).

Table 8.1 Topography of the brain involvement in various types of dementias

Area in brain	Type of dementia
Amygdaloid body	AD, LBD
Body of callosum	AIDS
Brain stem and pons	CJ
Cerebellum	CJD
Cingulate gyrus	FTD
Cortical and leptomeningeal vessels	AM
Frontal lobe	AD, FTD, PICK, PSP, HUN, MCI, CJ
Globus pallidus	PSP
Hippocampus, hippocampal gyrus	AD, VD, MCI, LBD, MCI, PICK, PSP
Inferior parietal lobule	HUN
Internal capsule	AL
Locus ceruleus	AD, PSP, LBD
Occipital	AD
Parietal	HUN
Putamen, claustrum, globus pallidus	AL, AD, PICK, FTD, PSP, CJD, AIDS
Substantia nigra	FTD, PSP, AD, LBD
Subthalamic nulei	PSP
Superior, middle, inferior temporal	AD, FTD, PICK, PSP, MCI
Thalamus	AD, PSP, CJ, AIDS

(AD: Alzheimer's disease; AL: Arteriopathy and leucoencephalopathy; AM: Amyloid angiopathy; CJD: Creutzfeldt-Jakob's disease; FTD: Frontotemporal dementia; HUN: Huntington; LBD: Lewy body disease; MCI: Mild cognitive impairment; PICK: Pick's disease; PSP: Progressive supranuclear palsy; VD: Vascular disease (Binder and Haughton, 1979; Mirra et al. 1993)

Neurofibrillary tangle (NFT): (H&E): Basophilic thready masses in the cytoplasm of neuron, intensely argyrophilic with silver stain (Hirano, 1988).

Granulovacuolar degeneration (GVD): (H&E stain, silver stain) 5–6μ vacuoles in the cytoplasm of pyramidal neurons. Vacuoles contain 1–2 granules. Clusters of vacuoles cause neuron to bulge and displace nucleus to eccentric location (Hirano, 1988).

Hirano bodies: Eosinophilic, paracrystalline, cytoplasmic or juxtaneuronal rod-like bodies.

Perivascular amyloid deposit: Amyloid is homogeneous pink deposit which stains red with Congo red stain and fluorescent by thioflavin S fluorescent stain. Amyloid deposits are seen around blood vessels and in SP (Mirra et al 1993).

Pick bodies: Swollen or ballooned neurons containing silver staining cytoplasmic inclusion called pick bodies of 10–12 micron size.

Lewy bodies: Intraneuronal cytoplasmic eosinophilic inclusions are seen surrounded by halo. Inclusion is PAS +ve and ubiquitin + (Mirra, et al., 1993).

Spongiform change: Large vacuole in neuropil of neocortex with loss of neuron and reactive astrocytic gliosis are seen (Hansen and Crain, 1995).

Dystrophic neuritis: Short, thread-like, argentophilic, degenerating axon and dendrites of neurons with tangles. Thioflavin S +ve fibres stain identical to NFT and SP neuritis (Hirano, 1988).

Neuronal loss in the following regions:
- Pyramidal neurons of temporal and frontal lobe are lost
- CA I and subiculum of hippocampus
- Amygdala
- Cholinergic nucleus basalis of Meynert
- Septal nuclei

- Noradrenergic—locus ceruleus, raphe complex, central region projecting to the temporal and parietal cortex
- Serotonergic—dorsal raphe nucleus, superior central nucleus and dorsal segmental nucleus

Neuronal changes: Apical and basal dendritic spines undergo degeneration and dendritic plasticity is reduced resulting in decreased capacity for protein synthesis.

Synaptic loss: Around 50% synaptic loss occurs in neocortex.

PROTEINS AND DEMENTIA

Amyloid Precursor Protein

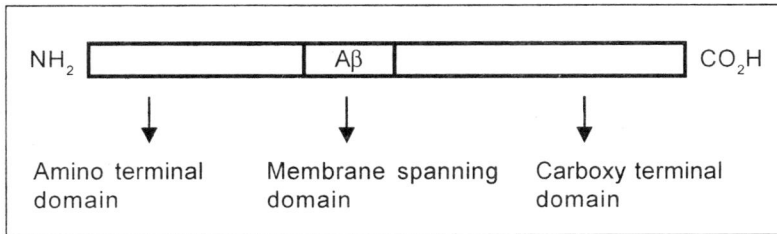

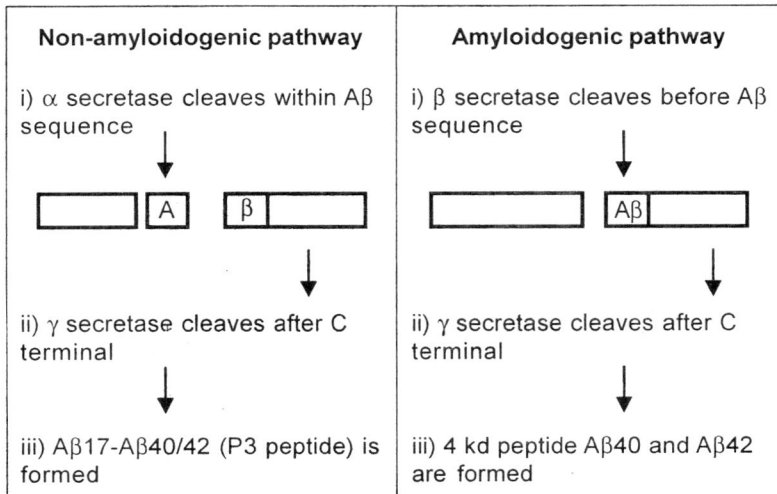

Non-amyloidogenic pathway	Amyloidogenic pathway
i) α secretase cleaves within Aβ sequence	i) β secretase cleaves before Aβ sequence
ii) γ secretase cleaves after C terminal	ii) γ secretase cleaves after C terminal
iii) Aβ17-Aβ40/42 (P3 peptide) is formed	iii) 4 kd peptide Aβ40 and Aβ42 are formed

Fig. 8.1 Normal metabolism of amyloid precursor protein
(Presenilin 1 controls γ secretase.) (Hedera and Turner, 2002)

Mutations of APP Gene

Amyloid Precursor Protein (APP) gene is located on long arm of Chromosome 21 (Hedera and Turner, 2002). Its mutations are depicted in Figure 8.2.

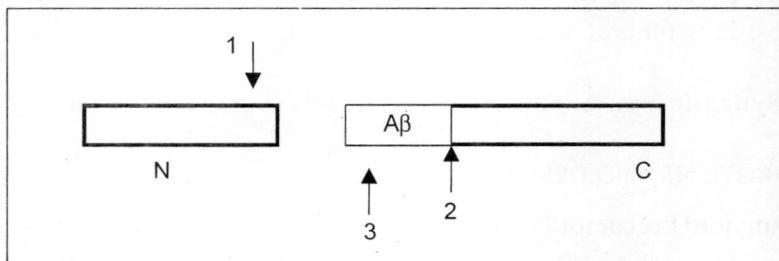

Fig. 8.2 Mutations of APP gene

1. Double missense mutations near 770 isoform of APP near β secretase cleavage site produce increase in Aβ40 and 42.
2. Single missense mutations near γ secretase cleavage site produces increase in Aβ42.
3. Mutation within Aβ sequence at position 692, 693 and 694 near γ secretase cleavage site produce mutated Aβ40 which causes vascular amyloid deposit and Aβ42, which is deposited in senile plaque.

Presenilin 1 mutation on chromosome 14 alters γ secretase cleavage to produce Aβ42–43. Above mutations cause early onset or autosomal dominant familial Alzheimer's disease. Apolipoprotein E mutation on chromosome 19, polymorphism on α -2 macroglobulin and low density related receptor protein seen on CH_{12} produce late onset sporadic Alzheimer's disease.

Role of Apolipoprotein E in Dementia

Apolipoprotein E is produced by glia and has receptors in the neuron. It mediates phospholipid, cholesterol mobilisation, membrane remodelling and maintains synaptic plasticity. It functions in reelin signaling pathway (Lovestone and McLoughlin, 2002), which is essential for migration of developing neurons. ApoE has 3 normal alleles e2, e3 and e4. All carry 2 copies of Apo-e gene. e3 is 80% prevalent. e3/4 genotype has 3 fold increase in Alzheimer's disease and e4/4 has 8 fold increase with early onset. e 4/4 allele is associated with decreased hippocampal insulin degrading enzyme resulting in decreased clearance of Aβ. Apo-e 4 has great avidity for Aβ42 and low efficiency for interacting with tau. e4 increases in senile plaque but not in NFT (Cook et al., 2003).

Role of Tau Protein in Dementia

Tau is microtubule associated protein and the gene MAPT has 16 exon on Ch 17q.21 (Delacourte and Buee, 2002). Tau is normal component of neuronal cytoskeleton, present in axons, assembles tubulin into microtubules, binds and stabilises microtubules for fast axonal transport. It promotes microtubule polymerisation. Tau expression is regulated by alternate splicing of exon 2, 3 and 10 resulting in 6 isoforms with 352–441 amino acids. Depending upon whether exon 10 is included or excluded, tau has 3 or 4 microtubules binding repeats, 3r tau or 4r tau. Mutation leads to disruption of normal regulation of tau expression and incorporation of exon 10 resulting in excess of 4 tau, which binds with microtubules with higher affinity than 3 tau isoforms. Proteomic regulation of tau function is by phosphorylation. More phosphorylated and unphosphorylated tau fails to bind and stabilise microtubules. Mutation in chromosome 17 produces autosomal tauopathies. Intronic mutation disrupts splicing of tau and missense mutation alters the function of tau.

Interaction of APP, ApoE and Tau in the Pathogenesis of Dementia (Fig. 8.3)

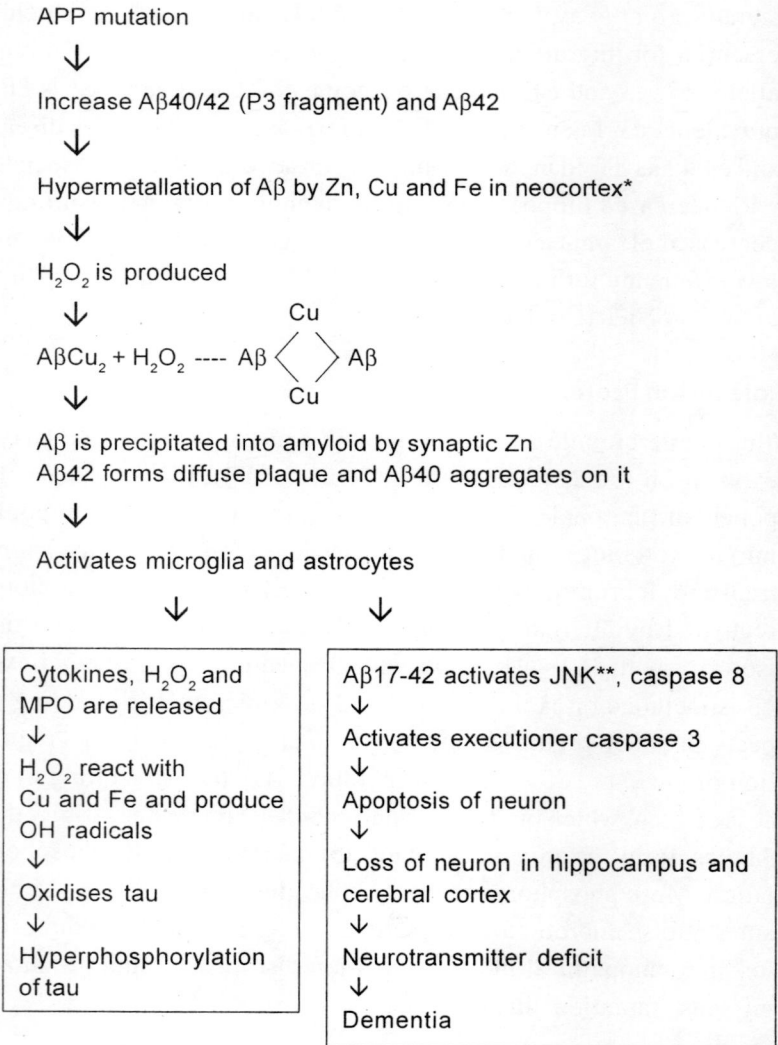

APP mutation
↓
Increase Aβ40/42 (P3 fragment) and Aβ42
↓
Hypermetallation of Aβ by Zn, Cu and Fe in neocortex*
↓
H_2O_2 is produced
↓

$$A\beta Cu_2 + H_2O_2 \ ---- \ A\beta \underset{Cu}{\overset{Cu}{\diamondsuit}} A\beta$$

↓
Aβ is precipitated into amyloid by synaptic Zn
Aβ42 forms diffuse plaque and Aβ40 aggregates on it
↓
Activates microglia and astrocytes

↓   ↓

Cytokines, H_2O_2 and MPO are released ↓ H_2O_2 react with Cu and Fe and produce OH radicals ↓ Oxidises tau ↓ Hyperphosphorylation of tau	Aβ17-42 activates JNK**, caspase 8 ↓ Activates executioner caspase 3 ↓ Apoptosis of neuron ↓ Loss of neuron in hippocampus and cerebral cortex ↓ Neurotransmitter deficit ↓ Dementia

Fig. 8.3 APP and pathogenesis of dementia
(*Bush, 2003; Lovestone and McLoughlin, 2002, **Wei, et al., 2002)

ApoE ε4

1. Promotes or stabilizes β sheet confirmation of Aβ
2. Decreases the activity of insulin degrading enzyme, which normally clears Aβ secreted by neurons and microglia in hippocampus. So Aβ deposits are not cleared
3. Reelin binds to ApoE receptor on neuron, phosphorylates disabled −1 intracellular adaptor protein. Defect in this pathway causes hyperphosphorylation of tau (Lovestone and McLoughlin, 2002).

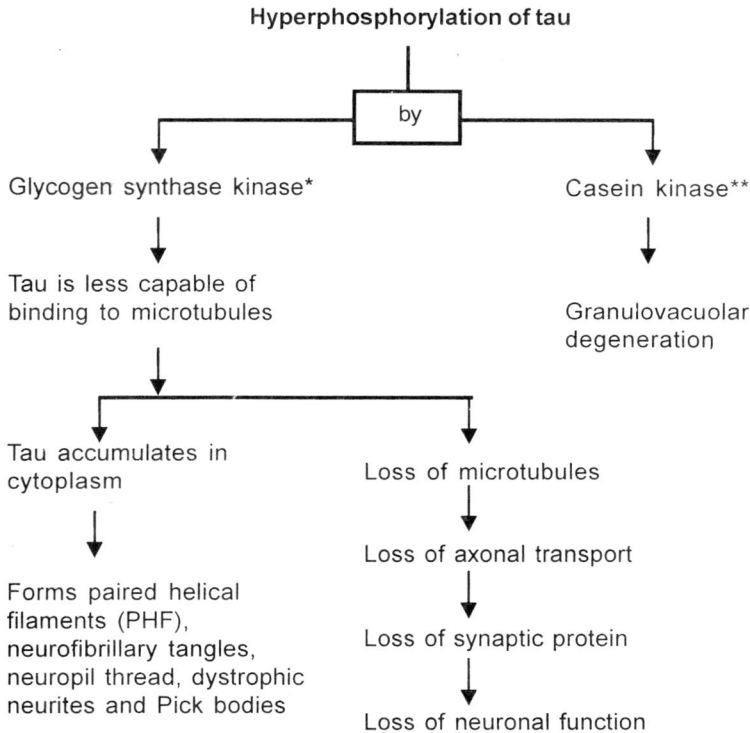

Fig. 8.4 Hyperphosphorylation of tau
(*Lovestone and McLoughlin, 2002; **Ghoshal et al., 1999)

PATHOLOGICAL DIAGNOSIS OF ALZHEIMER'S DISEASE

Gross findings: There is marked atrophy of frontal, temporal and occipital lobes, symmetrical enlargement of ventricles, large subarachnoid space, arteries widely patent and brain weighs 1000 g (Hirano, 1988).

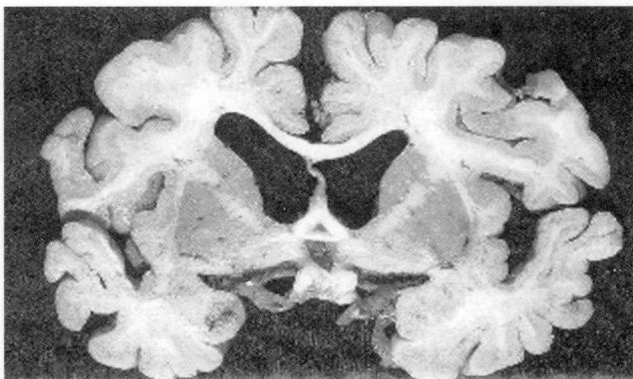

Fig. 8.5 Gross atrophy of brain

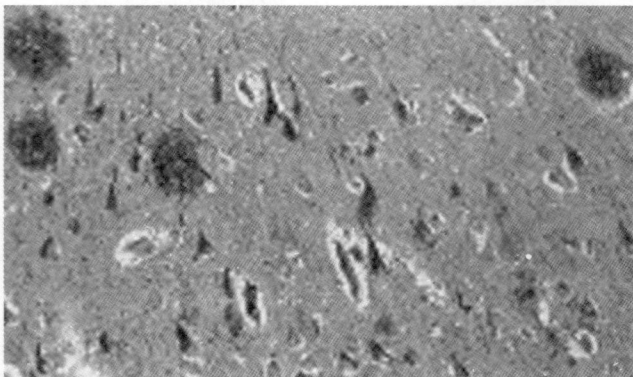

Fig. 8.6 Neurofibrillary tangles and senile plaques

Microscopically Salient Features

- Senile plaques
- Neurofibrillary tangles
- Granulovacuolar degeneration
- Loss of neurons and amyloid angiopathy

Senile Plaques

SP are present in neuropil. They are composed of soluble, aggregated fibrillar and non-fibrillar β-amyloid, surrounded by abnormal neurites, microglia and astrocytes.

Types of Senile Plaque (Scinto and Daffner, 2000)

- *Primitive SP:* Some amyloid as demonstrated by electron microscope and dystrophic neurites only
- *Classical SP:* Compact amyloid core surrounded by abnormal neurites
- *Burnt out or compact SP:* Large mass of amyloid, no neurites

Classification Based on Immunostaining by Specific Antibodies to Aβ

1. *Diffuse senile plaque:* Aβ immunostain: Round or amorphous deposits of aggregated non fibrillary Aβ with a granular reactive product without clear border (Janssen et al., 2000)
2. *Compact senile plaque:* Aβ positive compact plaque
3. *Cored senile plaque:* Clearly defined central round deposit of fibrillar Aβ called cored plaque (Janssen et al., 2000)
4. *Neuritic senile plaque:* Cored plaque with dystrophic neuritis— thick black neurites surround brown amyloid core. Presence of dystrophic neurites is specific for Alzheimer's disease.

Neurofibrillary Tangles

NFT are argentophilic, thioflavin T positive. Immunostain demonstrates antibody against paired helical filaments (PHF) and abnormally phosphorylated tau. Electron microscopically, PHF are 200 Å width, constricted at 800 Å interval to a width of 100 Å. Some straight filaments are also present. NFT are present in large neurons of cortex, limbic and paralimbic area. Neuropil threads are short, thread-like argentophilic, thioflavin T positive fibres composed of degenerating axons and dendrites (Janssen et al., 2000).

Granulo vacuolar Degeneration Bodies

GVD bodies in the neuron are large vacuoles measuring 5 μ in diameter, containing dense cored granules.

Cki δ Immunoreactive Bodies

These correspond to GVD. They contain casein kinase, which increases following transport defect due to hyperphosphorylated tau and microtubule dissolution.

Pathological Variants of Alzheimer's Disease

Tangle only variant: This type occurs in late onset non-AD type of dementia. Only NFT is present in limbic, paralimbic and temporal cortex. NFTs are absent in neocortex. No neuritic SP is present. Rarely Aβ positive diffuse SP may be present (Scinto and Daffner, 2000).

Neocortical plaque only variant: It clinically presents with AD type dementia of late onset. SP is present only in neocortex. NFT is present in limbic and paralimbic regions but not in neocortex. More diffuse SPs and fewer neuritic SP are seen (Scinto and Daffner, 2000).

Lewy body variant: NFT are rare in neocortex and present in the limbic and paralimbic regions with lower density than found in AD. Non-neuritic and diffuse variety of SP are abundant in neocortex. Lewy body is diffusely distributed in cortical non-pyramidal neurons of the layers V and VI (Scinto and Daffner, 2000).

AUTOPSY DIAGNOSIS OF ALZHEIMER'S DISEASE

CERAD Neuropathology Protocol for Diagnosis of Alzheimer's Disease

Gross findings: Weight of the brain is taken and gross abnormalities in the brain, spinal cord, meninges and blood vessels are noted to rule out any other pathology (Mirra et al., 1991; 1993).

Neocortical atrophy and ventricular enlargement are graded as none, mild, moderate and severe. Presence of atrophy of hippocampus and entorhinal area is recorded. Cerebral vessels are inspected for atherosclerosis, aneurysm and other abnormalities. Lacunar and large infarcts are noted for the number, size, frequency, distribution and laterality. Sections are taken from superior frontal gyrus, mid-frontal gyrus, caudate lobe, putamen, ventral thalamus, substantia nigra, hippocampus, parahippocampal gyrus, subiculum, superior temporal gyrus, mid-temporal gyrus, and inferior temporal gyrus (Mirra et al., 1991; 1993).

Staining: H and E, fluorescent thioflavin S preparation under UV light, Congo red stain viewed under polarized light and modified Bielschowsky silver stain are done and 10 random microscopic fields at 100X magnification are studied. Neuritic SP are counted in temporal neocortex and Brodman area 20 and graded as: None - less than 1/field, Rare - 1/field, Sparse - 2-5/field, Mild - 6–15/field, Moderate - 16–50/field, Severe ->50/field (Mirra et al., 1991; 1993).

NFT is evaluated in hippocampal formation and temporal neocortex with modified Bielschowsky's silver stain. Ten random microscopic fields at 200X magnification are counted and graded as: None: nil; Rare: 1 NFT/field; Mild: 1–2 NFT/field; Moderate: 3–10 NFT/field; Severe: more than 10 NFT/field (Braak and Braak, 1991).

NIA Consensus Criteria

Sections are taken from neocortex, amygdala, hippocampus and entorhinal region. Sections (5–15 micron) are cut and previously mentioned special stains are done. 200 microscopic fields are examined and scored as follows (Khachaturian, 1985):
- Less than 50 yrs: 2–5 SP or neuritic SP and NFT/field in neocortex
- 50–60 yrs: 8 or more SP/field, NFT may be present
- 66–75 yrs: More than10 SP/HPF, NFT may be present
- More than 75 yrs: More than 15 SP, no NFT in neocortex.

NIA-RI Criteria

Sections are taken from superior temporal lobe, middle frontal, inferior parietal, occipital, hippocampal formation at the level of lateral geniculate nucleus, substantia nigra and locus ceruleus.

AMYLOID OR CONGOPHILIC ANGIOPATHY-CAA (CEREBRAL AMYLOID ANGIOPATHY)

Mutation in Aβ sequence in codon 692 (Roks et al., 2000), 693 and 694 near χ cleavage site produces increase in Aβ40. Glutamic acid to glutamine mutation at codon 693 of APP is associated with cerebral haemorrhage with amyloidosis of Dutch type. Mutated Aβ40 and Aβ42 are produced. Aβ40 is deposited in small to medium sized leptomeningeal and cortical vessel walls and Aβ42 in senile plaque (Singh et al., 2002). ApoE ε4 increases risk for amyloid angiopathy. ApoE ε2 allele increases vasculopathic changes such as cracking of amyloid laden vessel wall, paravascular leakage of blood, vascular ectasia, microaneurysm, inflammation and fibrinoid necrosis (Greenberg et al., 1998).

Lesions are graded as follows:

0 = Amyloid absent
1 = Trace or occasional vessels affected
2 = One or few vessels with deposit around the circumference
3 = Widespread involvement of the vessels with deposit around the circumference
4 = As in 3 along with haemorrhage, occlusion and recanalisation.

VASCULAR DEMENTIA

Multi-Infarct and Diffuse White Matter Dementia or Binswanger's Disease – Small Vessel Disease

Gross findings: White matter infarcts present as cystic cavity with ragged edge. Gray matter infarct is cystic or slit like or present as gliotic foci without neuron.

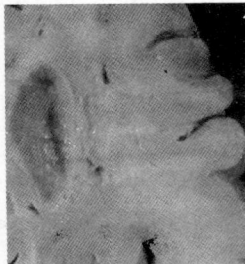

Fig. 8.7 White matter infarct

Small vessel associated disease was semiquanitatively scored as follows (Esiri et al., 1997):

0 = No widening of perivascular spaces or hyaline thickening of arterioral wall or perivascular pallor of myelin staining, loosening of tissue, or attenuation of nerve fibres, or gliosis in white matter, or loss of nerve cells and gliosis in deep gray matter.

1 = Widened perivascular spaces, or hyaline thickening of arterioral walls, or a few perivascular macrophages, but none of the other features mentioned above, occurring in one or more sections of white matter or deep gray matter.

2 = Widened perivascular spaces, or hyaline thickening of arteriolar walls plus mild or moderate perivascular pallor of myelin staining, or loosening with attenuation of nerve fibres with gliosis in white matter or loss of nerve cells and gliosis in deep gray matter in one or more sections.

3 = Widened perivascular spaces, hyaline thickening of arteriolar walls, severe perivascular and some more widespread pallor of myelin staining and nerve fibre attenuation with gliosis in white matter or loss of nerve cells and gliosis in deep gray matter in more than one section. These findings are equivalent to those of Binswanger's disease.

Microscopically, hyline thickening of vessel wall, widening of perivascular space, haemosiderin-laden macrophages around white matter blood vessels and loss of perivascular white matter have been described (Kril et al., 2002).

CADASIL – Cerebral Autosomal Dominant Arteriopathy with Subcortical Infarct and Leukoencephalopathy

Notch-3 gene on Ch19q 13.1 contains 34 EGF (epidermal growth factor) domain in the extracellular part of the protein. EGF domain contains 6 cysteine residues. Mutation in the notch-3 gene leads to accumulation of notch-3 cleavage product containing all EGF domains in the cytoplasmic membrane of vascular smooth muscle resulting in the deposit of PAS-positive, eosinophilic material, which is negative for amyloid stain. Electron microscopically osmiophilic granules deposit between smooth muscle cells or within thickened basal lamina producing vascular thickening of the media and reduction in the lumen of small and medium sized penetrating arteries leading to multiple strokes. Leptomeningeal vessels and vessels of various organs are involved. Skin biopsy is diagnostic (Hedera and Turner, 2002).

DEGENERATIVE DISORDERS ASSOCIATED WITH TAU MUTATION

Following disorders have been described to be associated with tau mutation (Brun et al, 1994; McKeith et al, 1996):
1. Familial frontotemporal dementia and parkinsonism
2. Familial progressive subcortical gliosis
3. Progressive supranuclear palsy
4. Corticobasal ganglionic degeneration
5. Familial multiple system tauopathy with presenile dementia

FRONTOTEMPORAL DEMENTIA

It is due to intronic and exonic mutation in MAPT gene on Ch 17q21 affecting alternate splicing of exon 10, resulting in increased 4r tau, which impairs the ability of tau to bind to microtubules resulting in microtubular assembly and tau filaments deposits.

Gross findings: Symmetrical convolutional atrophy in frontal and anterior temporal lobe, frontal widening of ventricular system are seen. No atrophy of striatum, amygdala or hippocampus are there usually. Occasionally, it may be severe in these areas (Brun et al., 1994). Microscopically, lesions are seen in the cortex of frontal, orbitofrontal, anterior third of temporal, anterior and rarely posterior cingulate gyrus. Superior temporal lobe is spared.

Lesions in gray matter: Tau positive inclusions in neurons, microvacuolation, mild to moderate astrocytic gliosis of lamina I-III layers, atrophy and loss of neurons in lamina II and III, mild atrophy of lamina V and mild loss of pigmented neurons in substantia nigra.

Microscopically, tau filament in temporal cortex, tau deposit stained by antibody AT 8 in the inner molecular layer and granular cells of dentate gyrus have been described (Spillantini et al., 1998).

White matter lesions: Mild to moderate astrocytic gliosis in subcortical U fibres and deeper white matter, loss of myelin and mild ischaemic attenuation of white matter are seen. Some cases of frontotemporal dementia show swollen neurons with inclusion bodies, which are due to 3R tau than 4R isoform. Families with frontotemporal dementia have been described where neuronal inclusions are tau negative and glial inclusions are positive. Ubiquitnated neurites are found in all FTD. Filamentous cellular inclusions composed of abnormal tau protein are hallmarks of all tauopathies. In the electron microscope they appear as paired helical filaments and straight filaments. Paired helical filaments are 20 nm in diameter that narrow to 8 nm at cross over point at every 80 nm.

PICK'S DISEASE

Pick's disease is due to class III tauopathy due to increase in 3R tau (McKhann et al., 2001; Delacourte and Buee, 2002).

Gross findings: Frontotemporal lobar and limbic atrophy, wide sulci, knife edged and walnut like gyri, sometimes disproportionately asymmetric temporal lobe atrophy with sparing of superior temporal gyrus are observed. Basal ganglia are involved. There is neuronal loss, spongiosis and gliosis extending into subcortical white matter.

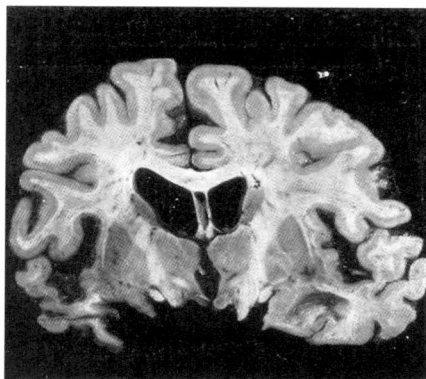

Fig. 8.8 Asymmetric temporal lobe atrophy with sparing of superior temporal gyrus in a patient with Pick disease

Microscopically (silver stain), ballooned neuron containing silver staining inclusions called Pick bodies are seen in large neurons of II and IV layers of neocortex, dentate gyrus, neurons of hippocampus and selected brain stem nuclei. It is abnormal 3r tau, 64–68 doublet, biochemically.

Electron-microscopically PHF are 10–12 micron straight and constricted fibrils, 10 nm neurofilaments and 24 nm straight tubules. Pick bodies are silver+, tau, neurofilaments and ubiquitin immunoreactive. Brain also may contain amyloid plaque, granulovacuolar change and NFT.

CORTICOBASAL DEGENERATION

Cerebral cortex, deep cerebellar nuclei and substantia nigra are involved. There is asymmetric frontoparietal atrophy severe in pre- and postcentral region. There is depigmentation of substantia nigra. Temporal lobe is spared. Neurons are enlarged with eccentric nucleus and loss of Nissl. Argyrophilic tau positive inclusions are seen in oligodendrocytes (Feany and Dickson, 1995). Amyloid is negative in cortical plaque. Microscopically, there is neuronal loss, spongiosis pale cortical neurons with eccentric nucleus, achromatic ballooned neuron, basophilic subcortical neuronal inclusions and corticobasal bodies. Ballooned neurons are intensely positive for tau.

Thinner intermediate filaments 10–15 nm in diameter are seen with electron microscope. Granular material and neuropil thread in gray and white matter of cortex are tau positive.

PROGRESSIVE SUPRANUCLEAR PALSY

There is atrophy of basal ganglia, subthalamus and brain stem (Stanford et al., 2000; Hauw et al., 1994). An increase of tau 4r occurs by 11 tg dinucleotide repeat in intron 9 and silent mutation S305S in exon 10 of tau gene.

Microscopically, there is neuronal loss, gliosis, increased neuropil thread and shrinkage of globus pallidus. NFT are round and globose. Abundant glial fibrillary tangles in astrocytes (tufted astrocytes) and oligodendrocytes (coiled bodies) are seen.

Wide PHF or 10–15 nm straight filaments are seen in electron microscope. NFT are tau positive and ubiquitin may or may not be positive. NFT are found in subcortex of subthalamus, globus pallidus, substantia nigra, locus ceruleus, periaqueductal gray matter, superior colliculus, oculomotor nuclei and neocortex.

DIFFUSE LEWY BODY DISEASE

Alpha synuclein is presynaptic membrane associated protein responsible for synaptic maturity, transport of vesicles and synaptic plasticity (Dickson, 2001; McKhann et al., 2001). It forms non-amyloid component of amyloid plaque. α synuclein is coded by SNCA gene on Ch4. Mutation of α synuclein on chromosome 4q results in protein that self-aggregates more readily than wild type synuclein. It acts as nidus for aggregation of wild type and mutant synuclein forming fibrillar inclusion bodies in dendrites. This forms Lewy body resulting in 70% reduction in dopamine concentration in putamen (Lippa et al., 1999). Loss of dopamine cell is accompanied by loss of dopamine transporter presynaptic receptors. Synucleopathies are (i) multiple system atrophy, (ii) Parkinson's disease, and (iii) dementia with Lewy body disease.

In diffuse Lewy body disease, Lewy body is present in CA2 of hippocampus, amygdala, periamygdala cortex, 8 and 9 regions of frontal lobe, locus ceruleus, basal forebrain and neurons of nucleus of Meynert. It is present in substantia nigra in Parkinsonism. Intraneuronal cytoplasmic inclusions are discrete, homogenous, spherical, push the nucleus to the periphery, pale eosinophilic, PAS positive, and contain epitope recognised by antibody against phosphorylated and nonphosphorylated neurofilament protein, ubiquitin and presynaptic protein α synuclein. Electron-microscopically it is straight neurofilament of 7–20 nm with surrounding amorphous material.

Criteria for diagnosis: Three or more cortical fields at 250x with 4 or more ubiquitin positive Lewy bodies are required to meet CDLB neocortical score of more than 6.

HUNTINGTON'S DISEASE

Huntingtin is intracellular transport protein present in the cytoplasm of striatal neurons in high concentration. Mutation of the Huntingtin gene in chromosome 4 results in expansion of polyglutamine tract in N terminus of Huntingtin (Lovestone and McLoughlin, 2002). Truncated N-terminal fragments of Huntingtin with expanded glutamine repeats result in defect in mitochondrial function, increased ubiquitinated intraneuronal and perineuronal lesions producing nuclear inclusions and dystrophic neurites. Nuclear aggregates cause apoptosis and death of neurons. Neurons that contain gamma aminobutyric acid, enkephalin and dynorphin are decreased. These are medium sized spine neuron in caudate and putamen. Intranuclear inclusions stain with antibody to polyglutamine. Large cholinergic neurons are spared.

In Huntington's disease, symmetric dilatation of frontal horn of lateral ventricle is seen. Caudate and putamen are atrophic. In the initial stages neuronal loss and gliosis are moderate and more diffuse throughout the caudate nucleus (CN) sparing only most ventral and paracapsular region. Later, nerve cell depletion and fibrillary astrocytosis are severe and diffuse throughout the caudate and putamen.

Table 8.2 Pathological grading of Huntington's disease

Grades	Description
Grade 0	No discernible neuropathological abnormalities, suggesting that the anatomical changes lag behind the development of clinical abnormalities
Grade I	Neuropathological changes are recognised only microscopically. Grossly, brain is normal. Microscopically, mild neuronal loss and astrocytic gliosis in medial paraventricular region of CN, tail of CN and dorsal region of putamen. Neuronal loss 50%. Relative preservation of the lateral half of the head of the caudate.
Grade II	Atrophy in the head of CN, convex outline at the lateral ventricle is retained. Astrocytes are greatly increased. Relative preservation of the lateral half of the head of the CN.
Grade III	Ventricular outline of head of CN is a straight line. Astrocytes are greatly increased.
Grade IV	CN is shrunken with medial concavity. Putamen and internal capsule are atrophic. Neuronal loss 95%.

(Myers et al., 1988; Vonsattel et al., 1985)

DEMENTIA OF PRION PROTEIN AND TRANSMISSIBLE SPONGIFORM ENCEPHALOPATHIES

Prnp gene on short arm of chromosome 20 codes for prion protein. Human prion protein PrP is 253 amino acid membrane associated glycoprotein present in the neurons and astrocytes (Greicius et al., 2002; Lovestone and McLoughlin, 2002). PrPc is antioxidant, protects against copper toxicity and plays a role in synaptic function. Increased β sheet content at the tertiary and quaternary structure of PrPc converts it to PrP scrapie (PrPsc) which converts normal PrPc to pathogenic PrPsc. Confirmational difference allows PrPsc with the ability to convert host PrPc at a late posttranslational event either at the cell surface or after endocytosis of PrPc. PrPsc is protease resistant, aggregates more and is present in amyloid.

Point Mutations and Insertions in Prnp on Chromosome 20

1. P102L mutation: Gerstmann-Straussler-Scheinker syndrome (GSSS)
2. D178N: Fatal familial insomnia, Creutzfeldt- Jakob disease
3. E200K: CJD like disease in Libyan Jews
4. Methionine valine polymorphism in codon 129 of PrP-sporadic (methionine) and iatrogenic (valine) CJD
5. 80% sporadic, 15% familial, 1% iatrogenic

Pathology

CJD: Diffuse vacuolation of gray matter, gliosis, neuronal loss, few Prp amyloid plaques are seen.

GSSS: Less vacuolar and spongiform change, extensive PrP amyloid plaque, mild cerebral and cerebellar atrophy are noticed. NFT may be present.

Fatal familial insomnia: Neuronal loss, gliosis in thalamus, inferior olive and cerebellum are observed. Vacuolation is seen.

New variant of CJD: There is diffuse vacuolation and dense core Prp containing plaque surrounded by halo of vacuolar spongiform change called florid plaque. Tonsil biopsy is positive for PrPsc. Prp deposits around neurons and capillaries. Perineural and periaxonal Prp accumulate in basal ganglia. CJD suspected tissue should be fixed in formic acid fixation. Well fixed 4–5 mm thick tissue is put in 50–100 mL of 90–100% formic acid for 1 hour and 10% formalin for 2 days.

AIDS-DEMENTIA COMPLEX

It is frontotemporal subcortical dementia involving white matter and basal ganglia. HIV virus coat Gp120 binds to CD4 receptor on macrophages, internalises, activates macrophages to replicate and release neurotoxins like glutamate-like molecules, free radicals, arachidonic acid metabolites and cytokines. There is overstimulation of N-methyl-D-aspartase receptor with increased influx of calcium ions in the neurons and injury to neurons. Induction of pathogenic sets of nearly 98 genes such as osteopontin and others enhance monocyte accumulation, activation of microglia and astrocytes, which release toxic factors like IL-1b and IL1c, GM-CSF etc. Activated macrophages and astrocytes lead to CNS dysfunction by direct damage to neuron (Roberts et al., 2003; Rosenbaum, 1990; Lipton and Gendelman, 1995).

Gross findings: Cortical ribbon is intact or mildly thin. White matter is decreased in volume and poorly demarcated from gray matter. White matter shows grey mottling. In children, weight is reduced. Calcification of basal ganglia and periventricular white matter is present. Ventricle shows mild to moderate dilatation.

Microscopically, there is diffuse astrocytosis, spongy vacuolation, pallor, decreased staining intensity of white matter due to myelin sheath involvement and dissolution of astrocytic process. Astrocytosis extends to basal ganglion and thalamus. Vascular mineralisation is present in basal ganglia. Proliferative leptomeningeal arteriopathy with infarct is seen. Cerebral cortex is spared. Cerebral white matter, corpus callosum, basal ganglia and ventral pons are involved. Perivascular loose inflammatory infiltrate composed of foamy, lipid-laden macrophages and a few lymphocytes are seen. In putamen and pallidus, haemosiderin is seen. Critical to diagnosis are multinucleated giant cells similar to Touton or Langhan's type, some having overlapping of nuclei. Polykaryotic cells are diagnostic. Demyelination is present.

Axons are preserved. Sponginess of parenchyma, astrocytosis and isolated multinucleated cells are diagnostic.

MILD COGNITIVE IMPAIRMENT

MCI is memory loss greater than that for the age but not enough to meet the clinical criteria of dementia. NFT is present in hippocampus, entorhinal areas, SP in neocortex and neuronal loss in CA1 of hippocampus. Medial temporal lobe atrophy predicts AD in patients with minor cognitive impairment (Peterson et al., 2001; Visser et al., 2002; Du et al., 2001).

Earliest change is NFT in hippocampus and entorhinal area and later it involves lateral temporal cortex. Senile plaques occur later on. Volumetry of hippocampus, parahippocampus and medial temporal lobe show atrophy. Neocortex shows high total plaque density of diffuse plaque sub-type and NFT. There is decreased hippocampal neuronal count.

NORMAL-PRESSURE HYDROCEPHALUS

There are enlarged lateral ventricles, little or no cortical atrophy, upward stretching of corpus callosum and it is communicating. Aqueduct of sylvius is patent. It is due to delay in the absorption of cerebrospinal fluid (CSF), overconvexity and partial obstruction to the flow of CSF probably following scarring due to basilar meningitis, subarachnoid haemorrhage and trauma. The pathophysiology is thought to be related to disruption of neural function either through stretching of periventricular fibres or through disruption of the pressure differential between the ventricular and subdural spaces, compromising neuronal function by altering cerebral blood flow.

REFERENCES

- Binder GA, Haughton VM. (1979) *Computed tomography of the brain in axial, coronal and sagittal planes.* Boston: Little Brown and Company.
- Braak H, Braak E. (1991) Neuropathological staging of Alzheimer related changes. *Acta Neuropathologica,* 82, 239–259.
- Brun A, Englund B, Gustafson L, et al. (1994) Clinical and

neuropathological criteria for frontotemporal dementia. *Journal of Neurology, Neurosurgery and Psychiatry,* 57, 416–418.

- Bush AI. (2003) The metallobiology of Alzheimer's disease. *Trends in Neurosciences,* 26, 207–214.
- Cook DG, Leverenz JB, McMiller PJ et al. (2003) Reduced hippocampal insulin degrading enzyme in late onset Alzheimer's disease is associated with Apolipoprotein E e4 allele. *American Journal of Pathology,* 162, 313–319.
- Delacourte A, Buee L. (2002) Tau pathology a marker of neurodegenerative disorders. *Current Opinions in Neurology,* 13, 371–376.
- Dickson DW. (2001) α synuclein and Lewy body disorders. *Current Opinion in Neurology,* 14, 423–432.
- Du AT, Schuff N, Amend D, et al. (2001) Magnetic resonance imaging of the Entorhinal cortex and hippocampus in mild cognitive impairment and Alzheimer's disease. *Journal of Neurology, Neurosurgery and Psychiatry,* 71, 441–447.
- Duvernoy HM. (1991) *The Human Brain Surface: Three-Dimensional Sectional Anatomy and MRI.* New York: Springer-Verlag Wien.
- Esiri MM, Wilcock GK, Morris JH (1997) Neuropathological assessment of the lesions of significance in vascular dementia. *Journal of Neurology, Neurosurgery and Psychiatry,* 63, 749–753.
- Feany MB, Dickson DW. (1995) Widespread cytoskeletal pathology characterises corticobasal degeneration. *American Journal of Pathology,* 146, 1388–1396.
- Ghoshal N, Smiley JF, De Maggio JA et al. (1999) New molecular link between the fibrillar and granulovacuolar lesions in Alzheimer's disease. *American Journal of Pathology,* 155, 1163–1172.
- Greenberg SM, Van Sattal JPG, Segal AZ. (1998) Association of Apolipoprotein E e2 and vasculopathy in cerebral amyloid angiopathy. *Neurology,* 50, 961–965.
- Greicius MD, Geschhwind MD, Miller BL, et al. (2002) Presenile dementia syndrome, an update on taxonomy and diagnosis. *Journal of Neurology Neurosurgery and Psychiatry,* 72, 691–700.
- Hansen LA, Crain BJ (1995) Making the diagnosis of mixed and non-Alzheimer's dementia. *Archives of Pathology and Laboratory Medicine,* 119, 1023–1031.
- Hauw JJ, Daniel SE, Dickson D, et al. (1994) Preliminary NINDS Neuropathologic Criteria for Richardson-Olszewski Syndrome (Progressive Supranuclear Palsy). *Neurology,* 44, 2015–2019.
- Hedera P, Turner RS. (2002) Inherited dementias. *Neurologic Clinics,* 20, 779–808.
- Hirano A. (1988) *Colour Atlas of Pathology of the Nervous System.* 2nd edition. Tokyo: Igaku-Shoin.
- Janssen JC, Hall M, Fox NC et al. (2000) Alzheimer's disease due to

an intronic presenilin-1 intron 4 mutation. *Brain,* 123, 894–907.

- Khachaturian ZS. (1985) Diagnosis of Alzheimer's disease. *Archives of Neurology,* 42, 1097–1105.

- Kril JJ, Patel S, Harding AJ, Halliday GM. (2002) Patients with vascular dementia due to microvascular pathology have significant hippocampal neuronal loss. *Journal of Neurology Neurosurgery and Psychiatry,* 72, 747–751.

- Lippa CF, Schmidt ML, Lee VM. (1999) Dementia with Lewy bodies. *Neurology,* 52, 893.

- Lipton A, Gendelman HE. (1995) Dementia associated with the acquired immunodefeciency syndrome. *The New England Journal of Medicine,* 332, 934–940.

- Lovestone S, McLoughlin DM. (2002) Protein aggregates and dementia: Is there a common toxicity? *Journal of Neurology Neurosurgery and Psychiatry,* 72,152–161.

- McKeith IG, Galasko D, Kosaka K. (1996) Consensus guidelines for the clinical and pathologic diagnosis of dementia with Lewy bodies (DLB). Report of consortium on DLM internal workshop. *Neurology,* 47, 1113–1124.

- McKhann GM, Albert MS, Grossman M, et al. (2001) Clinical and pathological diagnosis of frontotemporal dementia. Report of work group on frontotemporal dementia and Pick's disease. *Archives of Neurology,* 58, 1803–1809.

- Myers RH, Vansattel J-Page, Steven TJ, et al. (1988) Clinical and neuropathologic assessment of severity in Huntington's disease. *Neurology,* 38, 341–347.

- Mirra SS, Heyman A, Mc Keel D, et al. (1991) The consortium to establish a registry for Alzheimer's disease (CERAD) Part II. Standardisation of neuropathologic assessment of Alzheimer's disease. *Neurology,* 41, 479–486.

- Mirra SS, Hart MN, Terry RD. (1993) Making the diagnosis for Alzheimer's disease. A primer for practising pathologist. *Archives of Pathology and Laboratory Medicine,* 117, 132–144.

- Petersen RC, Doody R, Kurz A. (2001) Current concepts in mild cognitive impairment. *Archives of Neurology,* 58, 1985–1992.

- Roberts ES, Zandonatti MA, Watry DD, et al. (2003) Induction of pathogenic sets of genes in macrophages and neurons in Neuro AIDS. *American Journal of Pathology.* 162, 2041–2057

- Roks G, Van Harskamp F, DeKoning I. (2000) Presentation of amyloidosis in carriers of codon 692 mutation in the Amyloid Precursor Protein gene (APP 692). *Brain,* 123, 2130–2140.

- Rosenblum MK. (1990) Infection of the central nervous system by the human immunodeficiency virus type I. Morphology and relation to syndrome of progressive encephalopathy and myelopathy in patients with AIDS. *Pathology Annual,* 25, Part 1, 117–169.

- Scinto LEM, Daffner K. (2000) *Pathological diagnosis of Alzheimer's disease. Early diagnosis of Alzheimer's disease.* Totowa, New Jersey: Humana Press.
- Singh SK, Cras P, Wang R, et al. (2002) Dense core senile plaque in Flemish variant of AD are vasocentric. *American Journal of Pathology,* 161, 507–520.
- Spillantini MG, Crowther RA, Kamphorst W, et al. (1998) Tau pathology in microtubule binding region of tau. *American Journal of Pathology,* 153, 1359–1363.
- Stanford PM, Halliday GM, Brooks WS. (2000) Progressive Supranuclear Palsy pathology caused by a novel silent mutation in exon 10 of tau gene. Expansion of the disease phenotype caused by tau gene mutation. *Brain,* 123, 880–893.
- Vonsattel JP, Myets RH, Stevens TJ, Ferrante RJ, Bird ED, Richardson EP Jr. (1985) Neuropathological classification of Huntington's disease. *J Neuropathol Exp Neurol,* 44 (6), 559–577.
- Visser PJ, Verhey FRJ, Hofman PAM. (2002) Medial temporal lobe atrophy predicts Alzheimer's Disease in patients with minor cognitive impairment. *Journal of Neurology Neurosurgery and Psychiatry,* 72, 491–497.
- Wei W, Norton DD, Wang X, et al. (2002) Ab 17-42 in Alzheimer's disease activates JNK and caspase 8 leading to neuronal apoptosis. *Brain,* 125, 2036–2043.

9

Course and Outcome of Dementia

KS Shaji, Srikala Bharath, David Jolley

Introduction

In a minority of people with dementia a treatable, reversible cause can be identified and corrective action taken. But most people with dementia will experience a progressive decline of cognition and other abilities, perhaps complicated by the emergence of additional symptoms, over a period of months or years. This deterioration may be described over a continuum or as a series of stages. It is punctuated by the possibility of placement in some form of residential/institutional care and terminates in death.

SIGNIFICANCE OF THE NATURAL HISTORY

Knowledge of the likely course and outcome of dementia is immensely important in planning services. The stage and severity of the condition often determine the type and intensity of service, which will be needed. This understanding of the natural history of the condition also underpins the evaluation of any type of intervention, which might be offered, be it medical, psychosocial or behavioural. Delay in the progression, reversal to an earlier stage, improved quality of life for the patient or carer, are appropriate targets.

For an individual person and his family, information about the likely course and outcome of dementia is useful for the following reasons:

- To confirm the diagnosis and understand the biological nature of the condition.
- To plan for the future: taking into account arrangements, which may be needed to provide safety through care and attention to the legal protection and management of individual and family affairs.
- To be aware of treatment options and the advantages and hazards associated with particular modes of management.

For professionals working with people with dementia, knowledge of the likely course and outcome of dementia is useful:
- To underline their responsibility to share this information with patients and families.
- To share with patients, families and other carers, the task of making comprehensive, realistic plans and proposals for the future.
- To temper their own suggestions for particular interventions with a balanced understanding of their costs and likely effects.
- To work with planners and those who commission and provide services, to generate an affordable infrastructure of care, which will meet the predictable needs of populations.

For those responsible for public services, knowledge of the likely course and outcome of dementia is important:
- To inform them in providing training to equip a workforce to complement the efforts of families in providing care.
- To inform them in generating a balanced infrastructure of services, which meets the needs of the population, not only for assessment, investigation and treatment, but also for support and care, including care in the terminal stages of dementia.

HISTORICAL DEVELOPMENTS AND THE CURRENT WORLD CONTEXT

Sir Marin Roth's studies of outcome amongst older people admitted to a mental hospital in the England of the 1950s (Roth, 1955), demonstrated that discharge of patients with dementia was unusual. Fifty-five percent were dead within six months; 80 percent were dead within two years. Yet the population of patients admitted to psychiatric care is a function of service configuration at the time, and their outcomes relate to factors intrinsic to each individual and to the conditions of care they receive.

In many parts of the world, all but a small fraction of people with dementia live and die within the community of ordinary households. In the UK, Europe and North America, which have generated much of the literature on the natural history of dementia, the context of care has changed during the past 60 years. Large mental hospitals have been closed and emphasis has been placed upon Care in the Community (Department of Health, 2001). Yet, within these countries, the proportion of patients with dementia living within normal household has fallen from 80 percent (Kay, Beamish and Roth, 1964) to 50 percent (O'Connor, 1992). Extrapolating the specific rates of deterioration, rates of institutionalisation or death from one country to another, would be a flawed exercise. There is much to be gained from careful, modest studies of these matters within individual countries, with note of the care configurations in place at the time. Never the less, general themes can be extracted from experience and publications, which are available. These can be applied usefully, if cautiously, within a given context.

CHANGES DURING LIFE WITH DEMENTIA

Two main approaches can be identified to describe the course of dementias:

- Global staging systems
- Change in psychometric test scores.

Staging Systems

The course of Alzheimer's disease, for instance, can be divided into stages based on the progression of clinical features (Table 9.1) (Cummings and Jest, 1999). The divisions are arbitrary and overlap significantly.

Table 9.1 Stages of Alzheimer's Dementia

Mild dementia (0-2 years) →	Moderate dementia (2-5 years) →	Severe dementia (4-7/9 years)
Short-term memory affected Recall of recent information affected	Severe impairment of recent memory. Inability to recall any recent information	All cognitive functions severely impaired
Long term declarative memory not much affected	Long term declarative can show evidence of being affected	Even personal information may not be recalled
Remote information and personal information are recalled with more ease	Living in the past is seen Sometimes mistakes in the recall of the past information also	
Communication – No significant aphasias, reduced vocabulary. Occasional word naming and semantic difficulties observed	Language – nominal aphasia, paraphasia present Circumstantial and repetitive speech Writing and reading deteriorate	Single phrases or words, later mutism
Visuospatial difficulties are present – leading to misplacing objects and losing ways	Visuospatial disorientation - finding way in known places	Aimless wandering or lying on the bed due to apathy
Routine ADL not affected More complex demands in ADL like planning, organizing, judgement calls are difficult	Difficulties in ADL observed due to apraxias. Reasoning, planning and judgement more affected and obvious Apraxias lead to difficulties in ADL – dressing, cooking, eating, using regular appliances Agnosias – lead to difficulty in identifying known people	Needs help in all ADL as the deficits are very severe Apraxias may lead to difficulty in chewing, swallowing and drinking Often doubly incontinent

Depression may be present	Agnosias could lead to delusions of misidentification Hallucinations could be present Behavioural symptoms worsen – agitation, restlessness due to disorientation and agnosias are seen	Simple motor stereotypes, wandering, restlessness may be present, and/or apathy
Neurological symptoms are mainly primitive reflexes	Neurological signs present	More neurological symptoms – seizures, myoclonus may be present Parkinsonian symptoms may be present – rigidity Severe primitive reflexes like snouting and grasping may interfere with feeding and dressing
Independent living is possible	Independent living is impossible – needs supervision and a good care plan to be in the community Significant burden to a carer	May need institutional care with significant inputs from multidisciplinary approach

A number of global staging systems have been proposed. The two in widest use are:

- Washington University Clinical Dementia Rating Scale (CDR) (Hughes et al., 1982; Morris, 1997)
- Global Deterioration Scale (GDS) (Reisberg et al., 1982; 1986)

Both the scales reflect functioning of the affected person as observed by a carer. They reflect the influence of the cognitive deterioration on the daily functioning and behaviour.

Clinical Dementia Rating Scale (CDR)

CDR incorporates information for 6 areas of functioning: memory, orientation, judgement and problem solving, community affairs, home and hobbies, and personal care. Scoring is done for each area as: 0 – normal, 0.5 – questionable, 1 – mild, 2 – moderate, and 3 – severe.

All the scores are added up and the similar scores with similar definitions are used to stage the dementia. Table 9.1 has been prepared based on the stages of CDR. CDR has been standardized with interrater reliability (0.91). It correlates well with other scales like the ADL, Blessed Dementia (BDS) (r – 0.53). CDR is widely used as a valid global assessment measure for AD. It is not sensitive to short term change.

Global Deterioration Scale (GDS)

GDS divides AD into seven clinically identifiable stages (GDS1 – Normal Cognition; GDS 7 – Severe Dementia). Staging is based on a combined assessment of history and objective mental status examination including cognitive functioning. Hence, it has high correlation with clinical objective scales of cognitive functioning like the Mini Mental Status Examination (MMSE) ($r = 0.9$; P: 0.001) and the cognitive BIMC ($r = 0.8$; P: 0.001) (Reisberg et al., 1989).

Stages 1–3 are the pre-dementia stages. Stages 4–7 are the dementia stages. Beginning in stage 5, an individual can no longer survive without assistance.

Psychometric Tests/Cognitive Tests

Commonly used scales include:

- Blessed Information Memory Concentration Test (BIMC) (Blessed et al., 1968)
- Mini Mental State Examination (MMSE) (Folstein et al., 1975)
- Dementia Rating Scale (DRS)
- Alzheimer's Disease Assessment Scale (ADAS) (Rosen et al., 1984)
- Cambridge Cognitive Examination (CAMCOG) (Roth et al., 1986)

Institutional Care

A move away from home to life within an institution, is very significant and not one which many anticipate with enthusiasm. In constructing the protocol for the AD 2000, the authors listed a move to institutional care as an end point (Courtney et al., 2004). They assumed that life beyond that threshold was of less value than life in the community. In this they were reflecting, in a formal way, a view which many hold in private. Yet it is a move made by most individuals who survive into the more debilitated or disturbed stages of dementia. Dementia renders an individual progressively less able to care for themselves socially and eventually compromises their biological integrity, destabilising basic homeostatic mechanisms.

Thus, follow-up studies find few people surviving alone with dementia for more than a few months (Kay et al., 1970). Even when effort is made to provide good care at home, it may flounder. Some would suggest that effort and resource should be concentrated on more hopeful scenarios where the person with dementia is supported within a family (Bergmann et al., 1978). Thus it is that in the residential and nursing homes of Europe, North America and Australasia, 40 percent of clients and more are affected by dementia. The presence of particular symptoms makes admission more likely. These include: incontinence, irritability, wandering, inability to walk, inability to talk or communicate, loss of ADL – bathing, grooming, hyperactivity or aggression, sleeplessness and nocturnal behavioural problems (Sanford, 1975; Bowman et al., 2004).

Yet beyond these, the most powerful determinants are social: living alone with insufficient social support or at risk of exploitation by a hostile community, living with a frail and dependent partner or bereaved and alone as consequence of the death or hospitalisation of a main supporter.

DEATH

Studies are consistent in demonstrating that a diagnosis of dementia is associated with earlier death compared with controls of the same age, living at the same time and in similar circumstances (Jolley and Baxter, 1997). Reduced longevity is most marked amongst younger subjects but is evident even within the very elderly. Both institutional and community populations in Europe appear to live longer with dementia when given a better environment and more enlightened care (Wood et al., 1991; Office of Health Economics, 1979).

Many people with dementia die from conditions which are common amongst the elderly population at large. They usually die in circumstances which do not differ from their non-demented contemporaries. In Europe, North America and Australasia, most such deaths occur in general hospitals. The presence of dementia as a co-pathology may or may not be appreciated by the medical team providing treatment in this terminal admission. It may, or may not, be mentioned on the death certificate. Thus, it is believed that dementia is massively underreported as a significant factor amongst pathologies at death.

When individuals have lived for many months or years with dementia, or their symptoms arising from the condition have been severe or complicated, their experience of dying and mode of death may be very uncomfortable (Black and Jolley, 1990). It is important that services are equipped to deal with this great challenge. A hospice approach is recommended (Volicer, 1986). Cause of death in these circumstances is often given as 'bronchopneumonia', and post-mortem studies usually confirm the presence of this terminal pathology (Burns, 1992; Tench et al., 1992), though the real cause of death is dementia.

FACTORS RELATING TO OUTCOMES

Progression of symptoms in dementia is erratic and variable so that reliable estimates of change require that measurements are taken over periods longer than a year. Some of the factors that have been found to influence the progress and longevity include:

- Severity of the cognitive symptoms at time of entry to studies or involvement with services: severe cognitive impairment usually indicates faster rate of progression and earlier death (Gale et al., 1996).
- Lower neuropsychological scores indicate faster cognitive progression and lower non-verbal neuropsychological scores predict faster functional deterioration (Mortimer et al., 1992).

- Aphasia (Faber-Langendoen et al., 1988) and parietal lobe dysfunction (Burns et al., 1991) carry a poor prognosis.
- Brain scan evidence of atrophy or attenuation densities is associated with progress and early death (Burns et al., 1991; Cogan, 1985)
- Gender: findings are inconsistent and controversial. While many have shown that the progression is not related to gender, others have shown slower progression in men (Corey-Bloom, 2000) or women (Barclay et al., 1985). Certainly women survive longer with dementia than do men (Jolley and Baxter, 1997)
- Level of education: findings are not conclusive.
- Higher social class may predict longer survival (Magnusson, 1989)
- Better nutrition, including vitamin C intake, predict a better outcome (Gale et al., 1996)
- Physical ill-health and/or disability are strongly predictive of early death (Diesfeldt et al., 1986, Ballinger et al., 1988; Burns et al., 1991; Pietier et al., 1992)
- Age of onset: earlier onset may be associated with rapid deterioration, but younger people survive longer with dementia than do older people. This means they often experience much more severe and advanced symptoms.
- Associated extrapyramidal symptoms (EPS) are not predicative of the rate and type of progression, if dementia of Lewy Body disease and the use of conventional neuroleptics are excluded (Larson et al., 2004).
- Associated psychotic symptoms or behavioural disorder indicate faster cognitive decline (Stern et al., 1994; Barclay et al., 1985).
- Associated depression may denote a greater functional deficit, but is not predictive of cognitive decline, nor early death (Lopez et al., 1990).
- Presence of apolipoprotein E4 allele: Conflicting results over different studies. In essence, not associated with rate of progress, nor longevity (see Corey-Bloom, 2000).
- Use of non-steroidal anti-inflammatory medication: Extensive use over many years is associated with lower incidence and slower progression of Alzheimer's disease, as may oestrogen therapy (Rich et al., 1995; Yaffe et al., 1998).

- Diagnosis: more information is available about progress and death rates in Alzheimer's disease than in other dementias. The balance of evidence suggests that prognosis in Lewy Body dementia is not greatly different from that in Alzheimer's (Mitra et al., 2003; McKeith et al., 2004). The course of vascular dementia is more erratic and associated with more periods of hospital care, especially when large vessels are affected. Longevity is also more variable but, on average, less than in Alzheimer's (Molsa et al., 1995). Frontal lobe dementia is usually slowly progressive and longevity greater than in the other main dementia illnesses (Munoz and Kertesz, 2002)

REFERENCES

- Ballinger B, McHarg A, MacLennon W, Ogston S. (1988) Dementia, psychiatric symptoms and immobility: a one-year follow up. *International Journal of Geriatric Psychiatry,* 3(2), 125–129.
- Barclay L, Zemcov A, Blass J, McDowell F. (1985) Factors associated with survival in Alzheimer's Disease. *Biological Psychiatry,* 20, 68–93.
- Bergmann K, Foster EM, Justice AW and Matthews V. (1978) Management of the demented elderly in the community. *British Journal of Psychiatry,* 132, 441–449.
- Black D and Jolley D. (1990) Slow euthanasia? The deaths of psychogeriatric patients. *British Medical Journal,* 300, 1321–1323.
- Blessed G, Tomlinson BE, & Roth M. (1968) The association between quantitative measures of dementia and of senile change in the cerebral grey matter of elderly subjects. *British Journal of Psychiatry,* 114, 797–811.
- Bowman C Whister J Ellerby M. (2004) A national census of care home residents. *Age and Ageing,* 33(6), 608–611.
- Bracco L, Gallato R, Grigoletto F, et al. (1994) Factors affecting course and survival in Alzheimer's disease: A 9-year longitudinal study. *Archives of Neurology,* 51(12), 1213–1219.
- Burns A. (1992) Cause of death in dementia. *International Journal of Geriatric Psychiatry,* 7, (7), 461–464.
- Burns A, Lewis G, Jacoby R, Levy R. (1991) Factors affecting survival in Alzheimer's disease. *Psychological Medicine,* 21, (2), 363–370.
- Colgan J. (1985) Regional density and survival in senile dementia. *British Journal of Psychiatry,* 147, 63–66

- Corey-Bloom J. (2000) The natural history of Alzheimer's disease. In *Dementia* (eds: O'Brien J, Ames D & Burns A), 2nd edition, Part 2, Chapter 34, p405–416. London: Arnold.
- Courtney C, et al. (2004) Long-term donepezil treatment in 565 patients with Alzheimer's disease. *Lancet,* 363, 2105–2115.
- Cummings JL & Jeste DV (1999) Alzheimer's disease and its management in the year 2010. *Psychiatric Services,* 50 (9), 1173–1177.
- Department of Health (2001) National Service Framework for Older People. London. www.doh.gov.uk/nsf/olderpeople.htm.
- Diesfldt HF, van-Houte LR, Moerkens RM. (1986) Duration of survival in senile dementia. *Acta Psychiatrica Scandinavica,* 73(4), 366–371.
- Faber-Langendoen K, et al. (1988) Aphasia in senile dementia of the Alzheimer type. *Annals of Neurology,* 23, 365–370.
- Folstein MF, Folstein SE, & McHugh PR. (1975) Mini mental state. A practical method for grading the cognitive state of patients for the clinician. *Journal of Psychiatric Research,* 12, 189–198.
- Gale C, Martyn C, Winter P and Cooper C. (1996) Cognitive impairment and mortality in a cohort of elderly. *British Medical Journal,* 312, 608–611.
- HelmerC, Joly P, Letenneur L, Commenges D, Dartigues JF. (2001) Mortality with dementia: Results from a French prospective community-based cohort. *American Journal of Epidemiology,* 154, 7, 642–648.
- Heyman A, Peterson B, Fillenbaum G, Pieper C. (1996) The consortium to establish a registry for Alzheimer's disease (CERAD). Part XIV: Demographic and clinical predictors of survival in patients with Alzheimer's disease. *Neurology,* 46, 3, 656–660.
- Jolley D and Baxter D. (1997) Life expectation in Organic Brain Disease. *Advances in Psychiatric Treatment,* 3, 211–218.
- Kay D, Beamish P and Roth M. (1964) Old age disorders in Newcastle upon Tyne I. *British Journal of Psychiatry,* 110, 146–158.
- Kay D, et al. (1970) Mental illness and hospital usage in the elderly. *Comprehensive Psychiatry,* 11(1), 26–32.
- Larson E, et al. (2004) Survival after initial diagnosis of Alzheimer's disease. *Annals of Internal Medicine,* 140, 501–509.
- Lopez OL, Boller F, Becker JT, Miller M, & Reynolds CF. (1990) Alzheimer's disease and depression: neuropsychological impairment and progression of the illness. *American Journal of Psychiatry,* 147, 855–860.
- Magnusson H. (1989) Mental health of octogenarians. *Acta Psychiatrica Scandinavica,* Suppl. 349, 1–112.

- McKeith IG, Perry RH, Fairbairn AF, Jabeen S, Perry EK. (1992) Operational criteria for Senile Dementia of Lewy Body Type (SDLT). *Psychological Medicine,* 22, 911–922.
- McKeith I, et al. (2004) Dementia with Lewy bodies. *Lancer Neurology,* 3 (1), 19–28.
- Mitra K, Gangopadhaya PK, Das SK. (2003) Parkinsonism plus syndrome. *Neurology India,* 51(2), 183–188.
- Molsa PK, Marttila R, and Rinne UK (1995) Long-term survival and predictors of mortality in Alzheimer's disease and multi-infarct dementia. *Acta Neurologica Scandinavica,* 91, 159–164.
- Munoz DG and Kertesz A (2002) The fronto-temporal lobar atrophies: The Pick complex. In *Evidence-based Dementia Practice,* (eds: Qizilbash N et al.), Chapter 111.5 p 297–311. Oxford: Blackwell. www.ebdementia.info.
- Morris JC. (1999) Clinical presentation and course of Alzheimer's disease. In *Alzheimer's Disease* (2nd edition) – Terry RB, Katzman R, Bick KL, Sisodia SS (eds) Part II: Ch 2; p11–24. Philadelphia: Lippincot Williams & Wilkins.
- Morris JC. (1997) The Clinical Dementia Rating (CDR): a reliable and valid diagnostic and staging measure for dementia of the Alzheimer's type. *International Psychogeriatrics,* 9 (suppl.1), 173–176.
- O'Connor D. (1992) Current questions in the epidemiology of dementia. In: *Recent Advances in Psychogeriatrics 2,* (ed: Arie T.), Chapter 15, p173–186. London: Churchill Livingstone.
- Office of Health Economics (1979) *Dementia in old age.* OHE. London
- Pietier T, vanDijk HJ, et al. (1992) The nature of excess mortality in nursing homes patients with dementia. *Journal of Gerontology, Medical Science,* 47(2), 28–34.
- Reisberg B, Ferris S, De Leon MJ, & Crook T. (1982) The Global Deterioration Scale (GDS): an instrument for the assessment of primary degenerative dementia. *American Journal of Psychiatry,* 139, 1136–1139.
- Reisberg B. (1988) Functional assessment staging (FAST). *Psychopharmacology Bulletin,* 24, 653–659.
- Rich J, Rasmusson D, Folstein M, Carson K, Kawas C & Brandt J. (1995) Non-steroidal anti-inflammatory drugs in Alzheimer's disease. *Neurology,* 45, 224–232.
- Roth M. (1955) The natural history of mental disorder in old age. *Journal of Mental Science,* 101, 281–301.
- Rosen J, Mohs RC, & Davies KL. (1984) A new rating scale for Alzheimer's disease. *American Journal of Psychiatry,* 141, 1356–1364.

- Roth M, Tym E, Mountjoy CQ et al. (1986) CAMDEX: a standardized instrument for the diagnosis of mental disorder in the elderly with special reference to the early detection of dementia. *British Journal of Psychiatry*, 149, 698–709.
- Sanford JR (1975) Tolerance of debility in elderly dependents by supporters at home. *British Medical Journal*, 5981, 471–473.
- Stern Y et al. (1989) Predictors of disease course in patients with probable Alzheimer's disease. *Neurology*, 37, 1649–1651.
- Stern Y, Tang M, Denaro J & Mayeux R. (1995) Increased risk of mortality in Alzheimer's disease patients with more advanced educational and occupational attainment. *Annals of Neurology*, 37, 590–595.
- Tench D, Benbow S and Benbow E. (1992) Do old age psychiatrists miss physical illness. *International Journal of Geriatric Psychiatry*, 7, (10), 713–718.
- Volicer L. (1986) Need for hospice approach to treatment of patients with advanced progressive dementia. *Journal of the American Geriatrics Society*, 34(9), 655–658.
- Wood E, Whitefield E and Christie A. (1991) Changes in survival in demented hospital inpatients 1957–1987. *International Journal of Geriatric Psychiatry*, 6 (7), 523–528.
- Yaffe K, Sawaya G, Lieberburg I, & Grady D. (1998) Estrogen therapy in postmenopausal women: effects on cognitive function and dementia. *Journal of American Medical Association*, 279, 688–695.

10

Assessment Scales in Dementia

Rosie Jenkins

Introduction

For any clinician using an assessment tool, the point of the exercise must not only be to confirm that a suspected pathology is indeed present and causing symptomatology, but also to understand better the degree to which the patient is affected by the pathology. This in turn will greatly help decision making about the therapeutic interventions, care and support that may help the patient and those who are concerned about him. The mainstay for making diagnoses and treatment decisions will remain clinical, and this clinical judgement will grow with the pursuit of knowledge and experience. However, the more accurate the formulated diagnosis and prognosis, the better the ability to start appropriate treatment and prepare the patient and his carers for what lies ahead. In the field of Old Age Psychiatry this has become even more important with the relatively recent development of drug interventions for dementia syndromes. It falls beyond the remit of this brief chapter to exhaustively review all the available schedules, their strengths and cross-cultural shortcomings, but the following is intended as an introduction to some of the more commonly used and reliable tools being used in the area of dementia studies, and suitable for general clinical practice. Some of these assessments are already available in translation and work is ongoing to produce culturally sensitive and appropriate tools for use outside of western clinical practice.

SCREENING TOOLS

The use of assessment scales in the evaluation of people presenting with memory and related difficulties has become an integral part of day-to-day, routine clinical practice. To be useful to the clinician and the patient alike, though, the scales that are used in initial patient assessment especially, must be appropriate to the situation that presents and easy to perform: more extensive testing can always be undertaken later on. Scales have been developed in all cultures to aid in the screening of older people with cognitive difficulties, scales that are reliable and valid for such a purpose. This means that such tools should be appropriate for use by practitioners from any health discipline, as it is the questions that are being asked in the assessments, not the person asking the questions, that then becomes important. Even so, there is no absolute certainty about the interpretation of test scores and clinical judgement is still required. The greatest problem that presents itself in a work such as this is to recommend scales that are culturally and educationally relevant to the people they are to assess. The commonest screening tools in use in the UK and USA include the Mini-Mental State Examination (MMSE), the Mental Test Score (MTS), the Abbreviated Mental Test Score (AMTS) and the clock-drawing test. These tools examine general cognitive skills in a brief manner that can be easily managed in most settings.

Mini-Mental State Examination

Developed by Folstein et al (1975), the MMSE in particular is widely used by practitioners in community and care home settings as well as by specialist teams in other clinical situations. The format assesses the subject's ability to perform in tests of orientation (in time and place), registration and recall of 3 words, attention and calculation, language functions, and visual construction. Although there are versions in a number of languages including Hindi and Punjabi, the test does require the subject to be literate although not highly numerate: the translated versions often have substituted sections to get around any difficulties this may cause. A simple pen and paper test taking around 10 minutes to complete, the MMSE has been extensively used since its introduction in 1975 and so it has the advantage of a body of knowledge that has come from all these years of usage. Cut off scores are suggested for estimating early, moderate and severe dementia impairments, and as well as its use as a screening tool, the MMSE can be used to assess changes in cognitive abilities over time. This has value not only for charting the progress of the dementia, but also now in assessing response to treatment with cholinesterase inhibitors. Some authors have further suggested that if the MMSE is used along side a verbal fluency test, it may also have a role in the early diagnosis of Alzheimer's disease. It is, however, important to note that the MMSE is not designed as a diagnostic tool but allows the assessor to have a quantitative measurement of cognitive impairment. The reader is referred to the paper by Anthony et al (1982) in respect of the limitations of the use of the MMSE, and to other general information about the test (Tombaugh and McIntyre, 1992). There is also a standardised version of the MMSE available, and for both test schedules, some rater training is advised.

Mental Test Score

The MTS (Hodkinson, 1972) is another brief screening assessment tool. It has two forms, the 34-item test and the Abbreviated MTS (Qureshi and Hodkinson, 1974), which is composed of the 10 most highly discriminating elements of the original. The 34-item test assesses the subject's orientation in time and place, ability to register and recall new information, to recognise people within their environment and to recall personal and general information. Attention and concentration are measured by the subject reciting the months of the year in reverse order, and counting tests. Again its use is limited even in translation by these numeracy requirements, but the AMTS, which can be done in as little as 3 minutes only, has one short number-using subscale which could be approximately replaced by a non-numerical test of attention and concentration for routine clinical application. It is important to remember the difference between an adapted scale acceptable for use in clinical practice and a scale which has been validated, as a sensitive and reliable one.

Clock Drawing Test

The clock drawing test is somewhat more culture bound, but is a quickly performed and fascinating screening measure of dementia severity. Shulman et al. (1986) and Brodaty et al. (1997) provide interesting views on the use of this assessment which interprets the performance of patients asked to draw a clock and set the hands. The number and type of errors are scrutinised and a score given that reflects the likely severity of the patient's cognitive impairment.

DIAGNOSTIC GUIDELINES

Once there is evidence of probable cognitive decline, then the next step for the clinician is to ascertain the diagnosis, with the greater emphasis in respect of making this diagnosis on the clinical picture and the histories available from the patient and any informants. Such histories will give the assessing doctor important evidence as to the onset and progress of the cognitive decline: the presence of major risk factors for cerebrovascular disease and an episodic pattern of deterioration in skills and abilities may strongly suggest a vascular dementia, for example. The presence of marked, persistent visual hallucinations in the setting of a fluctuating cognitive impairment accompanied by Parkinsonian features would indicate the possibility of a dementia with Lewy bodies. A more gradual decline with more uniform, global cognitive difficulties might represent an Alzheimer's picture. Further physical examination and investigation will generally be required as part of the assessment process, and the formulation of the diagnostic picture will be facilitated by reference to diagnostic guides of worldwide repute, The International Classification of Mental and Behavioural Disorders (WHO, 1992) and the Diagnostic and Statistical Manual of Mental Disorders IV (American Psychiatric Association, 1994). The Neuropsychiatric Inventory (NPI, Cummings et al., 1994) is one assessment schedule that can be quickly completed (with the aid of a carer's information) that can help differentiate the possible causes of dementia, although some training of the observers is advised. The Ischaemic Score (Hachinski et al., 1975) may help to clarify the vascular elements of a dementia presentation, and is very quick and easy to perform once a thorough history and examination have been completed.

ASSESSMENT OF RESPONSE TO TREATMENT

As mentioned, there are now opportunities to intervene with drug treatments for some dementia sufferers, and there is therefore a need to be able to objectively assess the benefits (and any drawbacks) of such treatments in individual patients. The Alzheimer's Disease

Assessment Scale (ADAS) with its cognitive and non-cognitive sections (ADAS-Cog, ADAS-Non-Cog) can be extremely useful and bear transposing into different cultural settings. Devised by Rosen et al. (1984), it is widely used in drug trials but it can equally be applied to the assessment of an individual's response to treatment in a clinical setting. The assessment takes approximately 45 minutes, and the assessor must be trained in its use and the observations required. The MMSE can also be used as a longitudinal measure of ability, and the Clinician's Global Impression of Change (Guy, 1976) can inform on wider issues when done by a trained and experienced rater, as can a number of similar interview-based scales derived from it (see Knopman et al., 1994). As well as the cognitive changes, behavioural and emotional disturbances and disturbances in activities of daily living all combine to give depth to the understanding of the patient's experience of dementia, and scales exist to quantify all these areas and allow the evaluation of care interventions. It is important to remember that as well as many other scales available to the clinician, there are specific neuropsychiatry assessments usually undertaken by clinical psychologists who are invaluable colleagues in the dementia assessment process. As well as the ADAS-Non-Cog, one particular schedule that is finding an increasing role in the assessment of psychiatric symptoms and behavioural changes in patients with dementia is the Manchester and Oxford Universities Scale for the Psychopathological Assessment of Dementia, or MOUSEPAD (Allen et al., 1996). This scale not only records observations at the time of the test but also measures symptoms in the four weeks preceding the assessment. Results from this mini-battery can inform the clinician of a number of non-cognitive areas where changes may have occurred and be causing problems, or require intervention. The schedule does not, though, have any items for depression, and it has been recommended by various authors that where depression is a concern, the Cornell Scale for Depression in Dementia (Alexopoulos et al., 1988) can be a useful supplement, and indeed recommended by the MOUSEPAD's authors.

ASSESSMENT OF CARERS' BURDEN

Finally, it is most important to remember the carers of dementia patients, who experience a high degree of stress and care burden as they support the sufferers. The importance of acknowledging and relieving these stresses, where possible, is difficult to overestimate. A checklist approach to identifying difficulties can allow clinical teams to work with the carers to ease these burdens and safeguard the care situation for both the sufferers and carers alike. Examples of such lists are the Problem Checklist and Strain Scale (Gilleard, 1984) and the Ways of Coping Checklist (Vitaliano, 1985). The additional use of clinical case screening schedules such as the General Health Questionnaire (Goldberg and Williams, 1988) may highlight developing clinical problems in carers and allow for appropriate and timely therapeutic interventions.

REFERENCES

- Alexopoulos G, Abrahams R, Young R, et al. (1988) Cornell Scale for Depression in Dementia. *Biological Psychiatry,* 23, 271–284.
- Allen NHP, Gordon S, Hope T, Burns A. (1996) Manchester and Oxford Universities Scale for Psychopathological Assessment of Dementia (MOUSEPAD). *British Journal of Psychiatry,* 169, 293–307.
- American Psychiatric Association (1994) *Diagnostic and Statistical Manual of Mental Disorders,* 4th edition. Washington DC: American Psychiatric Association.
- Anthony J, LeResche L, Niaz U, et al. (1982) Limits of the "Mini-Mental State" as a screening test for dementia and delirium among hospital patients. *Psychological Medicine,* 12, 397–408.
- Brodaty H, Moore CM. (1997) The Clock Drawing Test for dementia of the Alzheimer's type: a comparison of three scoring methods in a memory disorders clinic. *International Journal of Geriatric Psychiatry,* 12, 619–627.
- Cummings JL, Mega M, Gray K, Rosenberg-Thompson S, Carusi DA, Gornbein J. (1994) The Neuropsychiatric Inventory: comprehensive assessment of psychopathology in dementia. *Neurology,* 44, 2308–2314.
- Folstein MF, Folstein SE, McHugh PR. (1975) "Mini-Mental State": A practical method for grading the cognitive state of patients for the clinician. *Journal of Psychiatric Research,* 12, 189–198.
- Gilleard CJ (1984) *Living with dementia: community care of the elderly mentally infirm.* Beckenham: Croom Helm.
- Goldberg DP, Williams P. (1988) *A User's Guide to the General Health Questionnaire.* Windsor: NFER-NELSON.

- Guy W (ed) (1976) Clinical Global Impressions (CGI). In: *Assessment Manual for Psychopharmacology.* US Department of Health and Human Services, Public Health Service, Alcohol, Drug Abuse and Mental Health Administration, NIMH Psychopharmacology Research Branch, 218–222.
- Hachinski VC, Iliff LD, Zilhka E, et al. (1975) Cerebral blood flow in dementia. *Arch Neurol,* 32, 632–637.
- Hodkinson M. (1972) Evaluation of a mental test score for assessment of mental impairment in the elderly. *Age and Ageing,* 1, 233–238.
- Knopman D, et al. (1994) The Clinician Interview-Based Impression (CIBI): a clinician's global change rating scale in Alzheimer's disease. *Neurology,* 44, 2315–2321.
- Qureshi K, Hodkinson M (1974) Evaluation of a 10 question mental test of the institutionalised elderly. *Age and Ageing,* 3, 152–157.
- Rosen WG, Mohs RC, Davis KL. (1984) A new rating scale for Alzheimer's disease. *American Journal of Psychiatry,* 141, 1356–1364.
- Shulman K, Shedletsky R, Silver I (1986) The challenge of time. Clock drawing and cognitive functioning in the elderly. *International Journal of Geriatric Psychiatry,* 1, 135–140.
- Tombaugh TN, McIntyre NJ. (1992) The Mini-Mental State Examination: a comprehensive review. *Journal of the American Geriatric Society,* 40, 922–935.
- Vitiliano PP, Russo J, Carr JE, Maiuro RD, Becker J. (1985) The Ways of Coping Checklist: revision and psychometric properties. *Multivariate Behavioural Research,* 20, 3–26.
- World Health Organization (1992) *The ICD-10 Classification of Mental and Behavioural Disorders: Clinical descriptions and diagnostic guidelines.* Geneva: World Health Organization.

11

Differential Diagnosis of Dementias

Jagadisha

Introduction

The term dementia generally evokes a nihilistic response not only from the patients and relatives, but also from the health care professionals. However, the fact remains that dementia is a syndrome, which can result from several aetiopathological processes and several of them are potentially reversible. The exact differential diagnosis of dementia has major implications in management and prognostication, as each disorder causing dementia has its own unique course and response to treatment. This can be achieved only through a meticulous clinical evaluation and pertinent investigation.

There is ample evidence from clinical experience and from literature reviewed by Lishman (1999) that a substantial proportion of people diagnosed with dementia actually suffer from other disorders. Among those who are confirmed to have dementia also, a substantial proportion suffers from disorders that can either be reversed or arrested from progressing. There are instances, where dementia co-exists with other disorders, which can aggravate the problems of dementia and treatment of these ensures substantial clinical benefit. The likelihood of confirming the absence of dementia in people suspected to have dementia in neurologic centers after careful inpatient evaluation is about 16%. Among dementias, the likelihood of finding non-Alzheimer's dementia, where the prognostic and management issues have considerable variation is about 40%. The numbers are higher in psychiatric settings – approaching 50% being not diagnosed as dementia and much lower in populations above 65 and even less in people over 80. These figures underline the need for a careful inpatient evaluation of patients with suspected dementia.

This chapter aims at answering the questions, which are likely to arise in a clinician's mind when faced with a patient with cognitive impairment. Is it dementia? If not, is it something similar to, but not dementia? What is the cause of dementia in this patient? Have I ruled out other possible causes? Initially, a clinical classification of dementias is presented. This is followed by a discussion of an approach to differential diagnosis of dementia. Finally, we present a section highlighting the clinical features of some dementias, where the cause is not very obvious – most of them are classically considered to be degenerative dementias.

DIAGNOSIS OF DEMENTIA

When a person comes with features of cognitive decline or when middle-aged or elderly people present with psychological or personality disturbances for the first time in their lives, the index of suspicion towards dementia should be high. First, one should try to *see if there is a syndrome of dementia*. The Diagnostic and Statistical Manual DSM IV defines dementia as development of multiple cognitive deficits manifested by both:
1) Memory impairment, and
2) One (or more) of aphasia, agnosia, apraxia and disturbance of executive functioning (planning, organizing, sequencing and abstracting)

Some general screening questions at history level, e.g., 'how is his memory?'; 'is he forgetting things off late?'; 'has he lost some valuables?'; 'would he forget the events of the day?'; 'does he forget his way?' would help in establishing memory impairment, which is meaningful clinically. Similarly, asking about his ability to name objects /persons' name would bring out early signs of aphasia; difficulty in communicating with the patient follows that. Difficulty in dressing up, taking bath, eating, etc., brings out apraxia, and using objects for purposes not meant for that brings out agnosia. Questions about ability to perform complex tasks like ability to manage household chores, running a business, managing money, independent of disabilities in other fields elicit executive dysfunction.

A *decline* from a previous level of cognitive functioning needs to be established. It is important to establish that both the above should be clinically meaningful, i.e., they cause *significant impairment* in social/occupational functioning. Generally, this is based on meticulous history taking and clinical examination – it is important to ask "how much problem the cognitive impairment is causing in his/her day-to-day life?" One would find both memory disturbance and executive dysfunction even in a young person with schizophrenia on neuropsychological examination, but these deficits seen in neuropsychological examination may not be clinically meaningful. Such a thorough enquiry establishes *global decline* and rules out other disorders of cognitive decline, which can mimic dementia: Korsakoff's syndrome, other amnestic disorders and aphasia, especially, angular gyrus syndrome, in which one finds specific disabilities vis-à-vis global decline. Demonstration of such a global cognitive deficit by routine clinical mental status examination (MSE) confirms the diagnosis of syndrome of dementia. Finally, if patient has delirium also, then establishing features of dementia during the periods when delirium is not present is important, as DSM IV diagnosis of dementia warrants that it should not be present exclusively during a period of delirium.

Before going on to enquire which type of dementia a person has, a few causes of pseudodementias – disorders, which resemble organic dementia, yet where a physical disease proves to be little if at all responsible for the picture – may need to be ruled out.

Depressive Pseudodementia

This is the kind of pseudodementia that is most commonly misdiagnosed. Frequent co-occurrence of dementia and depression is only part of the explanation for this. In addition to factors, which may prevent a person from performing a cognitive function adequately because of depressed mood – psychomotor retardation, preoccupation and inability to register and pessimistic thoughts about self-efficacy –

there seems to be a real cognitive dysfunction in depressed patients (Abas et al., 1990). Possible interaction between ageing brain and neurochemical changes due to depression has been thought to be the cause of this and the term *dementia syndrome of depression* has been coined to validate the "reality" of cognitive disability in them (Folstein and McHugh, 1978).

Several pointers suggest dementia syndrome of depression vis-à-vis "organic" dementia. Generally, it is of more acute onset, with a life event preceding in some cases; the patient may often utter depressive statements in the midst of seemingly incoherent speech of dementia. A depressed person complains of inability to perform task, as against an organically demented person, who tries to underplay his disability, giving excuses. "Don't know" answers of depressed patients typically contrast against the confabulation seen in organic dementias. Inconsistency in performance and striking absence of dyspraxias and dysphasias also give clues towards the diagnosis. Performance is worse in the mornings and better in the evenings in depressed patients, while sun-downing is typical in organic dementias. Drug assisted abreaction and sleep deprivation also help in differentiation. EEG changes typical of depression are seen in pseudodementia. Hypomania and schizophrenia also can cause significant confusion in diagnosis. However, discrepancy between the apparent cognitive dysfunction and the behaviour, which may reflect grossly intact cognitive functions, gives a major clue. Psychotic and mood symptoms also suggest the differential diagnosis by their predominance.

Ganser's Syndrome

This is very rare. It can be a syndrome by itself, but more commonly occurs in the course of another psychiatric disorder. The typical feature in this is that patient gives the answer, which though wrong, is never far wrong and bears a definite and obvious relation to the question, indicating clearly that the question has been grasped by the patient (approximate answer: e.g., "How many legs does a horse have"? "Five"). The other features are, second person auditory hallucinations, fluctuation of consciousness, clear-cut onset and offset and amnesia for the experience.

Dissociative Pseudodementia

This is the easiest to make out. Whereas patient's responses are grossly wrong or incoherent, his ward behavior, self-care, etc., easily indicate incompatibility between the cognitive impairment and disability. Wide fluctuations in cognitive abilities, suggestibility during testing and the presence of other dissociative phenomena clearly indicate the diagnosis. Disturbed personality or presence of significant stress is generally the case. It runs a fairly sustained but fluctuating course compared to the abrupt onset and offset with transient nature of Ganser's syndrome.

Simulated Pseudodementia

In this condition, in addition to the absence of disease, one gets a firm impression that the individual is consciously aware of both what he is doing and his motive for doing so; he is fixed in carrying out a purpose to a preconceived result. There is a definite purpose for feigning as demented. The discrepancy between observed behaviour and cognitive "impairment" is similar to dissociative pseudodementia. But the consistency in giving wrong answers clearly distinguishes this condition from other pseudoementias and organic dementias. For example, when a list of 20 words is read out and then patient is asked to identify them from a list of original and distracter words, simulators fall much below 50%. Pure dements and other pseudodements score nearly 50% by sheer chance. In Raven's progressive matrices, there are deficits even at the easy level. When inconsistencies arise, a simulator will try to explain it or gets angry when pointed out, whereas, other pseudodements remain apathetic towards it. Also, they resent any close enquiry into their deficits.

CLASSIFICATION OF DEMENTIAS

For clinical purposes, dementia is best classified based on the etiologies. This helps the clinician to clinically evaluate, investigate and plan management and prognosticate.

Table 11.1 Classification of dementias

1. Diffuse parenchymatous diseases of the central nervous system
   a. Alzheimer's disease
   b. Pick's disease
   c. Diffuse Lewy Body dementia
   d. Creutzfeldt-Jakob disease
   e. Parkinsonism-dementia complex of Guam
   f. Huntington's chorea
   g. Hallervorden-Spatz disease
   h. Spinocerebellar degeneration
   i. Progressive supranuclear palsy
   j. Parkinson's disease

2. Metabolic disorders
   a. Myxoedema
   b. Disorders of parathyroid glands
   c. Wilson's disease
   d. Liver disease
   e. Hypoglycaemia
   f. Remote effects of carcinoma
   g. Cushing's syndrome
   h. Hypopituitarism
   i. Uraemia
   j. Dialysis dementia
   k. Metachromatic leukodystrophy

3. Vascular disorders
   a. Arteriosclerosis
   b. Inflammatory disease of blood vessels
      i. Disseminated lupus erythematosus
      ii. Thromboangitis obliterans
   c. Aortic arch syndrome
   d. Binswanger's disease
   e. Arteriovenous malformation

4. Hypoxia and anoxia

5. Normal-pressure hydrocephalus

6. Deficiency diseases
   a. Wernicke-Korsakoff syndrome
   b. Pellagra
   c. Marchiafava-Bignami disease
   d. Vitamin B_{12} deficiency
   e. Folate deficiency

7. Toxins and drugs
   a. Metals
   b. Organic compounds
   c. Carbon monoxide
   d. Drugs

8. Brain tumours

9. Trauma
   a. Open and closed head injuries
   b. Punch-drunk syndrome
   c. Subdural haematoma
   d. Heat stroke

10. Infections
   a. Brain abscess
   b. Bacterial meningitis
   c. Fungal meningitis
   d. Encephalitis
   e. Subacute sclerosing panencephalitis
   f. Progressive multifocal leukoencephalopathy
   g. Creutzfeldt-Jakob disease
   h. Kuru
   i. Behcet's syndrome
   j. Lues

11. Other diseases
   a. Multiple sclerosis
   b. Muscular dystrophy
   c. Whipple's disease
   d. Kufs' disease
   e. Familial calcification of basal ganglia

DIFFERENTIAL DIAGNOSIS

Once one is clear about the syndrome of dementia and its "organic" nature, history taking should be directed towards arriving at a differential diagnosis, as to which type of dementia is the person having.

History: History of head trauma, however minor, must be asked about. In the elderly, atherosclerotic or alcoholics, even minor injuries can lead to subdural haematoma (SDH) and it can lead to such insidious onset of symptoms that one might miss the significance of head trauma. Such a history is important in causing normal pressure hydrocephalus also. History of seizures of recent onset, transient ischaemic attacks/stroke, headache, vomiting and visual disturbances would point towards tumours/infarcts or rarely, cerebral infections. History of recent loss of weight should raise the possibility of any malignancy or HIV infection or anaemia or uraemia, which might cause dementia by several mechanisms – secondaries in brain, nutritional deficiency or as a paraneoplastic syndrome. Nutritional deficiencies due to other causes like gastrectomy/gastrointestinal malignancy, chronic alcohol use needs to be probed specifically. History of cold intolerance, weight gain, constipation, hoarseness of voice should be asked to rule out hypothyroidism. Increased thirst or bone pain suggest parathyroid disorders. History of intravenous drug abuse and sexual exposure should be specifically probed to suspect HIV infection. Intravenous drug abuse should be specifically asked for when there are clear-cut fluctuations in clinical picture. Such a picture is also described in vascular dementia and diffuse Lewy body dementia. History of abnormal involuntary movements makes one consider Parkinson's disease or Huntington's disease or Parkinson's plus disorders; myoclonic jerks may point towards Creutzfeldt-Jakob disease (CJD).

Mode of onset: Abrupt onset is generally typical of vascular events, either solely responsible or complicating dementia. Similarly, a precise onset can be made out when some intracranial tumours cause dementia. Insidious onset is typical of all degenerative disorders. However, the exact sequence of symptoms may be different – starting with memory impairment is typical of Alzheimer's disease (AD). Other features of dementia follow memory deficits in months' time. In contrast, subtle changes in personality herald the onset of frontotemporal dementia, Pick's disease and subcortical dementias like Huntington's disease. Sometimes, diffuse Lewy body dementia (DLBD) presents only with extrapyramidal symptoms to start with. DLBD may also start with psychotic features, whereas this happens only in later stages of other dementias.

Steady progression is typical of degenerative disorders. If there is fluctuation in the course, a number of possibilities including DLBD, drug abuse, SDH, hypoglycaemic attacks and delirium due to any cause superimposing on dementia need to be considered and be evaluated for. Stepwise progression has been described as typical of vascular dementia, each deterioration corresponding to a vascular event.

Progression in degenerative disorders is generally slow and hence any dementia of shorter duration presenting with multiple cognitive disabilities should alert a clinician to look for treatable causes.

In *general examination*, pallor and features of vitamin deficiency indicate not only nutritional deficiency, but also makes the clinician think of causes of such deficiencies, which might have caused dementia on its own. Oedema, when pitting, suggests cardiorespiratory or renal pathology, which may be causing or exacerbating dementia. Myxoedema and obesity indicate hypothyroidism as possible cause of dementia. One should look for risk factors for vascular dementia, such as atherosclerotic thickening of arteries, bruits in the carotids and renal arteries, hypertension. Examination of lymph nodes may give clues to occult malignancy or HIV infection. Localizing neural signs generally indicate space-occupying lesions, infarcts or infections, though this can occur in the late stages of degenerative dementias. Though rare in recent times, one should look for Argyll Robertson pupils of neurosyphilis. Kayser-Fleischer ring indicates Wilson's disease. Extrapyramidal signs are of a lot of importance, as they may suggest dementia in Parkinson's disease, Huntington's disease, DLBD, progressive supraneuclear palsy and late stages of Alzheimer's disease. Chorea and myoclonic jerks point towards Huntington's disease and Creutzfeldt-Jakob disease. Presence of cerebellar signs suggest multi-system atrophy and may indicate consequences of chronic alcohol abuse, especially if also associated with signs of peripheral neuropathy.

Mental status examination, as already described, would be useful in differentiating dementia from pseudodementia and also to establish global impairment of cognitive functions.

Investigation

Routine estimation of haemoglobin percentage, TLC, DC, ESR, blood urea, serum creatinine, electrolytes, serum proteins, liver function tests and chest X-ray in all cases of dementia may show abnormalities, which may be complicating a dementing illness if not point to the exact aetiology. Presence of megalocytes would call for further examination of serum B_{12} and folate levels. Peripheral smear may show acanthocytes.

EEG shows loss of alpha and predominance of theta and delta waves in degenerative dementias, especially AD. Focal EEG abnormalities are observed in cases of tumours, or vascular insults. Repetitive spikes and classical triphasic sharp wave complexes are observed in CJD and hepatic encephalopathy. Though not diagnostic, routine use of EEG may help to pick up the presence of or suggest certain type of lesions.

Brain imaging: Either CT scan or MRI of brain should be done routinely in all cases of dementia. This helps greatly in differential diagnosis. Diffuse cerebral atrophy and ventricular dilatation is typical of Alzheimer's dementia, whereas selective atrophy of frontotemporal regions is seen in Pick's disease and frontotemporal dementias.

The following tests are done only when there is definite clue from history or examinations and not routinely: Serum ceruloplasmin to rule out Wilson's disease; arylsulfatase A for suspected cases of metachromatic leukodystrophy; skeletal muscle biopsy for the possibility of Kuf's disease, mitochondrial myopathy; lymph node or jejunal biopsy to rule out Whipple's disease; tonsillar biopsy for ruling out CJD; and angiography in suspected cases of granulomatous angitis are considered. Cerebrospinal fluid (CSF) examination is generally done if diagnosis remains uncertain, to examine for CSF VDRL, evidence of chronic meningitis like tuberculosis, cryptococcal infection. A positive immunoassay for protein 14-3-3 is deemed to be highly specific for

CJD. Brain biopsy may show pathognomonic signs of Alzheimer's disease and CJD, but at present, does not seem to figure in the list of clinically useful investigations.

CLINICAL FEATURES OF SOME DEMENTIAS

In this section the salient features of some of the dementias, whose differentiation generally is not very obvious are described. Most of them have been classically considered to be degenerative dementias or primary dementias.

Alzheimer's Disease

Traditionally, the term AD was used to describe patients, who have age of onset before 65 years. However, reflecting the increasing body of evidence that the conditions are likely to be identical, whether setting in before or after 65, the current international classificatory systems do not consider this age cut off of 65.

However, one is likely to find higher family history and more rapid progression of disorder when the age at onset is earlier than 65 years. It is rare to find age at onset earlier than 40 years. Male: female ratio is 1: 2–3. Invariably, the onset is insidious and difficult to date. Memory loss is the typical early feature. Changes in mood in the form of anxiety, hyperexcitablity, aspontaneity, though can present early, following memory changes. Generally, three stages are identified (Lishman, 1999). The first, lasting for 2–3 years is characterized by memory loss, inefficiency in work, spatial disorientation and subtle mood changes. From the second phase, there is an increase in rapidity of progress of disorder. Focal symptoms including dysphasia, apraxia, agnosia, acalcuclia appear in this phase. Majority of patients develop extrapyramidal symptoms (EPS) of typical Parkinsonian nature. Psychotic features – delusions and hallucinations – can predominate the picture. In the third stage, the patient is generally bed-bound, with frequent seizures, severe EPS and release reflexes. Patient becomes doubly incontinent. Appetite is generally preserved, but patient wastes rapidly. Kluver-Bucy like syndrome, focal – usually temporal lobe – seizures characterize transition from the second to third stage. EEG is generally abnormal in almost all – including early phases. Typical feature is reduction or absence of alfa activity. Diffuse theta waves and delta waves appear later. Paroxysmal and focal activities are rare. CT scan and MRI generally show diffuse cortical atrophy, though it is difficult to distinguish this finding from normal ageing, because of wide degrees of overlap. Hippocampal, parahippocampal atrophy seems to be more specific and sensitive early change (Seab et al., 1988; Kesslak et al., 1991). National Institute of Neurological and Communicative Disorders and Stroke and the Alzheimer's Disease and Related Disorders Association (NINCDES-ADRD) have laid down operational criteria for the clinical diagnosis of Alzheimer's disease for use in research (McKhann et al., 1984).

Diffuse Lewy Body Disease

Onset of DLBD is typically in the 60s or 70s. Mode of onset can be with cognitive impairment or extrapyramidal symptoms or psychotic features or confusion, depending on the setting. Almost all would present with a mixture of these at some periods of time, but rarely dementia alone might be present without other features.

Dementia is typically cortical in type, with progressive memory impairment and the development of dysphasia, dyscalculia and dyspraxia. Lucid intervals are also observed, when patient may not have any cognitive impairment. Extrapyramidal symptoms are typically Parkinsonian in type, with bradykinesia, rigidity, tremors and orthostatic hypotension. Frequent falls are also very common. Typically, these features may be induced by exposure to even low doses of neuroleptics. Loss of consciousness and deaths have been reported with use of even low neuroleptic medications.

Psychiatric manifestations are in the form of hallucinations, especially of visual and less commonly auditory types. Patient may develop persecutory and referential delusions. Severe depression is also not uncommon. Delirium-like picture with clouding of consciousness is present in almost 80% of patients. Neuropsychological assessments may reveal a pattern of deficits similar to AD, but with a predominance of deficits in visuospatial and frontal lobe functions (McKeith et al., 1995). CT scan may show mild diffuse cerebral atrophy. EEG shows non-specific slowing and CSF is generally normal. Operational criteria for the diagnosis have been suggested by McKeith et al. (1992).

Multi-infarct Dementia (vascular dementia)

Multi-infarct dementia (MID) has almost equal distribution between the genders. Generally, the age at onset is late 60s and 70s. Frequently, the onset is more acute than in AD – generally in the wake of a cerebrovascular event. When the onset is insidious, again, unlike in AD, where memory is the first to be impaired, the presenting complaints are emotional or personality changes or somatic symptoms like headache, dizziness, tinnitus, syncopes, etc., which would antedate intellectual impairment. However, because of patchy nature of deficits, personality, judgment and insight may be well preserved, until late, leading to anxiety and depression due to awareness of intellectual deficits.

When cognitive impairments are established, they typically tend to fluctuate from day-to-day or hour-to-hour because of frequent variations in levels and of clouding of consciousness, especially at nightfall. This is unusual in AD. The feature which differentiates MID from AD, is its typical course – stepwise increase in cognitive impairment, which accompanies neurological deficits like hemiparesis, visual impairment, dysphasia, due to cerebrovascular events. Lacunar infarcts would lead to a picture of pseudobulbar palsy, with lability of mood.

Examination reveals atherosclerotic changes in the periphery. Major or minor neurological abnormalities are evident invariably – Parkinsonian features are also common. Though EEG may be similar to that in AD, more often focal or lateralizing or paroxysmal abnormalities are observed, depending on the underlying brain insult. CT scan may show infarcts in cortical and basal regions, but generally it fails to distinguish AD from MID. MRI, by picking up lacunar infarcts in deep white matter and leukoaraiosis, can distinguish MID from AD better. Neuroepidemiology branch of the National Institute of Neurological Disorders and Stroke and Association Internationale pur la Resherche et l'Enseignement en Neurosciences (NINDS-AIREN) have proposed diagnostic criteria for vascular dementia, synthesizing both clinical and neuroimaging information (Román et al., 1993).

Pick's Disease and other Frontotemporal Dementias

Generally there is female preponderance. The age at onset peaks between 50s and 60s. The most characteristic feature is the onset; early abnormalities are of changes in character and social behaviour. Either the drive is diminished and the person becomes indolent or lack of restraint leads to episodes of grossly insensitive behaviours like stealing, sexual adventures. Mood remains to be one of fatuous euphoria or apathy with bouts of overactivity or aggression. Early appearance of Kluver – Bucy syndrome is characteristic. The next striking feature is speech abnormalities with perseveration and prominent reduction in vocabulary, leading on to jargon and periods of mutism. Memory impairment sets in and rarely apraxias and agnosias may develop. Testing reveals more severe memory deficits than activities of daily living reveal. Neurological abnormalities are rare, excepting frontal release reflexes.

Neuropsychological evaluation reveals prominent abnormalities in card sorting tests and other frontal lobe tests. EEG is generally normal; CT scan and MRI are typical with severe atrophy of anterior frontal and temporal lobes. Frontal horns are prominent. Other sulci and parts of ventricular system are near normal.

Subcortical Dementia

At this stage, it is useful to discuss about *subcortical dementia*, a concept proposed by Albert et al. (1974). In patients with progressive supranuclear palsy, Parkinson's disease, Huntington's disease, normal pressure hydrocephalus, Wilson's disease, etc., where subcortical rather than cortical structures are involved, though memory seems to be impaired, it can be seen that the patient would produce the correct answer if given a longer time to respond and if given a lot of encouragement. Thus, memory is not truly impaired, but the recall is slow; with cues and encouragement, patient may perform well on tests of memory. Patients do poorly on tasks requiring verbal manipulation or perceptual-motor skills under normal pressures. However, when given extended time, they do perform adequately. Dysphasia, agnosia and apraxia, which indicate dysfunction of higher cortical areas are absent.

Huntington's Disease

Dementia generally starts insidiously as inefficiency in work and management of daily affairs – this may appear even when testing may not show cognitive deficits. Since early days, cognitive processes are slowed. Poor concentration, disorganized thoughts are prominent. Memory impairment is a late development and is not as conspicuous as in AD. Typically, memory disorder is due to retrieval difficulty and not due to acquisition difficulty (recall is good with cues). Retrograde amnesia is severe and equally impaired across decades. Implicit memory is more severely affected than explicit memory. Language disorder is characterized by severe word finding difficulty and typical dysphasia, dyslexia, apraxia and agnosia are seldom found. Judgement is impaired severely, but insight may be present till late, leading to depression with suicidal risk. Ultimately, patient becomes apathetic or fatuously euphoric. He/she may show aggression and irritability. Akinetic mutism like picture characterizes terminal phases.

Age at onset is from childhood to extreme old age, but generally is in the fourth or fifth decade. Almost all would develop both neurologic and psychiatric manifestations, except a few, who might develop either of them without the other. One may precede the other in equally half of the cases. Neurologic manifestations may range from mild clumsiness or gait difficulty to typical choreoathetoid movements – psychiatric manifestations may be in the form of typical depression or schizophrenia like picture or just a change in personality.

Progressive Multifocal Leukoencephalopathy

This JC Papova viral disorder generally appears in immunocompromised patients like in AIDS, leukaemia, lymphoma, sarcoidosis etc. Persons between 30–60 years of age show progressive dementia with focal neurological abnormalities like paresis, ataxia, dysphasia and visual field defects. The progression is rapid with death within a few weeks or months. CT scan is typical with low-density lesions in the central and convolutional white matter with "scalloped" appearance to their lateral borders.

Primary Progressive Aphasia

This syndrome is characterized by progressive dysphasia, without any other cognitive impairments, save dyspraxias and dyscalculia. Onset is in 50s or 60s. Male to female ratio is 2:1. Starting as word-finding difficulty, the disorder gradually progresses to fluent/non-fluent dysphasias, with fairly intact reading and writing. Patient later progresses into mutism and loses all abilities of communication. CT scan or MRI shows atrophy of perisylvian region of left side and widening of left frontal horn. EEG shows asymmetrical slowing on the left. PET/SPECT scans show decreased blood flow and metabolism in left frontotemporal regions.

Semantic Dementia

This syndrome of loss of meaning of words and objects can easily be confused for AD because of apparent "memory loss". Speech is usually fluent and with normal syntax, with restricted content because of loss of nominal terms. Patient would show profound comprehension difficulty and has difficulty naming or pointing towards objects. Verbal fluency is seriously compromised. In contrast, repetition is intact (similar to transcortical sensory dysphasia). Prosopagnosia and visual agnosia are also prominent. Orientation and episodic memory are well preserved. Non-verbal memory is normal. Insight is preserved; so is social conduct. Only in late stages frontal lobe symptoms might appear. EEG is normal. Imaging shows focal temporal lobe atrophy.

REFERENCES

- Abas MA, Sahakian BN and Levy R. (1990) Neuropsychological deficits and CT scan changes in elderly depressives. *Psychological Medicine,* 20, 507–520.
- Albert ML, Feldman RG and Willis AL. (1974) The 'subcortical dementia' of progressive supranuclear palsy. *Journal of Neurology, Neurosurgery and Psychiatry,* 37, 121–130.
- Folstein MF and McHugh PR. (1978) Dementia syndrome of depression. In *Alzheimer's Disease: Senile Dementia and Related Disorders, Aging,* Vol. 7, eds Katzman R, Terry RD and Bick KL; pp 87–93. New York: Raven Press.
- Kesslak JP, Nalcioglu O and Cotman CW. (1991) Quantification of magnetic resonance scans for hippocampal and parahippocampal atrophy in Alzheimer's disease. *Neurology,* 41, 51–54.

- Lishman WA. (1999) *Organic Psychiatry. The Psychological Consequences of Cerebral Disorder.* Oxford: Blackwell Scientific Publication.
- McKeith IG, Galasko D, Wilcock GK and Byrne EJ. (1995) Lewy body dementia - diagnosis and treatment. *British Journal of Psychiatry,* 167, 709–717.
- McKeith IG, Perry RH, Fairbairn AF, Jabeen S and Perry EK (1992) Operational criteria for senile dementia of Lewy body type (SDLT). *Psychological Medicine,* 22, 911–922.
- McKhann G, Drachman D, Folstein M, Katzman R, Price D and Stadlan EM. (1984) Clinical diagnosis of Alzheimer's disease: report of the NINCDS-ADRDA work group under the auspices of Department of Health and Human Services Task Force on Alzheimer's disease. *Neurology,* 34, 939–944.
- Román GC, Tatemich TK, Erkinjuntti T, et al. (1993) Vascular dementia: diagnostic criteria for research studies. Report of the NINDS-AIREN International Workshop. *Neurology,* 43, 250–260.
- Seab JP, Jagust WJ, Wong STS, Roos MS, Reed BR and Budinger TF. (1988) Quantitative NMR measurements of hippocampal atrophy in Alzheimer's disease. *Magnetic Resonance in Medicine,* 8, 200–208.

12

Pharmacological Management of Dementia

Somnath Sengupta, Jisu Nath

Introduction

Dementia is a syndrome of gradual onset, sustained global cognitive impairment that particularly affects the elderly population. The most striking clinical features are forgetfulness and a variety of non-specific behavioural abnormalities without any impairment of consciousness (unlike delirium). Dementia can be divided into two types—irreversible and reversible—depending upon whether the cognitive decline is permanent or likely to improve after the underlying cause has been detected and treated. Alzheimer's disease (AD), first described by Alois Alzheimer in 1907, is the most common cause of dementia worldwide. It is a degenerative brain disorder characterized by progressive decline in multiple cognitive functions including memory, language, praxis, gnosis and disturbances of executive functions besides their secondary behavioural manifestations. Other causes of irreversible dementias are Lewy body disease (LBD) and frontotemporal dementia (FTD). In irreversible dementias like AD the improvement of the deficits is short-lived after a course of treatment. In contrast, reversible dementias are the cases where there is a specific cause for the cognitive deficits, such as hypothyroidism, which, when treated leads to continued improvement of the deficits.

AD is the prototype example of dementia. Therefore, discussion of management of dementia would generally follow its overall pattern. Specific differences shall, however, be pointed out as and when necessary. For simplicity, the symptoms of dementia can be divided into two types, cognitive and non-cognitive. The latter is also described as behavioural and psychological signs and symptoms of dementia.

Table 12.1 Common causes of dementia

1) Irreversible dementia
    a) Alzheimer's disease
    b) Lewy body disease
    c) Frontotemporal dementia

2) Reversible dementia
    a) Vascular lesions
    b) Parkinson's disease
    c) Head injury
    d) Normal-pressure hydrocephalus
    e) Alcohol dependence
    f) Hypothyroidism
    g) Vitamin B_{12} deficiency
    h) HIV/AIDS

The prevalence of AD increases as age advances, for example, it is 10.3% over the age of 65 (Evans et al., 1989) and it doubles after every five years. Given the ever-growing figure of elderly population and the number of people likely to be affected, the burden to the society is going to be colossal. Thorough assessment of a person who complains of forgetfulness is the first step before actual management begins. A detailed history should be taken from the patient as well as from a close relative focusing on nature of forgetfulness, duration, frequency, and its seriousness. Enquiry should also be made into difficulties in carrying out usual daily activities, handwriting, speech, and problems at work, sleep and appetite. Symptoms of depression, if any, are also to be looked into. For rapid cross sectional screening, a rating scale such as the Mini Mental State Examination (MMSE) is always indicated (Folstein et al., 1975). The score also gives an initial baseline for future comparison. This scale is simple for general practitioners and takes few minutes to administer. However, it should not be used for confirmation of diagnosis of dementia. A neuropsychological battery administered by a neuropsychologist may be used for confirmation and detailed evaluation of cognitive deficits.

Table 12.2 Role of investigations in dementia

- *Complete haemogram:* Baseline routine investigation, it can also detect anaemia, suggesting vit. B_{12} deficiency.
- *Blood biochemistry:* Baseline routine investigation. It rules out background metabolic disturbances, which may point towards a systemic condition and also has implication in drug side effect and monitoring.
- *Lipid profile:* Elevated lipid levels are associated with coronary and cerebral vascular diseases and have implication in vascular dementia.
- *ECG:* It is a baseline routine investigation and drug side effect monitoring.
- *Thyroid function test:* It rules out the most common reversible cause of dementia, i.e., hypothyroidism.
- *Serum vitamin B_{12}:* Confirmatory test for vit. B_{12} deficiency dementia. It requires clinical correlation. Peripheral smear can be normal in some cases.
- *HIV:* HIV/AIDS is associated with dementia and it is prudent to exclude this increasingly common viral pandemic.
- *CT or MRI brain:* Brain imaging is not routine. It rules out structural or vascular lesion easily. It requires careful interpretation in white matter lesions. Hippocampal sclerosis may be present in AD.
- *EEG:* It is not routine. It is helpful in rare cases such as prion-related dementias.
- *Lumbar puncture:* It is done in restricted cases such as to exclude chronic CNS infection etc.
- *Carotid Doppler:* For vascular dementia, it detects carotid stenosis.
- *SPECT brain:* It is not routine. It may aid in differentiating AD from frontotemporal dementia. It helps detecting abnormal blood flow pattern.

MANAGEMENT PRINCIPLES

Management of dementia is both pharmacological and non-pharmacological. Since caregivers frequently develop burn out syndrome, they often need counseling by trained professionals. In-patient management may be required for detailed assessment, for complications like delirium and in terminal care. Special nursing homes for dementia patient care are also there. Non-pharmacological strategies should always be attempted before starting any pharmacological treatment. This is particularly indicated for the non-cognitive symptoms.

The Quality Standards Subcommittee (QSS) of the American Academy of Neurology has suggested practice parameter for management of dementia where the investigators have extensively reviewed evidence-based support for various pharmacological as well as non-pharmacological methods in both cognitive and non-cognitive symptoms (Doody et al., 2001). Based upon the efficacy of various agents and procedures, different levels of recommendations have been advocated.

Recent advances in developing newer drugs for dementia have been mainly based on the understanding of the pathogenesis of AD. The molecules developed have also been tested in other commoner forms of the dementias like vascular dementia (VaD) and Lewy body disease (LBD).

PHARMACOLOGICAL STRATEGIES

Two broad strategies are currently in practice (clinical as well as research): replacement therapy and disease modifying therapy.

Replacement Therapy

This is based on the evidence of neurotransmitter deficiencies. This group includes cholinergic, monoaminergic (5HT, 5-hydrxytryptamine; NE, norepinephrine; DA, dopamine), neuropeptide (vasopressin; somatostatin; ACTH, adrenocorticotropic hormone; TRH, thyrotropin-releasing hormone) enhancers. Among all these, the cholinergic enhancers especially in the form of cholinesterase inhibitors have shown maximum promise so far. Three lines of evidences have drawn the scientific interest to the use of these drugs. Cholinergic projection from basal nucleus of Meynert to hippocampus and forebrain was found to be associated with consolidation of memory. Brain autopsy studies in AD have revealed differential atrophy of hippocampus and basal nucleus along with 50% reduction in cortical cholinergic levels (especially deficiency of the acetylcholine synthetic enzyme cholineacetyltransferase). Reduction in cholinergic levels in the brain was shown to correlate with cognitive deficits in AD (Etienne et al., 1986). Cholinergic enhancement has been attempted in three different ways:

- Precursor loading with choline and lecithin as dietary supplements has failed, as the precursor uptake mechanism in the affected neurons usually remains saturated in brains of AD.
- Use of muscarinic (M_1 receptors) and nicotinic cholinergic agonists has shown mixed results. Synthetic analogues are being prepared and used for clinical trials (Grundman et al., 2000).
- The most useful method of enhancing the brain cholinergic levels so far has been to use anticholinesterase drugs that inhibit the hydrolysis of extracellular acetylcholine by choline esterase (acetyl and butyryl). The first compound tested was physostigmine. Its therapeutic potential was limited by its narrow safety margin and transient clinical benefits.

Tacrine

Tacrine (tetrahydroaminoacridine, THA) was the first orally active reversible, cholinesterase inhibitor approved by Food and Drug Administration (FDA) in 1993. The clinical benefits were shown on dual outcome criteria required by FDA. This means that statistically significant treatment–placebo difference had to be shown in: (i) cognitive functions measured by the cognitive component of Alzheimer's Disease Assessment Scale (ADAS-Cog) (Grundman et al., 1984) in which a 4-point reduction was taken as a response criterion; (ii) global functions measured by Clinician Interview Based Impression of Change (CIBIC) (Knopman et al., 1994) or CIBIC plus with caregiver's input. Unfortunately, the findings of hepatotoxic effects in 30% recipients limited its popularity among the clinicians.

Donepezil

This is another specific reversible cholinesterase inhibitor that was approved for treatment of AD in 1996. It is a piperidine, well absorbed even when taken with food, extensively bound to plasma proteins with plasma half-life of 70 hours and so necessitating only single daily dosing. The drug is biotransformed in liver by cytochrome p450 system CYP 2D6 and CYP 34A and so its plasma levels may get altered by inhibitors (fluoxetine, ketoconazole, quinidine) or inducers (carbamezepine, phenobarbitone and phenytoin) of the microsomal enzyme system. Cholinergic side effects occur in only 5% of individuals when the drug is started at 5 mg and hiked to 10 mg after 6 weeks (Crismon et al., 1999).

Rivastigmine
It has two unique pharmacodynamic properties. It is a pseudo irreversible inhibitor of cholinesterase as the carbamate moiety of the drug makes a bond with the enzyme that lasts longer (10 hours) than that with donepezil. Secondly, the drug inhibits butyryl cholinesterase a mechanism that has been claimed to enhance extracellular cholinergic levels. It is rapidly absorbed orally; only 40% gets bound to plasma proteins, has a short elimination half-life and is converted to inactive metabolites at the site of action by cholinesterase itself. As it bypasses hepatic metabolic pathways it has few interactions with other drugs. Two types of doses have been used: low dose (1–4 mg/day) and high dose (6–12 mg/day). Cholinergic side effects (40%) and loss of body weight (24%) are reported in those receiving high doses. Slow escalation of the dose brings down the occurrences of side effects – 1.5 mg bid and 1.5 mg increase every two weekly (Jann, 2000).

Galantamine
This compound (galantamine hydrobromide) was originally isolated from plant products like daffodil bulbs but the synthetic drug is now available. The drug modulates the nicotinic acetylcholine receptor in addition to reversible inhibition of cholinesterase. The drug has high oral bioavailability, not highly protein bound and is metabolized by cytochrome P450 system to an active form 0-demethylgalantamine that specifically inhibits cholinesterase. The drug is started at a dose of 8 mg/day and increased once in 4 weeks up to 16–32 mg/day. Cholinergic side effects and loss of body weight are related to higher doses (> 24 mg/day; Tariot, 2001). The safety and efficacy of galantamine has been demonstrated in multiple randomized controlled trials of more than 2600 patients with mild to moderate AD (Denzig and Kershaw, 2004). The drug is undergoing trial in India but not yet available for clinical use. The drug is also useful in VaD and mixed dementia, i.e., AD with cerebrovascular disease (Erkinjuntti, 2002).

A number of multicenter studies (donepezil: Rogers et al., 1996; Rogers et al., 1998; Burns et al., 1999; rivastigmine: Corey-Bloom et al., 1998; Vellas et al., 1998; Roster et al., 1999; galantamine: Wilcock et al., 2000; Rockwood et al., 2001; Wikinson et al., 2001) have tested these drugs on more than 8000 patients till 2000. A modest improvement has been consistently shown in mild to moderate AD (MMSE score 10–26) (Crismon et al., 1999). For example, 25% to 30% of patients on drugs show improvement in cognitive function rated by clinicians and caregivers and by independent functional ratings whereas 10–15% do so on placebo. Moreover, these drugs also ameliorate non-cognitive symptoms like agitation, mood symptoms and delusion and hallucinations. The study period usually extends to six months but few studies have shown the benefits for one to two years. The treatment gains have been seen to decline to placebo treated levels within 3–4 weeks on discontinuation of drugs (Giacobini, 2000). The dose related cognitive enhancement is offset by dose related incidence of cholinergic side effects. So far there is no evidence that these drugs alter the natural history of AD. It is also being studied to find out if these drugs are able to prevent the onset of AD in patients with amnestic type of MCI. These drugs are also being tried in VaD (Chui, 2000), LBD (McKeith et al., 2000) and Parkinson's disease (McKeith, 2000) with beneficial results. In India, cost of these drugs tends to limit their generous use by the clinicians. Recently, the costs and consequences of donepezil versus placebo treatment in patients with mild to moderate AD were evaluated as part of a 1-year prospective, double-blind, randomized, multinational clinical trial by the Donepezil Nordic Study Group (Wimo et al., 2003). The positive effects on the efficacy outcome measures combined with no additional costs from a societal perspective indicated that donepezil is a cost-effective treatment.

Other cholinesterase inhibitors have also been shown to be beneficial in AD but some unique adverse effects had limited their clinical use. For example, metrifonate has a long half-life (up to 40 days) and has been associated with prolonged respiratory muscle weakness requiring respiratory support; similarly, epistagmine leads to dose dependent neutropenia in 6% patients. However, small studies have shown consistent benefits with an herbal ch I, called huperzine A.

Salvia officinalis is an herbal medicine that has in vitro cholinergic binding properties and modulates mood and cognitive performance in humans. This compound was assessed in patients with mild to moderate Alzheimer's disease in a 4-month, parallel group, placebo-controlled trial and significant improvement was found in the cognitive functions measured by ADAS-Cog and Clinical Dementia Rating (CDR) (Akhondzadeh et al, 2003).

Disease Modifying Therapy

The drugs in this strategy are intended to alter the anomalies at various steps in the pathogenesis of AD, for example, anti-inflammatory drugs, anti-oxidant drugs and oestrogen replacement therapy. Their use is based on both epidemiologic and pathogenic evidences.

Anti-Inflammatory Drugs

Epidemiological studies have shown that non-steroidal anti-inflammatory drugs (NSAIDs) may protect against developing AD (Stewart et al., 1994). Veld et al (2001) have shown low relative risk (RR) (0.05–0.83) of AD with long-term use of NSAIDs (cf. RR 0.7 to 1.29 with short term use). These observations are supported by the findings of immune and inflammatory responses in association with β - amyloid deposits in brain of AD. Trials with NSAIDs in mild to moderate AD have only shown non-significant trend in cognitive improvement. Indomethacin is not recommended for therapy in patients with AD at present (Tabet et al., 2002). Currently, lots of interests have centered on cycloxygenase-2 (Cox 2) inhibitors and one year long trials are in progress (Pasinetti, 2001).

Estrogen-Replacement Therapy

The epidemiological evidence of higher incidence of AD in women led to the hypothesis that postmenopausal fall in oestrogen levels could be related to increased rate of occurrence of AD in women. Further epidemiological observations (Tang et al., 1996) of the protective role of oestrogen against the development of AD had supported the rationale of trials with oestrogen-replacement therapy over one year in post-menopausal or hysterectomised women. However, such studies have not shown consistent results. In a recent study on postmenopausal women with AD there was no association between oestradiol and oestrone levels and cognitive functioning after either 2 or 12 months of treatment with conjugated equine oestrogen (Thal et al., 2003). The initial enthusiasm about female sex hormones has been further dampened by findings from two recent randomized, double-blind, placebo-controlled studies from the Women's Health Initiative Memory Study. The first study attempted to evaluate whether conjugated equine estrogen (CEE), either alone or in combination with medroxyprogesterone acetate (MPA), had an impact on the incidence of probable dementia in women aged 65–79 years. The authors concluded that use of hormone therapy for prophylaxis of dementia was not indicated and found that this treatment might even increase the risk of cognitive impairment or dementia (Shumaker et al., 2004). In the second study, the authors attempted to evaluate the impact of CEE on cognitive functioning in older women and concluded that in this study for women over the age of 65 years, hormonal therapy has a negative impact on cognition (Espeland et al., 2004). Both these studies thus indicate that women older than 65 years should not be treated with CEE with or without MPA to attempt to prevent dementia or enhance cognition. Further studies may help clear the picture convincingly.

Anti-Oxidants

Neurotoxic damage due to extracellular β - amyloid deposits has also been related to oxidative damage of the neurons. Epidemiological studies have shown that anti-oxidant vitamins protect against development of AD (Gale et al., 1996). The role of α - tocopherol 1000 IU twice daily has been successfully tested in double blind randomized controlled trial. The monoamine oxidase-A (MAO_A) inhibitor selegeline 10 mg /day has also been shown to delay the progress of AD (Sano et al., 1997). Gingko biloba extracts (flavonoids and terpenoids) are widely used in Germany for the treatment of cognitive disorders. The benefits have been tested in AD as well as in vascular dementia. Overall, there is promising evidence of improvement in cognition and function associated with Ginkgo. However, some modern trials show inconsistent results. The current view is that there is need for a large trial using modern methodology and permitting an intention-to-treat analysis to offer robust estimates of the size and mechanism of any treatment effects (Birks et al., 2002). Despite its initial promise as a potential neuroprotective agent, the role of selegiline in AD has proved insufficient. Although there is no evidence of a significant adverse event profile, there is also no evidence of a clinically meaningful benefit for sufferers of AD. There is currently no justification, therefore, of its use in the treatment of people with AD (Birks et al., 2003).

Antihypertensive Drugs
Results from the Systolic Hypertension in Europe (Syst-Eur) study showed that incidence of dementia is less in persons with systolic hypertension treated with antihypertensives, thereby indicating their role in prevention of dementia. This was applicable to both AD and non-AD dementia (Forette et al., 2002).

Anti-Amyloid Treatment
Amyloid cascade pathway is a crucial factor in the pathology of AD. Based on our current understanding, treatment strategies directed at the root cause of AD should reduce the production of amyloid beta (Aß), accelerate its removal, or prevent it from assembling into toxic fibrils. To this end, the biochemical mechanisms that generate Aß have been identified, and therapies directed at inhibiting Aß production are being developed. Three kinds of pharmacological strategies have been proposed in this regard:

i) Anti- amyloid vaccines are being developed that overexpress mutant type of Amyloid Precursor Protein (APP). Vaccination holds promise in the fight against Aß. This therapy has successfully passed initial tests on humans and is now being tested on a small number of volunteers who have AD. The vaccine trains the body's immune system to attack and dispose off Aß fibrils. In special AD mice, vaccination caused a dramatic reduction in the cognitive defects and the number of amyloid plaques. Whether this immunological model will also apply in humans is a matter of great debate but is being currently pursued with lot of zeal.

ii) α (alpha), β (beta) and γ (gamma) secretase (the proteolytic enzymes that cleave APP holoproteins to amyloid end products) inhibitors are being avidly developed by several pharmaceutical companies. Such drugs will stop the process of toxic amyloidogenesis and will avoid neurotoxicity.

iii) Chain-busting agents could be the molecules that will help lyse the amyloid deposits by inserting themselves into amyloid fibrils (St.George et al., 2001). Progress is also being made in isolating the genes that contain the code for the proteins that normally remove and degrade Aß.

Neurotrophic Agents
Nerve growth factors infused into the ventricles or given by gene therapy approach have been tested in animals and have been tested in small samples of patients with AD with beneficial results (Eriksdotter et al., 1998). Cerebrolysin is one of such tested neurotrophic agents. In a recent multicenter, randomized, double-blind, placebo-controlled, parallel-group study, patients were injected intravenously with placebo (ninety-five persons) or 30 mL cerebrolysin (ninety-seven persons) five days per week for four weeks. Effects on cognition and global function were evaluated with the Alzheimer Disease Assessment Scale - Cognitive Subscale (ADAS-Cog) and the Clinicians Interview-based Impression of Change with Caregiver Input Scale (CIBIC+) 4, 12, 24 weeks after the beginning of the injections. The treatment was well tolerated and found to be resulting in significant improvements in the global score two months after the end of active treatment (Panisset et al., 2002). They require further study.

Comparison of Recent Drugs with the Older Ones

The neurobiological basis of these drugs is purely evidence-based and not based on non-specific mechanisms like lack of cerebral activation, reduced cerebral metabolism or cerebral hypoperfusion. The anti-cholinesterase drugs are the mainstay in the pharmacotherapy of dementia. The role of anti-amyloid vaccine seems to have a high potential for future.

The research methodology testing the efficacy of the recent drugs is more rigorous than those for the older drugs. For example, previous studies were fraught with the problems of small sample of patients, open label uncontrolled or partially controlled designs using variable diagnostic criteria and instruments that measured limited items of cognitive functions. The results were mostly nonsignificant and the benefits could hardly translate into activities of daily life.

The beneficial results with the anticholinesterases have been consistently shown on cognitive and global outcome measures independently rated by the clinicians and caregivers. Both cognitive and non-cognitive symptoms have shown to be changed by these drugs. Several trials have also shown the cognitive improvement in non-AD dementias. Recognizing those at high risk of developing dementia is actively testing preventive role of these drugs.

Non-AD Dementia

Controlled trials of pharmacotherapy for mixed, vascular and other dementias are scanty. In one study, a group of mixed dementia patients were tried on propentofylline (a glial modulating agent), which showed improvement in various cognitive and global measures (Doody et al., 2001), but the same could not be replicated in a second study. For treatment of LBD, reduction or withdrawal of drugs with potential adverse effects is an essential first step. Neuroleptic sensitivity reactions appear less likely to occur with the newer atypical antipsychotics, such as olanzapine (Cummings et al., 2002), that have been shown to be useful. Cholinesterase inhibitors have been shown in open-label and one placebo-controlled study to be well tolerated and effective in treating cognitive and psychiatric symptoms of LBD and may be the first line of treatment (Barber et al., 2001).

Memantine

Memantine is a low affinity N-methyl-D-aspartate (NMDA) receptor antagonist that may prevent excitatory amino acid neurotoxicity without interfering with the physiological actions of glutamate required for memory and learning. In animal models, it protects cholinergic cells and prevents hippocampal injury due to ß-amyloid. It is a safe drug and may be useful for treating AD, VaD and mixed dementia of all severities. Memantine 20 mg daily has a beneficial effect for patients with moderate to severe AD on cognition and functional decline, but not in the clinical impression of change (Areosa et al., 2004; Wilcock et al., 2002). The drug can be combined with anticholinesterases without side effect.

Frontotemporal dementia does not have any specific treatment. Anticholinesterases are not beneficial; in fact, they may worsen cognitive deficits. VaD require control of vascular risk factors including control of hypertension. Low dose aspirin is usually prescribed without robust scientific evidence. At present, the balance of risks versus benefits of aspirin for the primary prevention of cardiovascular disease and vascular dementia has not been established in the elderly. Such studies are under trial and results likely to be out in next few years (Nelson et al., 2003).

Table 12.3 Drugs tested in mixed and VaD

■ Acetyl-l-carinitine	■ Nimodipine
■ Fluovoxamine	■ Piracetam
■ Ginkgo biloba	■ Oxiracetam
■ Glycosamine	■ Pyritonol
■ Memantine	■ Vincamine
■ Naftidrofuryl	■ Xantinolnicotinate
■ Nicergoline	

Drugs Used for Behavioural Symptoms

Details of the management of behavioural and psychological symptoms associated with dementia are given in a separate chapter in this book.

GUIDELINES OF PHARMACOTHERAPY

The Quality Standards Subcommittee (QSS) of the American Academy of Neurology has formulated a practice parameter for management of dementia where three levels of recommendations (Standard, Guideline and Practice option) have been suggested based upon strength of evidence (Doody et al., 2001). For example, in the "standard" level of recommendation, management strategies are to be based on evidence provided by well-designed randomized controlled trials. Similarly, the National Institute for Clinical Excellence (NICE), UK, in January 2001 has formulated a guideline for use of donepezil, rivastigmine and galantamine in AD (NICE, 2001). These guidelines are revised periodically based on accumulated new evidence and physicians should update accordingly.

Candidates

Not all patients of dementia would benefit from cholinergic drugs. These drugs are licensed for mild to moderate AD (MMSE score 10–26). They have not been tried in severe cases and it is doubtful that in such cases with advanced neuronal degeneration these agents have any role (Crismon et al., 1999); though recently memantine has been found to be effective in moderate to severe AD (Areosa et al., 2004).

Goal of Therapy

In the absence of any curative or disease reversing potential of any of these pharmacological agents, the primary goal becomes maintaining quality of life as long as possible. The secondary goal is to treat behavioural and psychological complications (Crismon et al., 1999). It is important to note that increase in MMSE score may not match with caregiver's perception of improvement. Listing problematic behaviours according to severity and following them up in the course of treatment would greatly enhance precision in management.

Choice of Agent

Clinically it is difficult to choose a particular agent from donepezil, rivastigmine and galantamine. All are equally efficacious and safe. They all have gastrointestinal side effect but these are not different when compared with placebo (Bullock, 2002). Donepezil may be started as a first line of treatment for mild to moderate AD (Crismon et al., 1999) and vitamin E may be combined with it as an adjuvant to slow the progression of the disease (Doody et al., 2001).

Dosage

Donepezil is started with 5 mg daily and increased up to 10 mg per day. For rivastigmine, two dose strategies have been employed—low dose (1–4 mg/day) and high dose (6–12 mg/day). Galantamine is started as 8 mg daily and increased once in a month up to 16–32 mg in a day. Slow titration is advisable for these drugs, to avoid side effects.

Duration of Treatment

There is limited data to recommend the exact duration of treatment for AD. All patients should receive an adequate duration of treatment, which may be up to 6 months. If improvement continues or remains at a baseline, the drug is to be continued longer provided the family members can afford (Bullock, 2002). In this regard the issue of cost-benefit analysis becomes important for the caregivers and the treating physician. Complex pharmacoeconomic calculations have been made in western countries without showing any consistent and conclusive outcome. The decision to terminate further cholinergic therapy depends upon persistent deterioration in the patient and economic burden to the family; the latter applicable particularly in Indian context. Cholinergic agents may be stopped when the MMSE score becomes less than twelve (NICE, 2001).

Monitoring Progress

Patients should start showing improvement within few months of starting cholinergic treatment. If they have not done so within a period of 3—6 months, they are unlikely to have any benefit from continuation of these drugs. All patients receiving treatment for dementia should be regularly (ideally every 6 months) assessed for improvement in the following domains—cognition (MMSE score), behavioural and psychological symptoms, activities of daily life, overall function and caregiver's perception. Associated medical problems, if any, e.g., seizure and side effects of the drugs, would also need appropriate intervention. Monitoring relevant investigations from time to time (like, liver function test for tacrine) is important.

FUTURE TARGETS FOR AD

At present, there is no cure for AD. The agents mentioned above can at best lead to partial symptomatic improvement. As the molecular basis of AD is unraveled, promise for more and specific pharmacological options are explored, which may ultimately alter the pathogenesis of this disease. The future agents thus would target the basic pathological processes of AD, namely, amyloid-β (beta) plaque, neurofibrillary tangles (NFTs) and neuronal death. Some of these agents are discussed in Table 12.4 and are expected to be available in near future (Bullock, 2004).

Table 12.4 Future agents for AD

Classes	Agents	Comment	Current status
Acetylcholinesterase inhibitor (AChEI)	Phenserine	Also binds to APP gene and reduces APP generation	Phase III clinical trial
Ā (gamma)-secretase inhibitor	Flubiprofen enantiomer	Does not have NSAID property	Phase II clinical trial
Mempasin-2 inhibitor	—	Mempasin-2 is a å-secretase	Under trial
AChEI+ Statin	Donepezil+ Atorvastatin	Statins enhance å-secretase activity	Under trial
GAG mimetics (glycosaminoglycan)	NC-758, NC- 531	Prevents amyloid-â fibrillogenesis	Phase II clinical trial
Chelating agent	Clioquinol	Has to be combined with vit.B_{12}	Under trial
Immunisation	—	Risk of meningoencephalitis	One phase II trial withdrawn
GSK-3 (glycogen synthase kinase 3) and CDK-5 (cyclidin- dependent kinase-5) inhibitors	Lithium (but too toxic)	Reduce tau phosphorylation	Animal study
Somatostatin- releasing agent	FK-960	Enhance cerebral blood flow and glucose uptake	Animal study
Stem cell therapy	—	Ethical controversy, but promising	Animal study

CONCLUSION

With the rapid increase in geriatric population the need for detection and proper management of old age problems are emerging as important issues. Management of dementia is one of these key issues having profound social implications. Non-pharmacological as well as pharmacological strategies are, therefore, constantly refined with the advent of scientific research findings. Clinical trials of drugs for treating AD are fraught with several constraints. The biggest problem in conducting clinical trials currently is the massive effort and cost of conducting periodic clinical evaluations. Research to develop more efficient assessment methods is clearly needed. Moreover, developing countries like India lack appropriate guideline for use of medications considering their fiscal positions. At the end, one can only dream for the day when disease-reversing agents are available to these unfortunate patients.

REFERENCES

- Akhondzadeh S, Noroozian M, Mohammadi M, et al. (2003) Salvia officinalis extract in the treatment of patients with mild to moderate Alzheimer's disease: a double blind, randomized and placebo-controlled trial. *J Clin Pharm Ther,* 28, 53–59.
- Areosa SA, Sherriff F. (2004) Memantine for dementia (Cochrane Review). In: *The Cochrane Library, Issue 3.* Chichester, UK: John Wiley and Sons, Ltd.
- Bains J, Birks JS, Dening TR. (2002) The efficacy of antidepressants in the treatment of depression in dementia. *Cochrane Database Syst Rev,* (4), CD003944.
- Barber R, Panikkar A, McKeith IG. (2001) Dementia with Lewy bodies: diagnosis and management. *Int J Geriatr Psychiatry,* 16 Suppl 1, S12–18.
- Birks J, Flicker L. (2003) Selegiline for Alzheimer's disease. *Cochrane Database Syst Rev;* (1): CD000442.
- Birks J, Grimley EV, Van Dongen M. (2002) Ginkgo biloba for cognitive impairment and dementia. *Cochrane Database Syst Rev,* (4), CD003120.
- Brodaty H, Ames D, Snowdon J. et al. (2003) A randomized placebo-controlled trial of risperidone for the treatment of aggression, agitation, and psychosis of dementia. *J Clin Psychiatry,* 64, 134–143.
- Bullock R. (2002) New drugs for Alzheimer's disease and other dementias. *Br J Psychiatry,* 180, 135–139.

- Bullock R (2004) Future directions in the treatment of Alzheimer's disease. *Expert Opin. Investig. Drugs,* 13, 303–314.
- Burns A, Rossor M, Hecker J, et al. (1999) The effects of donepezil in Alzheimer's disease: Results from a multinational trial. *Dement Geriatr Cogn Disord,* 10, 237–244.
- Chui H (2000) Vascular Dementia, A New Beginning: Shifting Focus from Clinical Phenotype to Ischemic Brain Injury in Dementia. *Neurologic Clinics,* 18 (4), 951–978.
- Corey-Bloom J, Anand R, Veach J. (1998) A randomized trial evaluating the efficacy and safety of ENA 713 (rivastigmine tartrate), a new acetylcholinesterase inhibitor, in patients with mild to moderately severe Alzheimer's disease. *Int J Geriatr Psychopharmacol,* 1, 55–65.
- Crismon ML, Eggert AE. (1999) Alzheimer's disease. In *Pharmacotherapy–A pathophysiologic approach,* fourth edn, Eds. Dipiro JT Talbert RL, Yee GC, Nmatzke GR, Wells BG, Posey LM. Stanford Connecticut: Appleton–Lange.
- Cummings JL, Street J, Masterman D, et al. (2002) Efficacy of olanzapine in the treatment of psychosis in dementia with Lewy bodies. *Dement Geriatr Cogn Disord,* 13, 67–73.
- Denzig AN, Kershaw P. (2004) The clinical efficacy and safety of galantamine in the treatment of Alzheimer's disease. *CNS Spectr,* 9, 377–392.
- Devanand DP, Pelton GH, Marston K, et al. (2003) Sertraline treatment of elderly patients with depression and cognitive impairment. *Int J Geriatr Psychiatry,* 18, 123–130.
- Doody RS, Stevens JC, Beck C, et al. (2001) Practice parameter: management of dementia (an evidence-based review) - Report of the quality standards subcommittee of the American Academy of Neurology. *Neurology,* 56, 1154–1166.
- Eriksdotter Jonhagen M, Nordberg A, Amberla k, et al. (1998) Intracerebroventricular infusion of nerve growth factor in three patients with Alzheimer's disease. *Dement Geriatr Cogn Disord;* 9: 246–257.
- Erkinjuntti T. (2002) Treatment options: the latest evidence with galantamine (Reminyl). *J Neurol Sci,* 203–204, 125–130.
- Espeland MA, Rapp SR, Shumaker SA, et al. (2004) Conjugated equine estrogens and global cognitive function in postmenopausal women: Women's Health Initiative Memory Study. *JAMA,* 291, 2959–2968.
- Etienne P, Robitaille Y and Wood P. et al. (1986) Nucleus basalis neuronal loss, neuritic plaques and choline acetyltransferase activity in advanced Alzheimer's disease. *Neuroscience,* 1919, 1279–1291.

- Evans DA, Funkenstein HH, Albert MS, et al. (1989) Prevalence of Alzheimer's disease in a community population of older persons. Higher than previously reported. *JAMA,* 262(18), 2551–6.
- Folstein MF, Folstein SE, McHugh PR. (1975) Mini Mental State: A practical method for grading the cognitive state of patients for the clinician. *J Psychiatr Res,* 12, 189–198.
- Forette F, Seux ML, Staessen JA et al. (2002) The prevention of dementia with antihypertensive treatment: new evidence from the Systolic Hypertension in Europe (Syst-Eur) study. *Arch Intern Med,* 162, 2046–2052.
- Gale CR, Martyn CN, Cooper C. (1996) Cognitive impairment and mortality in a cohort of elderly people. *Br Med J,* 312, 608–611.
- Giacobini E (2000) Present and future of Alzheimer therapy. *J Neural Transm,* Suppl, 59, 231–242.
- Grundman M and Thal L J. (2000) Treatment of Alzheimer's disease – rationale and strategies in Dementia: *Neurologic Clinics* ed. ST Dekosky, 18 (4), 807–828.
- Grundman M, Mohas RC, Davis KL. (1984) A new rating scale for Alzheimer's disease. *American Journal of Psychiatry,* 141, 1356–1364.
- Herrmann N, Mamdani M, Lanctot KL. (2004) Atypical antipsychotics and risk of cerebrovascular accidents. *Am J Psychiatry,* 161, 1113–1115.
- Jann MW. (2000) Rivastigmine: a new generation cholinesterase inhibitor for the treatment of Alzheimer's disease. *Pharmacotherapy,* 20(1).
- Knopman DS, Knapp MJ, Gracon SI, Davis CS. (1994) The clinical interview–based impression (CIBI): A clinician's global change rating scale in Alzheimer's disease. *Neurology,* 44, 2315–2321.
- Lee PE, Gill SS, Freedman M, Bronskill SE, Hillmer MP, Rochnon PA (2004) Atypical antipsychotic drugs in the treatment of behavioural and psychological symptoms of dementia: a systematic review. *BMJ,* 329, 75, doi:10.1136/bmj.38125.465579.55.
- McKeith IG. (2000) Spectrum of Parkinson's disease, Parkinson's dementia and Lewy body dementia in Dementia. *Neurologic clinics,* 18(4), 865–884.
- McKeith J, Del Ser T, Sapano P, et al. (2000) Efficacy of rivastigmine in dementia with Lewy bodies: a randomized, double blind, placebo-controlled international study. *Lancet,* 356(9247), 2031–2036.
- National Institute for Clinical Excellence (2001) *Guidance on the use of donepezil, rivastigmine and galantamine for the treatment of Alzheimer's disease.* London: National Institute for Clinical Excellence.

- Nelson M, Reid C, Beilin L, et al. (2003) Rationale for a trial of low-dose aspirin for the primary prevention of major adverse cardiovascular events and vascular dementia in the elderly: Aspirin in Reducing Events in the Elderly (ASPREE). *Drug Aging,* 20, 897–903.
- Panisset M, Gauthier S, Moessler H et al. (2002) Cerebrolysin in Alzheimer's disease: a randomized, double-blind, placebo-controlled trial with a neurotrophic agent. *J Neural Transm,* 109, 1089–104.
- Pasinetti GM (2001) Cyclooxygenase and Alzheimer's disease: implications for preventive initiatives to slow the progression of Clinical dementia. *Arch Gerontol Geriatr,* 33 (1), 13–28.
- Rockwood K, Mintzer J, Truyen L, Wessel T, Wilkinson D (2001) Effects of a flexible galantamine dose in Alzheimer's disease: a randomized, controlled trial. *J Neurol Neurosurg Psychiatry,* 71(5), 589–595.
- Rogers SL, Farlow MR, Doody RS, et al. (1998) A 24-week, double blind, placebo-controlled trial of donepezil in patients with Alzheimer's disease: Donepezil Study Group. *Neurology,* 50, 136–145.
- Rogers SL, Friedhoff LT. (1996) The efficacy and safety of donepezil in patients with Alzheimer's disease: Results of a US Multicentre, Randomized, Double-Blind, Placebo-Controlled Trial. The Donepezil Study Group. *Dementia,* 7, 293–303.
- Roster M, Anand R, Cicin-Sain A, et al. (1999) Efficacy and safety of rivastigmine in patients with Alzheimer's' disease: international randomized controlled trial. *Br Med J,* 318, 633–640.
- Sano M, Ernesto C, Thomas RG, et al (1997) A controlled trial of selegiline, alpha-tocopherol, or both as treatment for Alzheimer's disease: The Alzheimer's Disease Cooperative Study. *N Engl J Med,* 336, 1216–1222.
- Serfaty M, Kennell-Webb S, Warner J, et al. (2002) Double blind randomized placebo controlled trial of low dose melatonin for sleep disorders in dementia. *Int J Geriatr Psychiatry,* 17, 1120–1127.
- Shumaker SA, Legault C, Kuller L, et al. (2004) Conjugated equine estrogens and incidence of probable dementia and mild cognitive impairment in postmenopausal women: Women's Health Initiative Memory Study. *JAMA,* 291, 2947–2958.
- St. George-Hyslop P, Rossor M. (2001) Unraveling the disease process. *Lancet,* Suppl, 358.
- Stewart WF, Kawasc, Corrada M, et al. (1994) Risk of Alzheimer's disease and duration of NSAID use. *Neurology,* 48, 626–632.

- Tabet N, Feldman H. (2002) Indomethacin for the treatment of Alzheimer's disease patients. *Cochrane Database Syst Rev,* (2), CD003673.
- Tang MX, Jacobs D, Stern Y, et al. (1996) Effect of estrogen during menopause on risk and age at onset of Alzheimer's disease. *Lancet,* 348, 429–432.
- Tariot P. (2001) Current status and new developments with galantanine in the treatment of Alzheimer's disease. *Expert Opin Pharmacother,* 2 (12), 2027–2049.
- Thal LJ, Thomas RG, Mulnard R, et al. (2003) Estrogen levels do not correlate with improvement in cognition. *Arch Neurol,* 60, 209–212.
- Veld BA, Ruitenberg A, Hofman A, et al. (2001) Non-steroidal anti inflammatory drugs and the risk of Alzheimer's disease. *N Engl J Med,* 345(21), 1567–1568.
- Vellas B, Inglis F, Potkins, et al. (1998) Interim results from an international clinical trial with rivastigmine evaluating a 2-week titration rate in mild to severe Alzheimer's disease patients. *Int J Geriatr Psychopharmacol,* 1, 140–144.
- Wikinson D, Murray J. (2001) Galantamine: a randomized, double – blind, dose comparison in patients with Alzheimer's disease. *Int J Geriatr Psychiatry,* 16(9), 852–857.
- Wilcock G, Mobius HJ, Stoffler A. (2002) A double-blind, placebo-controlled multicenter study of memantine in mild to moderate vascular dementia (MMM500). *Int Clin Psychopharmacol,* 17, 297–305.
- Wilcock GK, Lilienfeld S, Gaens E. (2000) Efficacy and safety of galantamine in patients with mild to moderate Alzheimer's disease: multicentre randomized controlled trial. Galantamine International-I Study Group 55. *Br Med J 9,* 321(7274), 1445–49.
- Wimo A, Winblad B, Engedal K et al. (2003) An economic evaluation of donepezil in mild to moderate Alzheimer's disease: results of a 1-year, double-blind, randomized trial. *Dement Geriatr Cogn Disord,* 15, 44–54.

13

Management of Behavioural and Psychological Symptoms of Dementia

Nilamadhab Kar

Introduction

The approaches to behavioural and psychological symptoms of dementia (BPSD) involve pharmacological and non-pharmacological treatments, as well as structured activities and nursing care interventions. Treatment plan is individualized considering the need of the person, problematic behaviour and previous response and pre-morbid experiences. Combinations of interventions are usually tried. However, according to Profenno and Tariot (2004) only in emergent situations or when the non-pharmacological methods have failed should medications be deployed.

The key general elements in management of BPSD are clarification of target symptoms, ruling out delirium, and comorbid major psychiatric diagnoses and creatively addressing possible social, environmental, or behavioural remedies. It may be helpful to consider these questions (Cheong, 2004): 'What if he or she were a 2 or 3-year-old child—what would be causing this crying or agitation? How would I approach a small child in distress?'

NON-PHARMACOLOGICAL INTERVENTION

Non-pharmacological intervention aims at addressing the psychosocial and environmental underlying reason for the behaviour and is devoid of limitations of pharmacological treatment, namely, adverse effects and drug-drug interactions. There is another concern even when the pharmacological intervention is successful, it may eliminate the behaviour that serves as a signal for a need, which may not be picked up or attended to.

Social Contacts

One-to-one interaction: One-to-one interaction for 30 minutes per day for 10 days has been found to be effective in decreasing verbally disruptive behaviour by 54%, a reduction that is significantly larger than the control (Cohen-Mansfield and Werner, 1997). Interaction in the mother-tongue is better than in the learned language. Regularly prescribed period of intensive interaction with the patient providing skilled supervision helps in reality orientation.

Simulated presence therapy: This is simulated interaction. An example is playing an audiotape that contains a relative's portion of telephone conversation, and leaves pauses that allow the demented persons to respond to the relative's questions. Family videos will also help in the same way. Displaying photos and names of family and friends in the patient's living area help (Cohen-Mansfield, 2004).

Socialization can be further increased by group activity, conjoint tasks and simple games. Guidance and supervision from caregivers are helpful in this regard.

Pet therapy: Spending time with pets regularly has shown improvement in agitation. An intervention of one-hour daily visits with a dog for 5 days showed a trend towards improvement (Zisselman et al., 1996). Significantly lower level of agitation has been seen immediately after 30 minutes session with a dog than with 30 minutes sessions with only the researcher present. Presence of a pet at home was related to a lower prevalence of verbal aggression (Fritz et al., 1995).

Physical Stimulation

Outdoor walks, indoor exercises, helping patients to do stretching, exercise to music, other physical activities, and removal of restraints all help in reducing the inappropriate behaviour. In addition, adequate rest is also important.

Sensory Intervention

Music: It may be used for relaxation and sensory stimulation. Music interventions range from listening to a music tape (some preferring head phones) to music therapy session, which includes musical games, dancing to music, movement singing, and playing instruments. Music during bathing or dinner reduces agitation and aggressiveness. White noise is believed to induce relaxation and sleep and thereby decreases nocturnal restlessness.

Massage and touch: This is performed for few minutes, couple of times a day and can be coupled with verbalizations.

Sensory stimulation or enhancement: This is performed by combination of techniques where stimuli are delivered to different sensory modalities, including hearing, touch and smell. Aromatherapy and massage have been combined but no significant impact has been reported.

Environmental Interventions

The environment around the patient can be modified for a beneficial effect on the BPSD. Calm, non-taxing environments, prominent placement of frequently required objects, clocks, calendars, are helpful. Clear instructions, through visual means and repetition of instructions help. Clear direction to different rooms, e.g., lavatory, dining room, can be given through colour lines and pictures to improve orientation. Visual cues and labels on closets and doors serve as a helpful reminder. Brightly coloured tape may help to perceive dangerous situations. The environment should be maintained without frequent change; there should be minimum change of caregivers or staff. Simplifying the environment by using soft colour schemes, good lighting, non-abstract, non-threatening wall hangings, and avoidance of television, mirror and window reflections are beneficial.

Wall should be painted in soft colours, and floors should be covered with nonskid flooring or carpet. It is helpful to provide contrast between the wall, floor and handrails. Grids of masking tapes on the floor in front of the exit door may prevent wandering. A wanderer's lounge may be provided where agitated patients can move safely. Overhead paging, radios, and television are not recommended, and phones with a muted ring should be used at nursing station (Deutsch and Rovner, 1991).

Environmental interventions are often very effective in controlling BPSD. Environments can be natural, enhanced environments, or reduced stimulation environments, depending upon the needs. A natural environment consisting of recorded songs of birds, babbling brooks, or small animals, together with large bright pictures matching the audiotapes decrease agitation. In the nursing homes compared to usual décor, the simulated home environment, and a natural environment each composed of visual, auditory and olfactory stimuli decrease the chance of trespassing, exit seeking and other agitation behaviours (Cohen-Mansfield, 2004).

Reduced stimulation environments are designed with camouflaged doors, small dining tables, small group activities, neutral colours on pictures and walls, no televisions, radios, stereo players or telephones (except one for emergencies), a consistent daily routine, and an educational programme for staff and visitors concerning use of touch, eye contact, slow and soft speech and allowing residents to make choices (Cohen-Mansfield, 2004). This modification helps in decreasing agitation and use of restraint.

When the person is capable of going outside, access to outdoor area results in decreased agitation. Environment can be modified by installing adequate daytime lighting to improve sleep patterns in patients with disturbed sleep-wake cycles (Cohen-Mansfield, 2004).

Minimize the Impact of Sensory Deficits

Decrease risk of disorientation by providing needed corrective eyeglasses and hearing aids. It is helpful to put one item on the tray at a time at mealtime explaining where and what, if there are visual deficits and agnostic difficulties. This reduces confusion and agitation.

Medical and Nursing Interventions

Pain management: Managing pain promptly with medications and other appropriate methods helps in reducing agitation. Periodic routine medical examination and specific enquiries regarding pain are important in this regard.

Sleep interventions: Practice of sleep hygiene, leading to adequate sleep in the night can help reduce agitation. Increased daytime physical activity, decreased nighttime noise, and decreased sleep disruption by the nursing staff or caregivers result in a decrease in inappropriate behaviours during the day (Alessi et al., 1999).

Bright-light therapy: Agitation secondary to fatigue and circadian rhythm disturbances can be reduced by bright light (Cohen-Mansfield, 2004).

Hearing aids: Fitting of hearing aids has helped in decreasing inappropriate behaviour (Palmer et al., 1999) and one study reported decrease in yelling (Cohen-Mansfield, 2004).

Behaviour Therapy

The methods used are *extinction* (i.e., withholding of positive reinforcement during inappropriate behaviour), *differential reinforcement* (i.e., reinforcing either quiet behaviour or behaviour that is incompatible with the inappropriate behaviour, or successive approximations to desired behaviour) and *stimulus control* (i.e., teaching an association between a stimulus or cue and behaviour). Reinforcements include social reinforcements, food, touch, going outside etc. (Cohen-Mansfield, 2004). Sometimes, additional procedures like positive statements along with the other behavioural interventions help.

Structured Activities

Developing a daily routine, instituting pleasant activities are first step towards treating depression. A positive impact of activities has been reported (Cohen-Mansfield, 2004). The activities employed are various kinds such as: manipulative (e.g., bead maze), nurturing (e.g., doll), sorting (e.g., puzzles), tactile (e.g., fabric book), sewing (e.g., lacing cards), sound and music (e.g., melody bells), holding hands, singing etc. Outdoor activities like walks (with interpersonal contact during walk, especially for wanderers) are also helpful. Details of activities can be found in the chapter on occupational therapy of this book.

Day care may be enough to alleviate depression in many (Lyketsos and Lee, 2004) through various activities.

Encourage consistent daily routines: Schedule times for meals and for arising in the morning and going to bed at night to minimize disruptions and distress.

Spiritual and Religious Activities

These activities may continue to have significance for the patients. These help the patient remain engaged in ritualistic religious observations, which keep them calm and focused. Spiritual and religious activities help many to age gracefully.

Staff Training

Training the caregivers or caring staff about understanding inappropriate behaviours, improving verbal and non-verbal communication with dementia patients, and improving methods of addressing their needs has shown beneficial results. Ongoing training affects staff behaviour. The CARE programme (Calming Aggressive Reactions in the Elderly) involving six sessions that emphasized risk factors for aggression, preventive and calming technique, and protective intervention, utilizing videotaped vignettes, discussions and role plays, emphasizing non-verbal communications have been effective (Mentes and Ferrario, 1989).

The NACSP (Nursing Assistant Communication Skill Program) which includes 5 group training sessions and four individual conferences with nursing assistants, emphasizes enhancing residents' ability to use sensory input, effective and ineffective communication styles, utilization of memory aids and addressing residents' needs (McCallion et al., 1999). This program significantly decreased verbal agitation at the end of 3 months. Similar other programmes are abilities-focused programme of morning care, and emphasis on activities of daily living (ADL) (Cohen-Mansfield, 2004).

Communicating Clearly

Clear communication helps the patients in understanding their environments; and lack of it leads to frustration, anger and aggression. This sometimes leads to habitual calling out by the patients without goal. It is important to validate patients' statements, and then redirect any that may be inappropriate. Requests are to be given in stepwise fashion using clear and simple language.

Managing Caregivers' Problems

Dementia care giving is often provided by the family members who are not aware of the exact nature of the illness and are not familiar in care giving in chronic, progressively deteriorating illness with the patient requiring increasing levels of needs. Understandably, they experience difficulties in the process. The stress of care giving not only burdens caregivers but also affects their physical and psychological health and quality of life (Schulz and Martire, 2004). Often inappropriate, too much intrusive and excessive care giving, worsen the BPSD of the patient. So for both patients and caregivers managing caregivers' problems are important.

Education of Caregivers

It is an important strategy for reducing behavioural problem. Family members are less likely to interpret problem behaviours as deliberate and hostile if they understand about the illness. Education about dementia, and its symptoms, treatment options, both medicinal and non-pharmacological, the environmental modification required at home, the prognosis etc., should be provided. Families should be taught to approach the patient calmly, from the front, and to make eye contact by bending down if necessary. Families need to be told that comprehension may be difficult and patient may appear uncooperative, or may strike out in frustration. Aphasia is best handled by speaking slowly, observing nonverbal cues and asking yes/no questions. Visual and tactile cues may enhance communication (Deutsch and Rovner, 1991). Functional inability of the patients should be communicated to the families about the areas in which patient needs assistance. With the delusional patients, families should be told to reassure the patient rather than argue. Distraction is particularly helpful as concomitant memory loss may diffuse the situation once the patient is involved in something else. Inside locks, doorknob covers, routine walking with the patient, attending to emotional needs rather than only to reality orientation and use of restraint can help prevent wandering. For patients who may wander off, bracelets bearing information about them may help. Using a log of behaviours describing time of occurrence, duration, setting and the effect of particular intervention can make caregivers more knowledgeable about these behaviours to which they can respond more effectively. Greater understanding of patients' problems and clarification of the queries, and helpful tips regarding care giving can ease carers' problems.

Encouragement to Caregiver
Caregivers should make use of support groups and caregiver resources available in the locality. Consultation with attending psychiatrist or physician when psychosocial interventions do not adequately manage a patient's problem behaviour is an important step.

Problem solving skills of caregivers should be assessed and assistance in problem solving be provided. Caregivers may need help in learning skills of care-giving such as providing activities at home, and learning how to dress, groom, and bathe patients.

Further discussion on the caregivers' stress and resulting problems is given in a separate chapter in this book.

PHARMACOLOGICAL INTERVENTION

While considering pharmacological intervention it must be kept in mind that 'not every thing can be treated with medications' (Cheong, 2004). In addition, 'if it is not your first intervention (e.g., restraints and intramuscular injection of an antipsychotic) in a 3 to 5-year-old child throwing a tantrum, it probably should not be the first thing to try in a dementia patient with agitation and inappropriate behaviour. Behavioural techniques have been used successfully to reduce BPSD, and should be tried first; and such interventions may demonstrate even greater effectiveness when used in conjunction with pharmacological approaches (Bole and Malloy, 2004).

Medications in the conventional neuroleptic, atypical antipsychotic, cholinesterase inhibitor and serotonergic classes have been shown to ameliorate psychosis and behavioural symptoms in patients with dementia, although the evidence is not conclusive for many medications.

There are many concerns for the medicinal management in elderly. Side effects vary substantially across medication classes and modestly among individual patients. They are more vulnerable for adverse events for slower metabolism. There is a greater risk of fall and fractures, extrapyramidal symptoms (EPS) and tardive dyskinesia. So the dictum is 'start low, go slow, but go' (Cheong, 2004).

Cognitive Enhancers

Donepezil: It is a reversible and specific inhibitor of acetyl-cholinesterase. Randomised control trial (RCT) with behaviour as primary outcome comparing donepezil 5 mg to 10 mg vs. placebo found significant reduction in agitation in donepezil group (Tariot et al., 2001a). Improvement in agitation was noted in 28% with placebo and 45% with donepezil. Feldman et al. (2001) found significant difference at weeks 4 and 24 in donepezil group while the placebo group worsened.

Individuals with greater apathy, anxiety, agitation, delusions, depression, disinhibition and irritability at baseline are more likely to improve with treatment, indicating that donepezil may be most effective among individuals already exhibiting significant neuropsychiatric dysfunction (Mega et al., 1999).

Feldman et al. (2001) conducted a 6-month RCT of donepezil in Alzheimer's disease (AD) patients and found that the treated group showed significant reductions in apathy, anxiety and depression. Gauthier et al. (2002) conducted a 6-month double blind, placebo controlled trial of donepezil, and found significant reduction in scores for apathy, depression and anxiety. A subsequent analysis of only those patients with moderate AD (MMSE score 10–17) demonstrated significant reductions in apathy, delusions and aberrant motor behaviour following treatment. Additional evidence suggests that donepezil use is associated with a reduced need for psychotropic medications (e.g., antidepressants) in patients with AD (Small et al., 1998).

Galantamine: It is a slowly reversible, selective inhibitor of acetyl-cholinesterase. In a 5-month RCT of galantamine 16–24 mg/day vs placebo in 978 patients with mild to moderate AD it was found that patient receiving galantamine had no change in total Neuropsychiatric Inventory (NPI) score, whereas placebo patients worsened (Tariot et al., 2000a).

Rivastigmine: It is a slowly reversible, dual inhibitor of acetyl-cho-linesterase and butyrylcholinesterase (Giacobini, 2000). In an open-label, flexible dose, 2-year extension trial of 34 patients with AD it was found that the patients exhibited stabilization of aggressiveness, paranoia, and hallucinations (Rosler et al, 1988). It is important to mention that other studies have found no or limited effects on behaviour (Cummings, 2003).

A positive result was found by week 12, with symptoms of apathy, irritability, delusions and anxiety showing significant improvement among patients receiving active treatment with 3–12 mg of rivastigmine, as compared with placebo (Dartigues et al., 2002). There is also evidence that rivastigmine may reduce the need for other psychoactive medications (Rosler, 2002).

Memantine: It is a noncompetitive inhibitor of N-methyl-D-aspartate (NMDA) receptors that may permit normal memory formation but blocks their excitotoxic activation. As secondary outcome measures, no difference in change of NPI with memantine (NMDA receptor antagonist) monotherapy has been noted (Reisberg et al., 2003). Memantine augmentation of donepezil therapy resulted in a reduction in behavioural disturbances as measured by NPI (Tariot et al., 2004).

Antipsychotics

Haloperidol: There is insufficient evidence demonstrating that haloperidol is effective in controlling agitation. Haloperidol does decrease the aggression, but it should not be used indiscriminately for agitation. Side effects like EPS, somnolence and fatigue are more common (Lonergan et al., 2002).

Risperidone: In an RCT of 12-week fixed dose risperidone vs placebo in 625 nursing-home residents with dementia of which 70% completed the study (Katz et al., 1999) it was reported that reduction of behaviour score was noted in 33% receiving placebo, 45% receiving 1 mg/day dose (number needed to treat [NNT]—9) and 50% receiving 3 mg/day dose (NNT—7). Risperidone groups improved in scores of psychosis, aggression and total score. However, there were greater parkinsonian side effects with 2 mg/day dose and there were dose-related side effects like somnolence, EPS, and peripheral oedema.

In another study, there was 23% decrease in aggression in risperidone group compared to placebo and significant difference was noted in psychotic, affective and anxiety symptoms (Brodaty et al., 2003).

There is an increased risk of cerebrovascular adverse event with risperidone (4% versus 2% with placebo) (Wooltoton, 2002). However, a preliminary meta-analysis of clinical trials of atypical antipsychotics in dementia by Shneider and Dagerman (Profenno and Tariot, 2004) suggest a trend for death to be associated with randomization to *any* antipsychotic.

Olanzapine: Olanzapine 5 and 10 mg doses showed statistically greater improvement than placebo in a 6-week RCT on 206 AD patients, with more than 50% improvement (65% with 5 mg and 57% with 10 mg) (Street et al., 2000). In an 18-week open-label flexible-dose study efficacy persisted (Street et al., 2001). Injectable olanzapine can also be used to control agitation (Profenno and Tariot, 2004); it was found to be superior to placebo at 2 and 24 hours (Meehan et al., 2002).

Quetiapine: Possible behavioural benefit was noted in a dose range of 25–800 mg/day (median 100 mg); along with side effects like sedation (30%), orthostatic hypotension (15%), and dizziness (12%) (Tariot et al., 2000b). A decrease in delusion and aggression on NPI scores was observed in another open-label pilot study in outpatients diagnosed as probable AD, with quetiapine from 50–150 mg/day (Scharre and Chang, 2002). Davis and Baskys (2002) reported improvement of psychosis and agitation in outpatients with Lewy body dementia treated with 25–125 mg/day quetiapine.

Ziprasidone: Little data exist on use of ziprasidone in BPSD. However, a retrospective review reported decreased agitation, which also suggested that ziprasidone, is safe and effective in treating psychosis associated with dementia (Kasckow et al., 2004).

Aripiprazole: The available data is scanty. A randomized preliminary trial for 10 weeks with a mean aripiprazole dose of 10 mg/day compared with placebo suggested significant improvement in Brief Psychiatric Rating Scale (BPRS) psychosis subscale score, with improvement in akathisia and EPS. Somnolence was the most common side effect (Kasckow et al., 2004).

Clozapine: There are no placebo-controlled studies in patients with dementia, only case series. The usual starting dose is 12.5 mg/day, with maintenance doses 12.5–50 mg/day. Its toxicities, lack of efficacy data, limit its use in patients with dementia, although it has a legitimate role in patients with movement disorders, who have failed with other agents (The Parkinsons Study Group, 1999).

Improvement in agitation, aggression or other behaviours with antipsychotic medication treatment may not depend on distinct antipsychotic effects. In contrast, there is preliminary evidence that delusions and hallucinations may respond to treatment with medications outside the antipsychotic class (Sultzer, 2004).

Kasckow et al. (2004) suggest that safe treatment of BPSD depends upon three key factors: differentiating medical from psychiatric causes of patient's distress, using antipsychotics and other drugs as adjuncts to psychosocial treatments and to start low and go slow when titrating dosages. The dosages of first line medications suggested are: risperidone 0.5 to 1.5 mg; olanzapine 5 to 10 mg; quetiapine 25 to 350 mg per day. If antipsychotic monotherapy fails or if side effects limit dosing, adjunctive agents are required like valproate 125 mg bid or carbamazepine 100 mg bid, which can be titrated to effect and/or a cholinesterase inhibitor (if not already prescribed) like donepezil, 5 mg qd, which can be increased to 10 mg qd after 4 to 6 weeks; rivastigmine 1.5 mg bid which can be increased to 9 to 12 mg daily in divided dosage; and galantamine 4 mg bid which can be increased to 8 mg bid after 1 month, have been suggested (Kasckow et al., 2004).

Conventional antipsychotics are associated with side effects, e.g., akathisia, parkinsonism, tardive dyskinesia, sedation, peripheral and central anticholinergic effects, postural hypotension, cardiac conduction defects and falls, all of which cause considerable problem for the elderly. Significant extrapyramidal toxicity was observed in patients treated with 2–3 mg/day, illustrating the narrow therapeutic index of haloperidol in dementia (Profenno and Tariot, 2004).

Mood Stabilizers

Divalproex: Preliminary data suggest that valproate may be effective and safe for the treatment of agitation associated with dementia (Profenno and Tariot, 2004). With divalproex, trends for decreased scores on measures of agitation and psychosis was noted (in a 6-week placebo vs individual dose, mean serum level 45 microgram per mL; the results did not reach statistical significance) (Porsteinsson et al., 2001). Sedation, gastrointestinal symptoms and falls are common. No significant difference was noted in a short term (3 week) RCT of valproate 480 mg/day (Sival et al., 2002).

A multicenter RCT of divalproex sodium in patients with dementia and agitation, who also met criteria for secondary mania found no difference in mania features but significant change in agitation, a relatively high drop out rate, sedation in 36% and thrombocytopenia in 7% of drug group (Tariot et al., 2001b). Results from this trial were used to amend the package insert information, cautioning against use of similar doses and/or titration rates in the elderly. If valproate is used, the available evidence would suggest a starting dose of about 125 mg bid increased by 125–250 mg every 5–7 days, with a maximal dose determined by clinical response, or where there is uncertainty, a serum level of about 60–90 microgram/mL. The typical target dose is about 10–12 mg/kg/day (Profenno and Tariot, 2004).

Controlled studies involving lamotrigine, gabapentin, and topiramate are not available.

Carbamazepine: Significant decrease in BPRS was observed by Tariot et al. (1994 and 1998); however, Olin et al. (2001) did not find any. Hostility improved significantly in a RCT of carbamazepine 100 mg qid (Olin et al., 2001). Adverse events were reported as mild. Carbamazepine studies provide evidence that anticonvulsants have antiagitation efficacy (Profenno and Tariot, 2004).

Antidepressants

For depressive syndromes associated with dementia, nonpharmacological intervention should be the first step, particularly for milder depression, considering the safety advantage (Lyketsos and Lee, 2004). Cognitive behavioural and pure behavioural therapies for depression in patients with dementia have been developed (Teri et al., 1997).

Selective serotonin reuptake inhibitors (SSRI): In a RCT of sertraline as adjunct to donepezil, response rate was 60% for sertraline and 33% for placebo (Finkel et al., 2004). In a study comparing 25-50 mg sertraline vs haloperidol 1–2 mg, both groups showed significant improvement with no statistically significant difference (Gaber et al., 2001). Limited open label and case reports are available with no conclusive evidence.

Paroxetine (10–40 mg/day for 3 months) improved verbal agitation in dementia patients (Cohen-Mansfield, 1986; Ramadan et al., 2000).

Citalopram has showed significant benefit compared to placebo for agitation, lability and psychosis (Pollock et al, 2002). Information on the use of fluoxetine or fluvoxamine is not available; while that for other SSRIs are anecdotal. The side effect profile of this class includes gastrointestinal symptoms, sedation or insomnia, sexual dysfunction, hyponatremia, occasional neuromuscular sign and paradoxical agitation.

Initiation of citalopram or sertraline is recommended as the best first step, given the side effect profile of these agents; however, some experts consider venlafaxine or bupropion as first line (Alexopoulos et al., 2001). Studies suggest AD patients tolerate SSRIs better than tricyclic antidepressants (TCA). Low doses of sertraline (25 mg/day) or citalopram (10 mg/day) are the most appropriate to begin with which can be increased to a maximum of 150 mg of sertraline or 40 mg of citalopram. Sometimes higher dose and longer duration of treatment is required for response (Lyketsos and Lee, 2004).

Trazodone: Case series and open trials suggest benefit of trazodone in doses from 50–400 mg/day. Symptoms of irritability, anxiety, restlessness and depressed affect have been reported to improve in some cases, along with disturbed sleep, with side effects of sedation, orthostatic hypotension and occasional delirium (Profenno and Tariot, 2004). In a comparative study with haloperidol (mean 2.5 mg/day), trazodone (mean 220 mg/day) was better tolerated in addition to being equally effective for agitation (Sultzer et al., 1997). However, Teri et al. (2000) have reported negative results in a multi-center study contrasting trazodone, haloperidol, placebo and care giving. Trazodone is favoured for sleep disturbance primarily and as second or third line for 'mild' agitation. A typical starting dose would be 25 mg/day, with maximum doses usually of 100–250 mg/day (Profenno and Tariot, 2004).

Once the first agent is judged to be a failure or not tolerated, or if adding a second agent is not a good option, switching to another class of antidepressant should be considered. Considering the consistent neuropathologic evidence that depression in AD is associated with loss of the norepinephrine producing neurons of the locus ceruleus (Zubenko, 1992), preferred second line agents are antidepressants that lead to norepinephrine reuptake inhibition such as mirtrazepine, venlafaxine, secondary amine TCAs or monoamine oxidase inhibitors (Lyketsos and Lee, 2004).

Benzodiazepines

These are often used as rescue medicines. The major concerns are side effects like sedation, confusion and falls. There is little evidence supporting use or true safety. Lorazepam 1 mg IM is significantly more effective than placebo at 60 minutes and maintained through 2 hours; it was not significantly more effective at 30 minutes (Meehan et al., 2002). In a comparative study, 5% of patients with oxazepam (10–60 mg/day) improved versus 24% receiving haloperidol, a difference that was statistically not significant perhaps because of small sample size (Coccaro et al., 1990). Oxazepam and chlordiazepoxide were superior to placebo in many trials (Stern et al., 1991).

High rates of side effects with benzodiazepines, such as ataxia, falls, confusion, anterograde amnesia, sedation, light-headedness, tolerance and withdrawal symptoms are noted (Profenno and Tariot, 2004). So benzodiazepines are advocated for only limited use; time-limited acute, as-needed use and chronic use only when other agents have been proven ineffective. Drugs with simpler metabolism and relatively short half-lives, such as lorazepam (0.5 mg 1–4 times a day) are to be chosen; and long acting agents should be avoided.

Buspirone

There are no randomized, placebo-controlled double-blind trials of this agent in dementia patients. There are no relative benefits of this agent in comparison to trazodone and haloperidol. However, consensus statements tend to suggest a possible role for patients with mild agitation associated with anxiety or irritability, starting at 5 mg twice daily and increasing to a potential maximum daily dose of 40–60 mg/day (Profenno and Tariot, 2004).

Other Agents

Propranolol in low doses (30–80 mg/day) improves aggression in some patients; however, the likelihood of adverse reactions in this population including bradycardia, hypotension, worsening of congestive heart failure, or asthma, remained high (Shankel et al., 1995).

There are many published anecdotal reports of oestrogenic and antiandrogenic approaches, but these are not definitive (Profenno and Tariot, 2004).

Psychostimulants such as methylphenidate (Galynker et al., 1997) and dextroamphetamine have been shown to reduce symptoms of apathy in some studies (Marin et al., 1995). However, clinical observation indicates that the duration of positive effect may be short lived and traditional stimulants can cause agitation and irritability in dementia patients. Further research is needed to elucidate their utility.

Dopaminergic drugs, such as amantadine and bupropion, may be useful for reducing apathy in AD (Landes et al., 2001).

Table 13.1 Dosing strategies for medications for BPSD

Medication	Starting dose	Usual target dose	Major side effects
Antipsychotics			
Haloperidol	0.25–0.5 mg/day	2–5 mg/day	Extrapyramidal symptoms, orthostasis
Olanzapine	2.5–5.0 mg/day	10–15 mg/day	Sedation, weight gain
Quetiapine	25–50 mg/day	100–400 mg/day	Sedation, orthostasis, dizziness
Risperidone	0.25–0.5 mg/day	0.5–1.0 mg	Increased risk of cerebrovascular events
Ziprasidone	10–20 mg/day	20–40 mg/day	Sedation, dizziness
Clozapine	12.5 mg/day	50–200 mg/day	Agranulocytosis, seizures
Cholinesterase inhibitors			
Donepezil	5 mg/day	10 mg/day	Gastrointestinal distress
Rivastigmine	1.5 mg bid	6 mg bid	Gastrointestinal distress
Galantamine	4 mg bid	12 mg bid	Gastrointestinal distress
Tacrine	10 mg qid	30-40 mg qid	Risk of hepatotoxicity
Benzodiazepines			
Lorazepam	0.25–0.5 mg/day	1.0 mg 1–3 times /day	Falls, dependence
Oxazepam	5.0–7.5 mg/day	5.0–7.5 mg 1–3 times/day	Falls, dependence
Temazepam	15 mg at night	30 mg at night	Not recommended for use in day

Mood stabilizers and anticonvulsants			
Carbamazepine	100 mg bid	400 mg/day (serum level after 4 days: 4–12 microgram/mL)	P450 induction, aplastic anaemia, pancreatitis
Gabapentine	100 mg/day	600–1200 mg/day	Ataxia, dizziness, fatigue
Lamotrigine	25–50 mg/day	150–400 mg/day in divided doses	Rash (10% cases) Stevens-Johnson syndrome (0.1% cases)
Lithium	150 mg/day or bid	Serum level (0.4–0.8 mEq/L)	Tremor, tachyarrhythmias, seizures, renal toxicities, hypothyroidism
Valproic acid	125–250 mg/day or bid	500 mg/day (serum level after 3–5 days: 50–120 microgram/mL)	Gastrointestinal distress, ataxia, weight gain, liver enzyme elevation, alopecia

Clinically often the treatment of BPSD boils down to "treat what you see" relying more on experience. It should also be kept in mind that BPSD fluctuate in severity and type and interventions need to be tailored to that effect. About psychotropics there are understandably only a few studies. There is no evidence that one is superior to another. Overall, it appears that antipsychotics, mood stabilizers and SSRIs may be of benefit (details of their dosing are given in Table 13.1 adapted from Cheong, 2004).

ELECTROCONVULSIVE THERAPY

In dementia patients with treatment resistant severe depression, electroconvulsive therapy (ECT) should be considered especially when suicidality, dangerousness or violent thoughts are there (Lyketsos and Lee, 2004).

TREATMENT OF UNDERLYING MEDICAL ILLNESS

Identification and treatment of underlying medical illness should be given importance. A patient with dementia may be agitated because of a distended bladder or arthritis but unable to communicate his or her pain in words. Pacing and restlessness may be due to drug side effects. Delirium is a common trigger for BPSD. The causative factors can include acute illnesses such as a urinary tract infection or pneumonia, drug withdrawal, anticholinergic agents, medication changes, constipation, pain and dehydration.

SUMMARY GUIDELINES OF MANAGEMENT OF BPSD

General Principles
- Define specific target symptoms
- Consider possible aetiological factors
- Define a rational treatment endpoint prior to the intervention
- Have a long-term plan rather than short-term, temporary solutions
- Develop behavioural and environmental interventions
- Plan careful monitoring of interventions and effects
- Involve all caregivers and staff in the process
- Seek help from the specific helping agencies if there are any

Medicinal Treatment Principles
- Use medications only when necessary, preferably second-line after behavioural and environmental intervention
- Apply evidence-based treatment strategies
- Treat with doses that are conservative, but sufficient
- Avoid medications that are poorly tolerated by dementia patients
- Reconsider treatment strategy when response is incomplete

Managing Inadequate Response to Medications
- Confirm compliance to medications
- Review dose (consider increase if appropriate)
- Consider drug interactions that may inhibit response
- Review diagnosis (rule out delirium)
- Reconsider treatment goals
- Adjust appropriate behavioural and environmental interventions
- Consider cholinesterase inhibitors, if not already prescribed
- Switch to alternative medications
- Augment with additional medication

CONCLUSION

Effective management of BPSD understandably decreases the degree of morbidity of the patient and improves his quality of life. Caregivers will be immensely benefited by the above as it will decrease their burden. Non-pharmacological and pharmacological treatment approaches should be combined for better result; although more studies are required for the measure of their effectiveness.

REFERENCES

- Alessi CA, Yoon EJ, Schnelle JF, et al. (1999) A randomized trial of a combined physical activity and environmental intervention in nursing home residents: do sleep and agitation improve? *J Am Geriatr Soc*, 47, 784–791.
- Alexopoulos GS, Katz IR, Reynolds CF, Carpenter D, Docherty JP. (2001) *Pharmacotherapy of Depressive Disorders in Older patients. A Postgraduate Medicine Special Report.* Minneapolis, Minn: McGraw Hill.
- Boyle PA and Malloy PF. (2004) Treating apathy in Alzheimer's disease. *Dementia and Geriatric Cognitive Disorders*, 17, 91–99.
- Brodaty H, Ames D, Snowdon J, et al. (2003) A randomized placebo controlled trial of risperidone for the treatment of aggression, agitation and psychosis in dementia. *J Clin Psychiatry*, 64, 134–143.
- Cheong JA. (2004) An evidence-based approach to the management of agitation in the geriatric patient. *Focus: The Lifelong Learning in Psychiatry*, 2, 197–205.
- Coccaro EF, Krammer E, Zemishlany Z, et al. (1990) Pharmacologic treatment of noncognitive behavioural disturbances in elderly demented patients. *Am J Psychiatry*, 147, 1640–1645.
- Cohen-Mansfield J. (2004) Nonpharmacologic interventions for inappropriate behaviours in dementia: A review, summary, and critique. *Focus: The Journal of Lifelong Learning in Psychiatry*, 2, 288–308.
- Cohen-Mansfield J, Werner P (1997) Management of verbally disruptive behaviours in nursing home residents. *J Gerontol Med Sci*, 52A, M369–M377.
- Cohen-Mansfield J (1986) Agitated behaviours in the elderly. 2. Preliminary results in the cognitively deteriorated. *J Am Geriatr Soc*, 34, 722–727.
- Cummings JL (2003) Use of cholinesterase inhibitors in clinical practice: evidence based recommendations. *Am J Geriatr Psychiatry*, 11, 131–145.

- Dartigues JF, Goulley F, Bourdeix I, et al. (2002) Rivastigmine in current clinical practice in patients with mild to moderate Alzheimer's disease. *Rev. Neurl* (Paris), 158:807–812.
- Davis P and Baskys A. (2002) Quetiapine effectively reduces psychotic symptoms in patients with Lewy body dementia: An advantage of the unique pharmacological profile? *Brain Aging*, 2, 49–53.
- Deutsch LH, Rovner BW. (1991) Agitation and other noncognitive abnormalities in Alzheimer's disease. *Psychiatric Clinics of North America*, 14(2), 341–351.
- Feldman H, Gauthier S, Hecker J, et al. (2001) A 24-week, randomized double-blind study of donepezil in moderate to severe Alzheimer's disease. *Neurology*, 57, 613–620.
- Finkel SI, Mintzer JE, Dysken M, Krishnana KR, Burt T, McRae T (2004) A randomized placebo-controlled study of the efficacy and safety of sertraline in the treatment of the behavioural manifestation of Alzheimer's disease in outpatients treated with donepezil. *Int J Geriatric Psychiatry*, 19, 9–18.
- Fritz C, Farver T, Kass P, et al., (1995) Association with companion animals and the expression of noncognitive symptoms in Alzheimer's patients. *J Nerv Ment Dis*, 183, 459–463.
- Gaber S, Ronozoli S, Bruno A, Biagi A (2001) Sertraline versus small doses of haloperidol in the treatment of agitated behaviour in patients with dementia. *Arch Gerontol Geriatr*, 33 (suppl 1), 159–162.
- Galynker I, Ieronimo C, Minor C, et al. (1997) Methylphenidate treatment of negative symptoms in patients with dementia. *J Neuropsychiatry Clin Neurosci*, 9, 231–239.
- Giacobini E. (2000) Cholinesterase inhibitors stabilize Alzheimer's disease, *Ann NY Acad Sci*, 920, 321–327.
- Kasckow JW, Mulchahey JJ, Mohamed S. (2004) Using antipsychotics in patients with dementia. *Current psychiatry*, 3, 2, 55–64.
- Katz IR, Jeste DV, Mintzer JE, Clyde C, Napolitano J, Brecher M. (1999) Comparison of risperidone and placebo for psychoses and behavioural disturbances associated with dementia: a randomised, double blind trial. Risperidone Study group. *J Clinical Psychiatry*, 60, 107–115.
- Landes AM, Sperry SD, Strauss ME, Geldmacher DS. (2001) Apathy in Alzheimer's disease. *J Am Geriatr Soc*, 49, 1700–1707.
- Lonergan E, Luxenberg J, Colford J. (2002) Haloperidol for agitation in dementia. *Cochrane Database Syst Rev.* 2, CD 002852.
- Lytetsos CG, Lee HB. (2004) Diagnosis and treatment of depression in Alzheimer's disease: A practical update for the clinician. *Dementia and Geriatric Cognitive Disorders*, 17, 55–64.

- Marin RS, Fogel BS, Hawkins J, et al. (1995) Apathy: A treatable syndrome. *J Neuropsychiatry Clin Neruosci,* 7, 23–30.
- McCallion P, Toseland RW, Lacey D, et al. (1999) Educating nursing assistants to communicate more effectively with nursing home residents with dementia. *Gerontologist,* 39, 546–558.
- Meehan KM, Wang H, David SR, et al. (2002) Comparison of rapidly acting intramuscular olanzapine, lorazepam and placebo: a double blind randomised study in acutely agitated patients with dementia. *Neuropsychopharmacology,* 26, 494–504.
- Mega MS, Masterman DM, O'Connor SM, et al. (1999) The spectrum of behavioural responses to cholinesterase inhibitor therapy in Alzheimer disease. *Arch Neurol,* 56, 1388–1393.
- Mentes JC and Ferrario J. (1989) Calming aggressive reactions: a preventive program. *J Gerontol Nurs,* 15, 22–27.
- Olin JT, Fox LS, Pawluczyk S, Taggart NA, Schneider LS. (2001) A pilot randomised trial of carbamazepine for behavioural symptoms in treatment-resistant outpatient with Alzheimer's disease. *Am J Geriatr Psychiatry,* 9, 400–405.
- Palmer CV, Adams SW, Bourgeois M, et al. (1999) Reduction in care-giver-identified problem behaviour in patients with Alzheimer disease post hearing-aid fitting. *J Speech Lang Hear Res,* 42, 312–328.
- Pollock BG, Mulsant BH, Rosen J, et al. (2002) Comparison of citalopram, perphenazine, and placebo for the acute treatment of psychosis and behavioural disturbances in hospitalized demented patients. *Am J Psychiatry,* 159, 460–465.
- Porsteinsson AP, Tariot PN, Erb R, et al. (2001) Placebo controlled study of divalproex sodium for agitation in dementia. *Am J Geriatr psychiatry,* 9, 58–66.
- Profenno LA and Tariot PN. (2004) Pharmacologic management of agitation in Alzheimer's disease. *Dementia and Geriatric Cognitive Disorders,* 17, 65–77.
- Ramadan FH, Naughton BJ, Bassanelli AG (2000) Treatment of verbal agitation with a selective serotonin reuptake inhibitor. *J Geriatr Psychiatry Neurol,* 13, 56–59.
- Reisberg B, Doody R, Stoffler A, Schmitt F, Ferris S, Mobius HJ. (2003) Memantine in moderate to severe Alzheimer's disease. *N Engl J Med,* 348, 1333–1341.
- Reisberg B. (1986) Dementia: A systematic approach to identifying reversible causes. *Geriatrics,* 41, 30–46.
- Rosler M, Retz W, Retz-Junginger P, Dennier HJ. (1988) Effects of two-year treatment with the cholinesterase inhibitor rivastigmine on behavioural symptoms in Alzheimer's disease. *Behav Neurol,* 11, 211–216.

- Rosler M. (2002) The efficacy of cholinesterase inhibitors in treating the behavioural symptoms of dementia. *Int J Clin Pract Suppl,* 127, 20–36.
- Scharre DW and Chang SI. (2002) Cognitive and behavioral effects of quetiapine in Alzheimer disease patients. *Alzheimer Dis Assoc Disord,* 16, 128–130.
- Schulz R and Martire LM. (2004) Family care giving of persons with dementia: prevalence, health effects and support strategies. *Am J Geriatr Psychiatry,* 12, 240–249.
- Shankle WR, Nielson KA, Cotmn CW. (1995) Low dose propranolol reduces aggression and agitation resembling that associated with orbitofrontal dysfunction in elderly demented patients. *Alzheimer Dis. Asso Disord,* 9, 233–237.
- Sival RC, Haffmans PM, Jansen PA. Duursma SA, Eikelenboom P. (2002) Sodium valproate in the treatment of aggressive behaviour in patients with dementia - A randomized placebo-controlled clinical trial. *International Journal of Geriatric Psychiatry,* 17, 579–585.
- Small GW, Donohue JA, Brooks RL (1998) An economic evaluation of donepezil in the treatment of Alzheimer's disease. *Clin Ther,* 20, 838–850.
- Stern RG, Duffelmeyer ME, Zemishlani Z, Davidson M. (1991) The use of benzodiazepines in the management of behavioral symptoms in demented patients. *The Psychiatric Clinics of North America,* 14(2), 375
- Street JS, Clark WS, Kadam DL, et al. (2001) Long-term efficacy of olanzapine in the control of psychotic and behavioural symptoms in nursing home patients with Alzheimer's dementia. *Int J Geriatr psychiatry,* 16 (suppl 1), S62–S70.
- Street JS Clark WS, Gannon KS, et al. (2000) Olanzapine treatment of psychotic and behavioural symptoms in patients with Alzheimer disease in nursing care facilities: a double-blind, randomized, placebo controlled trial. The HGEEU Study Group. *Arch Gen psychiatry,* 57, 968–976.
- Sultzer DL. (2004) Psychosis and antipsychotic medications in Alzheimer's Disease: Clinical management and research perspectives. *Dementia and Geriatric Cognitive Disorders,* 17, 78–90.
- Sultzer DL, Gray KF, Gunay I, Berisford MA, Mahler ME. (1997) A double blind comparison of trazodone and haloperidol for treatment of agitation in patients with dementia. *Am J Geriatr Psychiatry,* 5, 60–69.
- Tariot PN, Cummings JL, Katz IR, et al. (2001a) A Randomised double blind placebo controlled study of the efficacy and safety of donepezil in patients with Alzheimer's disease in the nursing home setting. *J Am Geriatric Society,* 49, 1590–1599.

- Tariot PN, Erb R, Leibovici A, et al. (1994) Carbamazepine treatment of agitation in nursing home patients with dementia: a preliminary study. *J Am Geriatr Soc,* 42, 1160–1166.
- Tariot PN, Erb R, Podgorski CA, et al. (1998) Efficacy and tolerability of carbamazepine for agitation and aggression in dementia. *American Journal Psychiatry,* 155, 54–61.
- Tariot PN, Farlow MR, Grossberg GT, Graham SM, McDonald S, Gergel I. (2004) Memantine treatment in patients with moderate to severe Alzheimer disease already receiving donepezil: a randomized controlled trial. *JAMA,* 291, 317–324.
- Tariot PN, Salzman C, Yeung PP, Pultz J, Rak IW. (2000b) Long-term use of quetiapine in elderly patients with psychotic disorders. *Clin Ther,* 22, 1068–1084.
- Tariot PN, Shneider L, Intzer J, et al. (2001b) Safety and tolerability of divalproex sodium for the treatment of signs and symptoms of mania in elderly patients with dementia: Results of a double-blind placebo controlled trial. *Curr Ther Res,* 62, 51–67.
- Tariot PN, Solomon PR, Morris JC, Kershaw P, Lilienfeld S, Ding C. (2000a) A 5-month, randomised, placebo controlled trial of galantamine in AD. The Galantamine USA-10 Study Group. *Neurology,* 54, 2269–2276.
- Teri L, Logsdon RG, Peskind E, et al. (2000) Treatment of agitation in AD: A randomized, place-controlled clinical trial. *Neurology,* 55, 1271–1278.
- Teri L, Logsdon RG, Uomoto J, McCurry SM. (1997) Behavioural treatment of depression in dementia patients: A controlled clinical trial. *J Gerontol B Psychol Sci Soc Sci,* 52, 159–166.
- The Parkinsons Study Group (1999) Low dose clozapine for the treatment of drug-induced psychosis in Parkinson's disease. *N Eng J Med,* 340, 757–763.
- Wooltoton E. (2002) Risperidone (Risperdal): Increased rate of cerebrovascular events in dementia trials. *CMAJ,* 167, 1269–1270.
- Zaudig, M. (1996) Assessing behavioural symptoms of dementia of Alzheimer type: categorical and quantitative approaches. *International Psychogeriatrics,* 8 (Suppl 2), 183–200.
- Zisselman MH, Rovenoer BW, Shmuey Y, et al. (1996) A pet therapy intervention with geriatric psychiatry inpatients. *Am J Occup Ther,* 50, 47–51.
- Zubenko GS (1992) Biological correlates of clinical heterogeneity in primary dementia. *Neuropsychopharmacology,* 6, 77–93.

14

Nursing People with Dementia and their Families

Jenny La Fontaine

Introduction

Nurses' understanding of dementia in the UK, as with many westernised countries has been influenced by prevailing views of ageing. Although recognised by people such as Alois Alzheimer and colleagues in 1906, the concept did not fit with the prevailing view of mental health and illness at the time (Cheston and Bender, 1999). The predominant view at that time was that Alzheimer's disease and related dementias were a normal part of ageing. In the 1970s the UK, like many western nations began to realise that population ageing was occurring. With a predominantly negative view of ageing and older people evident in the UK, this increase was viewed with alarm. Concerns were expressed about costs of health and social care particularly in relation to those chronic conditions such as dementia, where cure wasn't perceived as a possibility.

This brought about the medicalisation of dementia; largely because alongside medicalisation came an increased research budget and recognition that it was an illness. However, care of people with dementia in the 1970s predominantly occurred in large and inhospitable institutions, either hospitals or homes where people were often admitted in the early stages and stayed until they died. In my first experience as a Nurse in 1979, I worked on a ward where 28 older women were cared for together. Those women were not seen as individuals; they were washed, undressed and put on the toilet together with no respect for their privacy or dignity. They were stripped of their humanity, skills and identity and labelled as "the babies". We as new recruits were told there was nothing you could do, you couldn't influence the inexorable decline that people experienced as a part of the dementia and there was no point in attempting communication because it wouldn't be understood. On that ward, I met a lady who challenged this view completely, she was dying and refused to eat or drink. I attempted to talk with her and she responded. Despite her difficulties she was listening and did understand some of what was said to her. I was trying to persuade her to drink. She clearly looked at me and said, "No, I don't want anything".

This and other experiences taught me that something different was possible. The prevailing belief that nursing older people was about purely basic care, and that you didn't need any skills as a nurse to work with older people was widely held and often still is. I didn't believe this and went on to work with older people with dementia and other mental health problems when I qualified. Huge leaps forward have occurred since then, and although there is always further to go, positive changes have taken place.

The purpose of this chapter is to assist the readers to understand a little of how nursing for people with dementia has developed. It is intended that this chapter will give nurses a taste of the models and care practices that have been developed and delivered in the United Kingdom. A reference list is included at the end in order that readers can source other literature, which can assist them on their journey of knowledge, attitude and skills development. To begin with, a theory of care with people with dementia and their families will be explored, as will the concept of nursing within this framework. A case study approach is then utilised to enable the reader to make sense of the model presented with regard to the different stages in the life of the person with dementia.

A Theory of Dementia Care and its Relationship to Nursing

In the early 1990s, a theory of dementia care began to emerge, developed in response to the negative care often experienced by people with dementia. Kitwood (1997), a social psychologist, was asked if he would assist some staff working in a hospital to develop the care offered to their patients, in the late 1980s. Kitwood had never worked with people with dementia, although he had some personal experience through a neighbour. He became increasingly interested and over the next 4 years began to question the received wisdom prevalent in care of people with dementia. Kitwood highlighted the absence of a theory of dementia care, and challenged the dominance of the biomedical model. He argued that the biomedical model could not provide all the answers to the experience of dementia, citing a number of reasons for this:

a) There was evidence in CT scans that some people had significant neuropathological changes to the brain with limited clinical presentation of dementia and vice versa.
b) People with dementia when placed in residential care deteriorated significantly.
c) Where people with dementia experienced stimulating and positive environments, their functioning seemed to improve.

Kitwood (1997) proposed that much of the care offered to people with dementia focused upon the illness rather than the person and didn't acknowledge the variety of factors influencing the way in which the illness progresses. He developed an integrative theory of dementia care, drawing on a number of theories and models that can assist us in understanding the experience of dementia for the person. His theory identifies that "Dementia = Neurological Impairment + Biography + Personality + Health AND Psychosocial Environment" (Kitwood, 1997).

He challenged us to believe that the person with dementia and his family are people with lives, histories and a future and that we should consider the meaning of this for our working practice. His theory involved a belief in the personhood of people with dementia, emphasising that the person with dementia is a person first, with dementia second. He defined personhood as, "To have concern for another person, above all else to experience a feeling, a movement of the soul in which the person's being is honoured and respected as if it were one's own" (Kitwood, 1997).

He argued that people with dementia are affected by the impact the illness has on them, but are also affected by the manner in which others treat them. The experience of the illness is for some a terrifying ordeal and a threat to who they are; as such, how others behave is important in helping a person to cope and live with the illness rather than just to exist. This is powerfully emphasised by this quote from a person with dementia:

"You don't understand. They don't need to tell me I'm dying with Alzheimer's disease. *I know that*... What they need to do, what *you* need to do, is help me to figure out how to *live* with it" (Spencer cited in Braudy Harris: 2002, p xiii, their emphasis)

In recent years, nurses have been challenged to consider the concept of personhood with regard to the practice of nursing. Henderson (1980) suggested that the essence of nursing was to provide humanistic care to neglected groups including older people. As Nolan (2000) indicates, this is still true today. People with dementia have long been a neglected group with regard to the development of nursing and Kitwood's (1997) theory provided a significant opportunity to address this neglect. Nursing incorporates a relational process, in which the individual nurse is challenged to understand the person in the context of his biography, agency, pattern of life and belongingness as well as the knowledge of the illness (Liaschenki, 1997).

Nursing people with dementia, using Kitwood's (1997) model requires the development of skills, which reflect the essential understanding and ability to develop this relationship in order to support the personhood of the individual experiencing dementia. People with dementia do not exist in isolation; they are affected by and relate within their psychosocial environment. This environment ranges from close family through to the wider society within which people live. It is necessary for nurses to address this if we are to provide effective care. In addition, dementia is an isolating and challenging ordeal; in these circumstances, the development of effective relationships through which the person can be supported to meet his needs is crucial.

Nursing people with dementia means working with the person and his family throughout the journey that is their life prior to, during and post diagnosis right until death. It involves a special relationship similar and different to that of family relationships, meaningful because the nurse can become a significant other. The contribution of nursing can be significant and meaningful at all stages in the person's journey. Nursing people with dementia in this context includes the need to develop a range of skills including such issues as effective assessment skills, communication skills, knowledge about the difficulties experienced and educative skills in order to assist the person with dementia and his family to cope. In addition, nursing skills should incorporate the ability to provide skilled family and individual counselling interventions where this is required. In the middle to later experiences of the illness, nursing interventions are required to support the person to maintain his practical, occupational and personal functioning and to carry out this care where the person is no longer able to do so independently. However, it is beyond the scope of this chapter to address all aspects of nursing practice that can be delivered utilising a person centred approach. The remainder of this chapter focuses on two possible interventions at different points in the experience of dementia for the person and his family, which serve to highlight the range of skills required.

Pre-assessment Counselling

Case Study 1

Anne and her husband John have lived in the same area for many years, having brought up their two children, who are now married, and having maintained close relationships with their families. Anne was working but was struggling with work and eventually went off sick. Her husband encouraged her to go to her doctor, who indicated that she was depressed and prescribed antidepressants. Some months later the depression had lifted leaving obvious difficulties with memory. Her family doctor referred her to a psychiatrist. Upon receiving the referral, a nurse was asked to see her and her husband to enable Anne to consider what she wanted to do next with regard to her memory difficulties, prior to assessment in the memory clinic. Anne was very distressed by her situation and when the nurse first visited, her anxiety was such that she could not describe her difficulties without becoming very tearful and clearly feeling overwhelmed. Through the process of pre-assessment counselling, Anne was able to acknowledge her fears and discuss her difficulties. She was able to make a choice about where and what assessments she was prepared to undergo, and finally how she wished to be told the diagnosis. The nurse involved in that process continued to work with Anne and her husband following the diagnosis.

Although fictitious, the above case study is typical of the referrals received for people under the age of 65 with suspected dementia. Older people too are increasingly being referred earlier in their experience of memory difficulties. One of the challenges facing people with dementia in the UK is that people are frequently not informed of their diagnosis (Audit Commission, 2001) and not given the option to consider what they wish to know and how, or even whether they wish to engage in the assessment process.

Cheston and Bender (1999) amongst others argue that this is unacceptable, that people with dementia have a fundamental right to decide how this happens and what they wish to know. They further suggest that person focused assessment should as a matter of course address these issues. Pratt and Wilkinson (2001) highlight in their research, that people with dementia want to know what is wrong, and that they want to be able to decide the process and approach used to assist them through this process. Various authors, including Clarke (2003), highlight the role that nurses can play in this process. As Clarke (2003) identifies, nursing practice in this area is common in other specialities, such as Parkinson's disease and palliative care. The nursing approach in this situation, using a person centred approach involves initially, the development of a therapeutic relationship. Through this relationship, a process can take place, which would include the following steps:

- Exploration of the current situation, the person's feelings surrounding the changes, which have occurred to necessitate a referral. Does the person already have an idea of what may be causing the changes?
- What will the assessment involve?
- What are the benefits of having an assessment?
- Exploration of the possibility of receiving bad news.
- Does the person feel emotionally prepared to undertake the assessment process?
- What support do they feel they need?
- What does the person understand about the possible illness and the diagnosis?
- Are there any treatments available?
- What are the alternatives?
- What are the risks?

With Anne in the case study, this would involve getting to know her and her current experience and perceptions of the situation she finds herself in. Pratt and Wilkinson (2003) highlight the importance of understanding the person's social context; it is also therefore important to establish, with Anne's permission, her husbands' perception too. This may need to occur over more than one visit. Anne would also need to know what she had been referred for and the nature of the service she had been referred to. Having established this, the nurses' role would also be to assist Anne and her husband to understand the process of assessment in order that they can make a decision about whether they wish to be assessed, where they want this to happen and what they wish to know.

The role of the nurse would also include ongoing support throughout the assessment process, to enable the person to express his views at each stage, including his willingness to continue to participate. It may be the case that people's views change as they experience the assessment; it is often described as a traumatic event, which further emphasises the reality of the difficulties being experienced (Keady and Gilleard, 2002). It is therefore crucial that the person with suspected dementia has the opportunity to express his views and to change his mind about any aspect of the process. An ongoing and therapeutic relationship based on honesty and trust is fundamental to this approach, which embodies person centred care.

Working with People whose Behaviour is Challenging

Case Study 2

Charles has a diagnosis of Alzheimer's disease and was referred because of his current difficulties. Staff were struggling to understand the reasons for his distress and his resulting behaviour. His family also understandably very distressed by his behaviour. He has been in long term care for 3 years, having had a diagnosis of dementia for 6 years. He and his family had been struggling with the difficulties associated with this for the past 10 years. Since his admission he has shouted and called out throughout the day; although initially this was more contained, it had increased significantly. He was very agitated, chair bound and appeared very distressed for much of the time. Other interventions tried by staff and family have worked for no more than a few days.

Kitwood (1997) amongst others highlight that using a person centred approach requires the nurse to view behaviour as an expression of unmet need. People whose behaviour is challenging are frequently unable to meet their needs independently and require support and understanding in order for these needs to be met. However, it is often such behaviour that alienates staff and can make their interventions task focused rather than person centred. The nurses' role in this is therefore to carry out a detailed and comprehensive assessment, which would assist the nurse and the staff group to understand what may be the cause of Charles's difficulties. This would then facilitate an agreed person centred approach to support Charles.

Assessment Processes

- Detailed observation of Charles using Dementia Care Mapping (Kitwood, 1997). This would be particularly important because Charles may be unable to communicate verbally
- Review of case notes
- Family meeting
- Biographical history
- Functional analysis

- Assessment of physical health
- Discussions with staff
- Making sense of his frame of reference
- Using different theoretical models to understand his difficulties

Having collated the assessment information, the nurses' role would be to facilitate discussion around the outcomes of the assessment, assisting staff to identify possible solutions to the person's difficulties. Assessment often identifies multiple pathways to understanding the person's experience and current difficulties. With Charles, these may include:

- Calling out to let people know he is there, and to maintain contact with the world around him
- Perseveration due to the frontal lobe damage
- Feelings of insecurity and isolation
- Irritability due to his difficulty in communicating his needs
- Loss of important and secure relationships

Interventions by nursing staff would need to address these issues and facilitate a greater understanding of the difficulties experienced by Charles. Interventions by nurses would include assisting his family on their regular visits to consider how to communicate with Charles in a meaningful manner and in addition, planning nursing interventions designed to support Charles to minimise his distress. This could include spending regular time with Charles; stimulating the senses he is still able to respond to, such as touch and hearing, using massage and enabling him to listen to music he used to enjoy. It would also involve consideration of the manner in which his personal care is given, and determining whether particular staff approaches appear to assist Charles to feel calm.

Conclusion

Nursing people with dementia using a person centred perspective is currently a very challenging and innovative area of practice for nurses in the UK. Many of the difficulties experienced by people with dementia and their families require the development of effective and stable relationships in which the nurse needs to be innovative and creative in the approaches utilised. Despite widely held negative views about working with people with dementia, more nurses are actively choosing to work with people who experience dementia, and their families.

Working with people with dementia is, as Liaschenko (1997) suggests, an area in which many different aspects of knowledge need to be brought into conscious use. Far from being an area where only basic care is delivered, it is increasingly recognised that nursing in this area of care practice needs to openly embrace the principles of therapeutic work with people with dementia, including counselling and psychotherapy, in order to build effective relationships. This is the basis of person centred nursing care, to be in a therapeutic relationship with the person and with his family. The opportunities for nurses to develop and offer a diverse range of skills and support are increasing. However, fundamental to this is the development of skills which enable the practitioner to not only reflect upon the interaction, but also to reflect on how this may affect them. Nursing people with dementia involves painful and personal feelings, which also require exploration if the nurse is to be able to care effectively.

REFERENCES

- Audit Commission (2000) *Forget Me Not, Mental Health Services for Older People.* London: HMSO.
- Braudy Harris P. (2003) *The Person with Alzheimer's Disease, Pathways to Understanding the Experience.* Baltimore: John Hopkins University Press.
- Cheston R and Bender M. (1999) *Understanding Dementia, The Man with the Worried Eyes.* London: Jessica Kingsley Publications.
- Clarke C. (2003) The Community Mental Health Nurse role in sharing the diagnosis of dementia. In *Community Mental Health Nursing and Dementia Care: Practice Perspectives* (eds: Keady, J. Clarke, CC and Adams T). Buckingham: Open University Press.
- Henderson V. (1980) Preserving the essence of nursing in a technological age. *Journal of Advanced Nursing,* 5, 245–260.
- Keady J and Gilliard J. (2002) Testing Times: The experience of neuropsychological assessment for people with suspected Alzheimer's disease. In *The Person with Alzheimer's Disease, Pathways to Understanding the Experience* (eds: Braudy Harris P). Baltimore: Johns Hopkins University Press.

- Kitwood T. (1997) *Dementia Reconsidered, The Person Comes First.* Buckingham: Open University Press.
- Liaschenko J. (1997) Knowing the patient. In *Nursing Praxis, Knowledge and Action* (eds: Thorne SE and Hays VE). Thousand Oaks: Sage Publications.
- Nolan M. (2000) Skills for the Future: The humanity of caring. *Nursing Management,* 7, 6, 22.
- Pratt R and Wilkinson H. (2001) *Tell Me The Truth: The effect of being told the diagnosis of dementia from the perspective of the person with dementia.* London: Mental Health Foundation.
- Pratt R and Wilkinson H. (2003) A Psychosocial Model for Understanding the experience of receiving a diagnosis of Alzheimer's disease. *Dementia,* 2,2:181–200.

Further Recommended Reading

- Berg A and Wellander-Hansson U. (2000) Dementia care nurses' experiences of systematic clinical supervision and planned nursing care. *Journal of Nursing Management,* 8, 357–368.
- Brechin A, Walmsley J, Katz J and Peace S. (1998) *Care Matters, Concepts, Practice and Research in Health and Social Care.* London: Sage Publications.
- Cheston R. (1998) Psychotherapeutic work with people with dementia: A review of the literature. *British Journal of, Medical Psychology,* 71, 211–231.
- Daker-White G, Beattie A, Means R and Gilliard J. (2002) Serving the needs of marginalized groups in dementia care: younger people and minority ethnic groups Dementia Voice [www.dementia-voice.org.uk/Projects_Marginalised_Groups.htm].
- Killick J and Allen K. (2001) *Communication and the Care of People with Dementia.* Buckingham: Open University Press.
- Kitwood T and Bredin K. (1992) Towards a theory of dementia care: personhood and well-being. *Ageing and Society,* 10, 269–287.
- Twigg J and Atkin K. (1994) *Carers Perceived, Policy and Practice in Informal Care.* Buckingham: Open University Press.

15

An Occupational Therapy
Perspective of Dementia

Shovan Saha, Sunitha Thomas

Introduction

Occupational therapy is the art and science of directing man's participation in selected tasks to restore, reinforce and enhance performance, facilitate learning of those skills and functions essential for adaptation and productivity, diminish or correct pathology and to promote and maintain health. Its fundamental concern is the capacity, throughout the life span to perform with satisfaction to self and others, those tasks and roles essential to productive living and to the mastery of self and the environment (Anonymous, 1972).

Occupational therapy has historically viewed human performance from a broad and holistic perspective. This philosophy of humane treatment was built on a set of beliefs attesting to the value of human relationships, the importance of a pleasant environment, and the value of purposeful activity (Fidler, 1997). From its inception, occupational therapy has viewed the human being as a complex mix of internal physical, psychological, social and cultural variables living within an equally dynamic environmental mixture of social, cultural, interpersonal, economic, and political variables (Kielhofner, 1985). The therapeutic use of activity and movement has been appreciated since the dawn of civilization. Before, it has been referred to by names like *moral treatment, work treatment, work therapy, diversional therapy, ergotherapy* and finally in the year 1914 the term Occupational therapy was coined by an American architect, George Edward Barton (Hopkins, 1983).

The uniqueness of the occupational therapy approach to psychosocial dysfunction lies in the philosophy of human being having the ability to influence his own health through occupation. Activity is basic to life and occupation; it releases tension, anxiety, and grief. For patients with mental illness, occupational therapy not only involves this normal aspect of life, but can strengthen resistance to breakdown through purposeful attainment and satisfying personal relationships by encouraging new skills, perfecting poorly used ones or relearning forgotten ones, resulting in restored self confidence and a more mature sense of responsibility.

Therapeutic activities enhance communication in two ways. They provide *non-verbal* communication and thus provide a means for bringing unconscious or unshared ideas to the level that they can be conveyed to others in ways that are not always possible through verbal communication alone. Secondly, these activities help the client to *communicate with self* as well. They provide an opportunity for the patient to select on some level of common recognizable, real or symbolic ways of expressing ideas and feelings that he is unaware of for one reason or another.

The term '*occupation*' from occupational therapy signifies two important aspects of the profession (Saha, 2001). The *first aspect* includes various performance skills and these are the skills that an occupational therapist tries to restore back on to the patient. These performance skills can be broadly classified as the following:
- *Activities of daily living (ADL)* – It is occupation that enables the individual to survive and that promotes and maintains health, including mental health. This includes activities like eating, grooming, dressing, shopping, etc.

- *Work* – It is any productive activity, whether paid or unpaid, that contributes to the maintenance or advancement of society as well as the individual. It becomes an important social role, giving him his position in society and a sense of his own value as a contributing member. Attitudes to supervision and authority, relationships with fellow worker are important aspects to assess.
- *Play and leisure activity* – It is an activity that is often used to satisfy individual needs that are not met by either self-care or work occupations.

The *other aspect* is known as therapeutic activity that forms the medium of occupational therapy intervention. These are goal-oriented tasks, which form the treatment tool. The conscious effort of the patient performing the activity is focused on the ultimate objective of the movement and not on the movement itself. The objective is planned or hypothesized by the therapist. For an activity to be purposeful the reason to be engaged in it should be apparent to the doer and is fundamental to optimal growth and development. These are the means whereby performance components are achieved. Participating in activities can help to prevent frustration, boredom and challenging behaviours. It helps the person maintain his or her independence in and around the home and improves self-esteem and thereby the quality of life.

While *analyzing a therapeutic activity*, an occupational therapist looks at its parts: the motions used; the procedure and the process; the interpersonal relations that influence the process and in turn are influenced by it; the context in which the activity occurs; its possible cultural meanings; the factor of age and gender; the performance components required and their relationship to occupational performance. This is a very important process as it facilitates in advising for right kind of activity at the right time and one of the essential components of this process is *simulation of activities*. These are those activities that an individual engages in within the confines of a clinical setting and are designed to develop skills that can be used in the community. Learning occurs through the experience in an initially protected environment where the individual is able to experiment with more adaptive modes of behaviour.

OCCUPATIONAL THERAPY EVALUATION

Dementia is a chronic, irreversible process accompanied by a progressive loss of cognitive and motor ability that results in severe incapacity. Of particular importance in evaluating clients with dementia are the identification of deficits and abilities in cognition that influence the individual's task performance and that includes observation and evaluation of patient's memory, language, problem solving skills, understanding of abstract concepts, orientation and executive functions. It also evaluates specific areas of sensory, perceptual and emotional-processing abilities that influence task performance and functional levels. Assessments are available to use in evaluating apraxia, aphasia and agnosia.

The occupational therapy evaluation begins by investigating the individual's functional levels in the *instrumental activities of daily living* (IADL) related to productive activities (work tasks, community mobility, home management and community safety), which are often of the greatest importance in the early dementia process. Task performance, the balance of activity, social support networks and the appropriateness of the work, leisure and living environments are also evaluated when gathering the baseline data necessary for planning occupational therapy interventions (Rogers, 1994). A variety of standardized assessment tools are used to evaluate various performance areas.

As dementia progresses, the occupational therapist evaluates function in *occupational performance areas* related to personal self care, mobility, home management, and relevant work and leisure areas. The level of assistance (independent, minimal, moderate, maximal, or dependent), type of assistance (supervision, type of prompt, modeling, guidance, or physical help), and adaptive equipment or environmental adaptations deemed necessა y to complete tasks in ADL and IADL are specified (Williams et al., 1998).

The *evaluation of sensory motor function* may include the assessment of gait, posture, balance, muscle tone, strength, gross and fine motor coordination, range of motion, and smoothness and quality of movement. An *evaluation of sensation* (particularly tactile involving superficial pain, light touch, deep pressure and position sense) should be considered in the overall assessment of the individual as it relates to safety and the potential of injury.

Emotional changes occur insidiously as dementia progresses. Monitoring for signs of depression and denials are an important component to evaluate during the early stages of dementia. During the later stages, observing and asking about the presence of inflexibility to changes, outbursts of uncontrolled crying or laughing, display of regressive and preservative behaviours in the individual with dementia are of great importance.

Finally, the *appropriateness of the home environment* is assessed for safety issues and to determine if modifications, adaptations or alterations are necessary in order to support the highest level of independence with ADL. The *individuals support network* is assessed to determine available resources, become informed of the needs and opinions of the caregiver and establish their degree of availability, knowledge, skills and health status.

In addition to serving as a guide for selecting the appropriate intervention modality or strategy, and as a baseline for such intervention, the assessment data may be used to facilitate and support decisions about level of care, placement and guardianship. Because of the progressive nature of dementias the assessment must establish a baseline and then become part of an ongoing monitoring process.

THEORETICAL FRAMEWORK

These are a set of concepts and assumptions for assessing a function-dysfunction and intervention strategies with well-defined outcomes. The following approaches are incorporated in occupational therapy intervention in dementia:

Model of human occupation (MOHO): According to model of human occupation, human being is seen as a dynamic and open system interacting with the environment in a series of cyclical processes. These processes are input, throughput, output and feedback (Bruce and Borg, 1987). In persons with dementia, the throughput is altered;

it is made easier by a less complex input of information producing an adapted output to the conditions of environment.

Behaviourist approach: In the learning of skills, the important feature is that the goal may be broken down into smaller and more manageable parts. These can be learned separately and then put back together again. A significant role of the therapist is to identify what in the environment serves to reinforce and therefore maintain specific patient behaviours, both adaptive and maladaptive.

Cognitive disability frame of reference: It provides a means for analyzing the relative difficulty of any desired activity in terms of requisite information processing demands. From this analysis, environmental factors can be identified that facilitate or constrain the production of each dimension of thought (Levy, 1993).

Sensory integration frame of reference: Sensory integration is the neurological process that organizes sensation from one's own body and from the environment and makes it possible to use the body effectively within the environment. The spatial and temporal aspects of input from different sensory modalities are interpreted, associated, and unified. As the behavioural expression of dementia is influenced by the physical and social environment, a stable appropriately organized environment can contribute to the demented person's adaptation and performance of activities in his or her environment (Robichaud et al., 1994).

Reality orientation: It is a technique to improve the quality of life of confused elderly people; it operates through the presentation of orientation information (e.g., time, place and person-related), which is thought to provide the person with a greater understanding of his surroundings, possibly resulting in an improved sense of control and self-esteem.

In occupational therapy, the *therapist-patient relationship* assumes enormous importance, as the process of rehabilitation continues over an extended period of time; and to retain a level of motivation in the course of the entire process there is a need for sharing a relationship that would foster the following aspects:

- Establish confidence and avoid situations that provoke symptoms, unless deliberately provoked in a group situation.
- Be friendly but decisive and give ample encouragement, as self-consciousness is often a serious hindrance to a therapeutic relationship.
- The therapist must adapt his approach to the patient's degree of understanding and grasp of situations.
- The staff attitudes must allow the elderly person's individuality as an adult with dignity, self-respect, choice and independence.

ROLE OF OCCUPATIONAL THERAPY IN VARIOUS PERFORMANCE AREAS

The occupational therapist is the rehabilitation specialist responsible for increasing the independence in various performance areas, which is the goal of rehabilitation in general and occupational therapy in particular for patients with dementia. Although the biological conditions causing dementia cannot be reversed, performance can often be improved by modifying task requirements and adapting the environment (Rogers, 1994). The intervention process addresses various components of the performance areas and when each component is put together it gives a larger perspective of the patient's functional life role. The essential *performance areas* considered are self-care activities, communication skills, leisure activities and productivity; the *performance components* are sensorimotor, cognition and psychosocial aspects.

Self- Care Activities

The impact of dementia on a person's ability to look after himself will vary from one individual to another. Washing, dressing and attention to personal care, all need to be approached in an orderly way. They involve skills which people with dementia sometimes find difficult. Lack of motivation, forgetfulness and inappropriate behaviour all have a serious effect on a person's ability to attend to their personal appearance and care. Common difficulties, which may be encountered, are as follows:
- A loss in personal appearance will result in inattention to cleanliness, grooming or to the appropriateness of dressing.

- The person with dementia may wear the same clothes day after day and refuse to change clothing and if challenged, may become irritable and uncooperative.
- There may be confusion over the order in which clothes should be put on and with fastenings such as zips and buttons.
- The patient may dress or undress at odd times or in inappropriate places.
- He may forget to wash, shave, comb hair, brush teeth and so on, or might perform certain activities repeatedly and neglect others.
- There is lack of awareness of personal safety when using hot water, electrical appliances, razors, wet floors and so on.
- The person may have sleep disturbances.
- Some patients will eat too much food because they can't remember their last meal and will start gaining weight. Some lose weight as they don't enjoy the food, have forgotten how to use cutlery; chewing and swallowing becomes a problem.
- A person with dementia may neglect oral hygiene, which can result in oral infections, inflammation and difficulties with chewing food.

If, after evaluation, it is determined that ADL training is to be initiated, it is important to establish appropriate short and long term objectives, based on the evaluation and on the patient's priorities for independence. The following principles form the essential components for developing an ADL training program by the therapist:

- Encourage independent performance of daily living activities as long as possible and select activities within the person's physical and mental capacity (Reed, 2001). Provide assistive devices and instructing and training in the use of the same.
- Structure the environment and cue the person to help him or her participate in self-care activities for a longer period of time.
- Instruct the caregiver on helping the person perform the daily living activities that the individual can no longer perform independently in a satisfactory or safe manner.

- Make sure the patient sits upright when eating to avoid problems with swallowing. Large handles, nonskid plates and later on spoons help the patient to feed himself. Offer many small meals throughout the day and pay attention to sufficient fluid intake, 1 to 2 liters daily.
- Grade self-care activities using environment modification and task simplification as the person's capacities decline. For example, serve the person one food at a time on a plate or in a bowl and provide the appropriate utensil. Keep other food out of view. When one food is finished, serve the next food.
- Increase physical comfort to promote relaxation and sleep.
- Simple, easily cared hair styles are best and choose a comb or brush, which is easy for the person to grasp.
- Oral hygiene can be improved by giving prompts, one step at a time throughout the process of cleaning teeth or dentures, to maintain independence as much as possible. For example, for brushing, the person needs to be reminded where the brush and paste are kept and need to be directed towards the wash basin.
- Choose clothing that is easy to wear and care for. Limit choice of clothing but continue to offer a choice if possible and lay items of clothing in the order to be worn. Clothing can be made more manageable by replacing hooks, buttons and zips with velcro fastenings. Dressing aids, such as long handled shoehorns, elastic shoelaces, may help to maintain independence and make it easier to help. Take away clothes that need washing to avoid them being worn again. If the person requires complete assistance with dressing, dress him or her in stages, dressing just the top or bottom half of the body at one time. If a person has a weakness on one side, it is easiest to put clothing on this side first and remove it last.
- Before bathing, check the water temperature. A shower unit is easier to use and use a stable seat. Safety aides including non-slip mats, support rails and bath seats may be used. Having a fairly regular routine in relation to bathing can be helpful. Carefully wash and dry skin folds and check for areas of redness, dryness, rashes or sores and then a favourite body oil or lotion may be used. Lay toiletries out in order of use.

- Changing over from the use of a blade razor to an electric shaver will be safer and can enable someone to shave himself for longer.
- Allow time for activities such as washing and dressing, make sure the room is warm and comfortable and try to make things as relaxed as possible.
- Provide the maximum degree of privacy, which safety will allow.
- When the person is trying to do things, give encouragement and compliments.
- Habit training may be necessary, and should aim at establishing for each patient a routine within his capabilities, which will give him a feeling of security by reason of familiarity. Good habits will be encouraged by the provision of suitable facilities, easy access to lavatories being one of the most important.

Toileting Skills

Toileting skills form an integral part of ADL training programme and needs a special mention as it has enormous psychosocial implication. The loss of *toileting skills* is often described as a major problem in the case of dementing people and they react differently to the experience of incontinence. Some find it very distressing and humiliating; other people appear to just accept it or may even be not aware of it. Occupational therapy intervention involves prompting, social reinforcement for toileting requests and for being dry and social disapproval for being wet. The important points, which are considered while laying a program to improve the toileting skills are:

- Remind the person to go to the toilet at regular intervals, before and after meals and before bedtime. Faecal incontinence can sometimes be managed by taking the person to the toilet at a set time, if their habits are regular.
- If the person is fidgeting, getting up and down or pulling at clothes it may be because he or she wants to go to the toilet.
- If the person is having trouble urinating, try giving a glass of water or running the tap. If the person is restless and will not sit on the toilet, let him or her get up and down a few times. Music may have a calming effect or try providing something to hold or look at to distract the person while he or she is on the toilet.
- A 'toilet' sign or picture on the door of the bathroom will remind the person where it is or leave the door to the bathroom open all the time, so that the person can see the toilet.

- Make sure that there are no obstacles, or doors which are hard to open, a clear path to the bathroom with suitable lighting and the toilet should be easy to identify and use.
- Help the person to avoid having too much to drink before going to bed. However, ensure that he or she has had enough to drink during the day, 6–8 glasses.
- Incontinence can lead to skin irritation and may make the person feel uncomfortable. If the person has become wet or soiled, help him or her to wash with mild soap and warm water and dry carefully before putting on fresh pads and clothes.
- Keep men out of women's rest room and vice versa, reclothing after toilet use, offer appropriate amount of assistance during toilet use by verbally and physically cuing and protect the privacy of the patient as best as possible (Hasselkus, 1992).

The person's general level of co-operation regarding personal care tasks may fluctuate considerably. It is pointless to argue and in a short time the person with dementia will forget the dispute. Try different approaches or choose a time of day when the person is usually most co-operative. Prompting includes verbal direction or a physical prompt such as handing the person a towel. Reinforcement used could be verbal praise, a wall chart for visual feedback on progress and a choice of bathing luxury as a reward for a set level of response. Perhaps skills are not being relearned, but rather the environment is restructured to elicit the person's remaining skills.

Communication Skills

As therapists interact with patients, signals come from both verbal and nonverbal aspects of the communication. Paying attention to both areas provides clues to the patient's internal frame of reference as well as to the therapist's thoughts, feelings, and reactions (Schwartzberg, 1993). Communication is a very complex process and many communication skills are lost when a person is suffering from dementia. Expression and comprehension are both affected in the following ways:
- The ability to think of the right word may be noticeably worse in the early stages. Later, only everyday words may be used and other words lost completely.

- Pronouncing letters and words is not affected until the very late stages.
- Putting sentences together is not much affected in the early and middle stages, but may get worse later.
- Knowing when to reply is not affected at first, but the person will tend to say things, which relate to him or her rather than respond to what has been said and may fail to pick up humour, sarcasm, or subtle messages.
- In the late stages, the person may say almost nothing, or keep repeating only one or two phrases or sounds, which makes no sense.
- Defective comprehension is likely to lead to misunderstanding.

Practicing effective communication skills like clarifying expectations, defining needs honestly and providing tactful and constructive feedback can decrease the number of stressful misunderstandings. The following are the essential components to be considered while structuring the intervention program for the patient:

- When we speak to someone with dementia we must try to send messages, which the person will understand.
- Make sure that the person is paying attention to the therapist and eye contact is maintained. Gently touching and calling the person's name can draw attention.
- Keep sentences short and simple. Make one point at a time. Stick to simple, familiar ideas rather than complicated new concepts.
- Avoid suggested or implied messages and use real names, not pronouns. This reminds the person of whom you are talking about and use concrete sentences.
- Do not ask questions which need a complicated answer. Questions, which can be answered with a word or two, are best.
- Information is not easily taken in. It helps to repeat the important parts of a message.
- Gestures, body language (how we use our hands, eyes and posture), touch and tone of voice are often understood right through to the late stages of the illness. Therapist should sit in a position where the patient can see him easily.

Productivity

It is a controlling mechanism and is the ratio between the output and the resources expended to obtain the desired output. A given level of quality is always implied for any output. The person with dementia may have loss of productive skills because of memory loss and other cognitive impairments and as a result may lose his or her job or be forced to take early retirement. The therapeutic measures as follows, are aimed at planning new programs, making personnel projections, balancing workloads, improving staff effectiveness and reducing or containing costs:

- Encourage the person to participate in productive activities (work, homemaking, volunteering) as long as possible; that is, as long as the person performs at a satisfactory level or meets an acceptable standard set by an employer or other person charged with establishing and maintain these criteria.
- Modify productive tasks if such changes will permit the individuals to continue productive activity at a level of performance that is satisfactory or meets an acceptable standard.
- Polishing, dusting, tidying stacks of magazines, sweeping, making the bed, folding clothes are all activities which can often still be done successfully. Try reminiscing at the same time, recalling how things were done in the early days and that can make tasks more meaningful and enjoyable.

Leisure

It is time whose content is oriented toward self-fulfillment and is outside the needs and obligations of a person's occupation, family and society. The reasons for satisfaction with leisure include the opportunity to recreate oneself; to gain new strength or to maintain good health, and to provide variety, self-actualization, self-reflection and contemplation. The person with dementia may lose interest in activities that used to be important leisure pursuits because of lack of motor coordination, lack of motivation, diminished cognitive and perceptual performance. Some useful measures to be considered as part of therapeutic intervention and which can enhance the leisure participation are:

- Modify leisure activities within the scope of the person's interests if original activities are no longer possible or practical.
- Listening to music, singing and dancing are other activities which can be enjoyed at home right through to the later stages of dementia. Listening to familiar music can be of great comfort and can calm and distract the person.
- Reading can become difficult for someone with dementia as the concentration and mental ability to read decreases as the illness progresses. If the person would still like to read papers, magazines and books, they can be helped by reading aloud and helping the person go through the paper.
- The person with dementia can enjoy quiz programs, old films and programs about the person's special interests.
- Dominoes, card games and jigsaws are also enjoyed by many people. There are special jigsaws with larger pieces available and specially designed cards for those whose eyesight may be failing or who have arthritic fingers.
- Remembering early childhood experiences is usually an enjoyable activity, and to some people with dementia it can be the only way that they can make contact with their own identity.
- The demented person may enjoy writing about school days, past holidays and family meetings if he or she has mild dementia.
- Producing artwork is often exciting and interesting. Remember that the end results do not have to look like 'works of art'.
- If the person has always knitted or done embroidery or tapestry, he or she may retain these skills for a long time. They need to be encouraged to start and might need help at each stage, but it is worth persevering.
- Gardening and daily walk provides a change of scene and will also ensure to get some fresh air and exercise. Some people enjoy swimming throughout the course of their illness.
- Taking the person out for a drive will often calm him or her down. Driving round the areas remembered during childhood, or where the person worked, will often stimulate memories.
- Help the person stay involved in community activities. For example, the person may have been used to going to the local community centers; let him continue to go if he wants to, as it is important to keep in touch with friends and maintain a normal routine. This will ensure the person with dementia remains as part of the community and the social contact is maintained.

Sensorimotor Skills

It is interesting to note how a patient interacts with his or her environment to enable him to function at a very basic level. The special and somatic sensory systems inform the person about the environment as well as about his own body and the interface between the two. In patients with dementia, there is interference with the interpretation and perception of the meaning of the sensory information. The following are the common pattern of presentation for a patient, whose sensorimotor functions are affected:

- The person usually has increasing loss of gross and fine motor skills, coordination, manipulation, balance and equilibrium reactions.
- The person may have gait disturbances such as stumbling, wide-based or shuffling gait.
- In advanced or terminal stages, because of loss of muscle strength and joint mobility the person may have contractures.
- The person may have increasing loss of sensory awareness, registration and processing, which at times may lead to over stimulation.
- The person usually has apraxia and thus has difficulty with motor planning activities.
- The person may lose binocular vision or visual accommodation, which affects depth perception.
- The person may wander around or pace without apparent sense of purpose or direction because of lack of spatial orientation.
- Problems with agnosia may involve anosognosia, stereognosis, prosopagnosia, autotopagnosia; these impairments are often frustrating and difficult for caregivers to understand.
- Slow speed of reaction, poor sight or hearing can put a person more at risk.
- Lack of initiation, poor self-control, changes in affect, lack of self monitoring, poor motivation, and problems in planning and carrying out activity.

Treatment involves education of different sensorimotor faculties and compensatory strategies to substitute for losses. The treatment to increase sensory experiences via the intact senses may be chosen to prevent further confusion and isolation. The following are the essential considerations for enhancing the sensorimotor skills of patients with dementia:

- Encourage exercise and participation in activities to maintain mobility and general fitness.
- Use more gross motor or large motor activities when fine motor activities become difficult or impossible. Examples are walking groups, musical chairs games, dancing, balloon volleyball, or exercise groups.
- Consider therapeutic exercises and splints to prevent contractures.
- Stimulate sensory systems regularly to maintain contact with the environment, but avoid overstimulation, which may cause agitation, confusion, and catastrophic reaction.
- Maintain balance and equilibrium reactions as long as possible to reduce possible falls and injuries. Examples are the use of vestibular boards, large balls or inflatable swings or seesaws.

Cognitive Skills

Following dementia the patient is left with various degrees of cognitive dysfunction. Cognitive deficits have been found to be significantly related to eventual independence in self-care. Occupational therapist, therefore, needs to focus attention on the evaluation and restoration of these abilities as prerequisites to the overall goal of occupational therapy, which is to function as independently as possible. The cognitive dysfunctions can present in several ways, as follows:

- The person usually has increasing memory loss, which begins with recent events (short-term memory) and increases to include remote events (long-term memory). Amnesia leads to endlessly repeated questions and demands for reassurances from the patient. The memory deficit in this stage is already so severe that it is difficult to keep patient occupied with any activities.

- Stressful event results in endlessly repeated requests from the patient for reassurances. Each request appears totally new for the patient, who shows no awareness of previous reply. With further progression of the illness, the patient begins to live in the past; the names of children may be forgotten, even fail to recognize them. He may start behaving like younger person and may talk about long dead parents. The patients may deny they are married causing embarrassment to the spouse.
- They have increasing disorientation, difficulty learning and remembering new information.
- The demented person will have lack of concentration, loss of abstract thinking skills and difficulty remembering the names of things.
- The person may have loss of judgement about personal safety, loss of sense of time.
- The person may experience the symptoms becoming worse at night.

The patients may attempt to organize the environment in order to maintain the sameness of their situation. In the early stages of illness, patients usually display some form of insight into their impairment, but even in mild stages, insight may be distorted by amnesia, perplexity or retain psychological defense mechanism. The occupational therapist does an initial screening of the various cognitive deficits and then depending on the patient's life style and goals, might work on a specific area in more depth and the following guidelines may be implemented:
- Maintain current level of attention and memory for as long as possible.
- The therapist should provide with structure, predictability and consistency in his approach.
- Use clear and concise instructions and person's habitual skills when possible to facilitate performance.
- Teach compensatory memory techniques, such as writing down a daily schedule and keeping a notebook of important personal information.
- In conjunction with sensory stimulation, have the person name the type of stimulation and review a past experience with the same or similar sensory input.

- Putting together a memory box is a good way of stimulating and drawing out memories. Put favourite objects, old photos, and items from the person's work in the box to be examined.
- Remember that many people with dementia have problems concentrating and may be unable to do certain tasks for any length of time. Plan for this by having a variety of activities he can do.

Psychosocial Considerations

Psychosocial sequelae resulting from changes in health and loss of physical function prevent patients from maximizing potential and re-engaging in life activities and also present barriers to a good quality of life within the community (Versluys, 1989). The psychosocial factors influence the outcome of rehabilitation in several ways:

- The person may become restless, especially at night; increasingly irritable, frustrated and combative if unable to cope. He or she may experience delusions and paranoid thinking because of memory loss. For example, the person may accuse someone of taking an object when actually the person put the object somewhere and now does not remember.
- The person usually becomes increasingly disoriented to time, place, or person and may experience mood and affect changes, especially apathy or lability and may appear depressed.
- The patient may have a catastrophic reaction or may overreact to seemingly inconsequential things or even to something the caretaker cannot identify.
- The experience of decreased ability to write or speak as a result of aphasia and loss of spontaneity is common.
- The person may withdraw from social situations or become very agitated.
- The awareness of some form of impairment in self encourages the adoption of the sick role, which results in psychological dependency.

The dementing person is to be treated as a person and not as an object or as a vegetable. If people are to live, then they must be allowed to have life of the highest quality with psychological needs met as well as the more basic physical needs. The objective of occupational therapy is to restore a sense of individuality and dignity and the determination of a lifestyle within society that provides enough satisfaction to motivate self-monitoring of physical and emotional health. While planning a therapeutic program, following considerations may help in overcoming the psychosocial problems:

- Orient the person to the environment through reality orientation sessions, including the name, place, date, day, and weather. Use memory aids if the person can read. A life storybook may help the person connect with reality and can become a source of self-expression and pride.

- Promote self-esteem and self-worth by praising the person for maintaining self-care skills (dressing and grooming) or for engaging in a leisure activity.

- Reduce anxiety by providing a structured, organized and scheduled environment, telling the person what is going to happen in advance and what behaviour is expected of him or her (e.g., wash hands before sitting at the table for lunch).

- Increase opportunities for and participation in socialization activities through such program as sing-alongs, field trips, show-and-tell session, get-together, and entertainment.

- Promote vocalization and interaction skills through such activities as word games, object identification games, or name that tune.

- Ingroup activities, assign one task or part of the process to each member so that each can contribute. Active involvement and human contact can decrease behavioural problems, discussion of current event and materials aimed at correctly orienting group members, perhaps making links with past, may be used.

- Reduce background noise levels to increase the social atmosphere.

- Remember that the person with dementia will gradually lose the ability to do some tasks as the illness progresses, but will retain other skills. Try and be aware of these changes and adapt activities to suit him. This will reduce the amount of distress and anxiety he feels as the dementia progresses.

- Try not to be critical of how he does things. The main aim of activities is to help the person with dementia achieve what he is capable of and ensure that he is stimulated and gains a sense of achievement and satisfaction.

INTERVENTION IN THE COMMUNITY

Under the present model of managed care, individuals with dementia are treated for short periods of time for a specific problem. Caregivers and persons with dementia often have ongoing needs that are not met through such short intervention periods or through the medical model. When developing a care plan for the patient with dementia and his or her family, the professionals must consider the type of services available in the community to provide the needed support. Referrals to community resources are provided by many different health professionals depending on the needs of the person. The treatment setting often shapes the role of occupational therapy intervention. Treatment will be discussed in terms of various treatment locations and how the environment, purposeful activity, and caregiver education are used therapeutically in each situation.

Managing Person with Dementia at Home

Families provide close to 90 percent of the primary care for the older adults diagnosed with dementia who live at home. The primary issues in home care are safety, promoting independence in self-care, increasing involvement in leisure activities, and caregiver education and support. The challenge faced by occupational therapists while handling someone with dementia is how to find the right balance between protecting him or her from risk for the sake of safety. Important issues associated with self-care in the mid to late stages of dementia include maintaining adequate nutrition, ambulating without falls and incontinence.

Home safety is assessed through direct observation of the individual's activities around the house and from caregiver reports. An evaluation of the neighbourhood environment will provide a broader understanding of safety issues, especially for individuals who continue to leave the house on their own. The home environment should be adapted to allow the individual as much mobility and freedom of function as possible without putting him or her at risk of injury. The following adaptations can help to facilitate safety in the home (Skolaski-Pellitteri, 1993).

- Assess the individual's ability to understand what he or she should do in case of an emergency, for example using the telephone.
- Lock up electrical tools, knives, medicines and poisonous materials.
- Install bells or alarms on doors or at the top of the stairs to alert the caregiver of the person's location.
- Use childproof doorknobs, cabinet locks and put new locks on doors that lead outside to prevent wandering. If the patient leaves alone, make sure that a set of duplicate keys is left with the neighbour.
- A person with dementia if liable to get lost while out alone, make sure he or she has identification like a card, bracelet or pendant with name and phone number to contact.
- Make sure that lighting is bright but not dazzling in places like halls and bathrooms and night-light in bedrooms, make sure there are no shadows or reflections.
- It is not suggested to stop smoking by the dementia patient, if it is something, which gives pleasure, but it needs to be supervised since it can be a fire hazard.
- The patient's ability to walk can be affected as he finds it difficult to judge the height of objects. A flat floor with a change in colour or floor covering may be misapprehended as a step or barrier. Check the home for anything that may cause a fall, such as loose carpets, especially on the stairs, broken stair rods, slippery and highly polished floors, loose mats, trailing flexes, unsteady furniture and general clutter. If stairs are a problem, you could fit a stair gate. A lot can be done to encourage safety through simple rearrangement and keep items for everyday use within easy reach. A handrail on both sides of the stairs and by the bath and the toilet will assist and give confidence.
- Supervise the taking of medicines and lock them away once they have been taken.
- Cooking can be a hazard. Make sure that somebody is present when he or she cooks. Safety locks for kitchen cupboards and fridges may be useful. Remove control knobs from the stove and hide stove burners.
- Since a dementia patient is likely to spend quite a lot of time sitting, use a firm, comfortable chair of right height so that it is easy to sit down in and to get up from.

Family involvement in treatment is important, not only to maintain consistency of care but also to give the family members skill for coping with their own reactions to the disease. Occupational therapists play an important role in providing on-going support and education for caregivers to help them develop the skills necessary to manage the patient.

Managing Person with Dementia in Adult Day Services

As the disease progresses, the caregivers may seek other services to relieve some of the strain of providing care. Adult day service is a type of program that may relieve the caregiver of the stress resulting from continuous support and care. Programs such as these allow persons with dementia to remain in their own community settings, thus delaying permanent institutionalization. It also allows time for the caregivers to work or simply relax and refresh themselves, so they can better care for their afflicted family members.

Adult day programs usually offer several hours a day of structured recreation ingroup settings plus a meal. These programs, much like special programs in long term care facilities, offer activities such as exercise, arts and crafts, music and discussions. They are designed to provide a meaningful, structured environment in which persons with dementia can be supported and helped to retain their cognitive and physical skills. These programs usually operate six to eight hours a day for two to five days a week. Clients are dropped off at facility by their caregivers or specially arranged transportation.

Most activities in adult day programs and long term care facilities are conducted in groups. When working in a group setting, the life experiences of a person with dementia must be considered in structuring the group and setting the atmosphere of the activities. Persons with dementia, who may fear that others may recognize their inadequacies, can sometimes perceive new activities as a threat. By allowing individuals to have meaningful roles, whether singing along to an old tune, socializing with friends, or washing dishes, their self-confidence can be increased. The therapist structures activities appropriate to each individual's level of understanding and may model playful behaviour to provide an atmosphere of acceptance and minimize the perceived consequences of failure. Social contacts have been shown to help those with dementia and without social contact it is thought that individuals with dementia decline at a much faster rate. When used appropriately, activities provide moment-to-moment satisfaction and raise self-esteem. Group activities in daily day care and long-term care are variable, depending on the interests and the needs of the clients. Activities may include, but are not limited to, reminiscence, reality orientation, poetry reading, music, physical activity, and grooming.

It is important to set up routines of exercise and to include meaningful engagement in exercise as a part of the daily program. Burns and Bruell (1990) at the Minnesota Veteran's Administration Medical Center, developed a day care program structured around work tasks such as folding towels, washing tables, and doing piecemeal work, which were available for two or three hours in each afternoon. Burns and Bruell (1990) report that people who participate in these work programs return home at night more calm and tranquil. They are less likely to wander or make extra demands on their families. Dementia deprives individuals of their ability to independently perform life role responsibilities. Without occupational roles to organize daily life, there may be no sense of structure or meaning in their daily existence, and feelings of incompetence, inadequacy, and low self worth can result.

Activity groups in adult day care need to include consideration of the individuals' past and present interests and life roles in the design of a social and physical environment that will promote participation. Occupational therapists may train the staff members in specific interaction skills to enable them to design more appropriate individual treatment programs for persons with dementia. The changes in personality and behaviour seen in persons with dementia can result in decreased social and interpersonal skills and they may become unable to behave appropriately in a social situation. Sometimes the person with dementia will be better able to interact socially in a one-to-one situation or in the home. Group activities that are not appropriately structured may overstimulate, distract or frustrate the individual with dementia resulting in acting out and disturbed behaviours. It provides activities based on individual needs and preferences: activity programming should be individualized. Instead of fitting the individual into the facility's activity calendar, each activity should be planned with the individual's interest in mind. The interest checklist (Matsutsuyu, 1969) is useful in identifying personal preferences and should be reviewed with the caregiver for accuracy. Too often the only choice offered to the person with dementia who is residing in long-term care setting is to attend or not attend an activity. The occupational therapist should work with demented person to identify the particular barriers (e.g., social and physical) that limit their participation in activities.

Ensure that activities are age appropriate: participating in activities intended for children often feels demeaning to adults with dementia. All too often, personnel in long-term care facilities include children's games in their activity programming because they feel that anything else would be too complex. Occupational therapists have the training to analyze and match activities to the abilities and preferences of the demented individual to ensure successful experiences.

Normalize activities; if possible, activities should be performed in the same manner as if the person were not in long-term care. Promoting activity selection and participation based on previous interests is one way to accomplish this. One example of a normalized activity is a dining program that eliminates institutional trays and instead uses place settings, tablecloths, and soft music. In these programs staff members are encouraged to eat with the residents, which help to increase socialization and decrease the feelings of distance between them. Emphasize active participation. This can have a noticeable effect on self-perceptions of control.

Managing Person with Dementia in Residential Long-Term Care

The burden of providing continual care is sometimes too much for caregivers, who then must place the impaired person in a facility with more specialized care. Relocation to a residential long-term care facility is traumatic for any older person, but it can be especially devastating for a person with dementia. Occupational therapists devise creative environment that make the transition to long-term care easier for persons with dementia. Environments are created that make it possible for them to reestablish and maintain their routines and to participate in meaningful activities on a daily basis. Occupational therapists have recommended environmental adaptations such as painting the room the same colour as the bedroom at home, arrange for the resident's furniture and personal possessions from home in an attempt to reconstruct a familiar, stable environment. Pictures of the resident and his or her family members can also provide a basis for reminiscence with the staff. Pictures also help the staff to perceive the resident as an individual who had a rich and fulfilling life prior to admission to the facility. Caregiver's training by occupational therapist should include an emphasis on the importance of allowing for individual differences in personalizing the resident's environment, which should be structured to support the person's personal needs while maintaining his or her safety. Occupational therapists must help the caregivers engaged in the care of the individuals with dementia to understand the significance of their routines and environmental cues.

In the later stages of dementia, individuals may have neurological deficits resulting in mobility limitations and dysphasia. If dysphagia is present, the occupational therapist will complete a clinical swallowing evaluation and then make recommendations regarding food and fluid consistencies and positioning techniques. The presence of individuals who occasionally act out in bizarre way can be very disturbing to the more cognitively intact individuals in the facility. The two approaches, going along with an individual's beliefs and viewing personal beliefs as a metaphor, accept the person's view of reality, are more responsive to his or her underlying need, and are generally more effective.

CONCLUSION

Occupational therapy has a critical contribution to make to the care of persons at all stages of dementia. The specific type of occupational therapy intervention depends on the stage of illness and the manner in which cognitive impairment is manifested in daily living activities and the needs of the family or social unit. Individuals with dementia may also have other medical and psychiatry diagnosis or age-related impairments that influence therapeutic programming. Occupational therapy practitioners work directly with persons with cognitive impairments as well as with their caregivers, who may be family members, friends, or paid personnel. They may also consult with health care providers about treatment approaches and environmental modifications. Occupational therapy includes the skillful application of principles, procedures, and interpersonal processes to assess, remediate, and/or compensate for the disabilities of a mental illness and to enable a more satisfying level of performance (Mosey, 1986). Thus, mental health as a specialty practice in occupational therapy is the application of both core and specialized knowledge to those individuals with a diagnosis of mental illness.

REFERENCES

- Anonymous (1972) Occupational Therapy: Its definition and function. *Am J Occup Ther,* 26: 204.
- Bruce MA, & Borg B. (1987) Model of human occupation. In Psychosocial Occupational Therapy Frames of Reference for Intervention (Eds: MA Bruce & B Borg), (pp.153–154). NJ: SLACK.
- Burns T, & Bruell J. (1990) Work program serves veterans with Alzheimer's disease. *OT Week,* 4(44), 7–14.
- Fidler G S. (1997) The psychosocial core of occupational therapy: Position paper. *Am J Occup Ther,* 51(10).
- Hasselkus BR. (1992) The meaning of activity: Day care for persons with Alzheimer disease. *Am J Occup Ther,* 46(3), 199–206.
- Hopkins HL. (1983) A Historical Perspective on Occupational Therapy. In *Willard and Spackman's Occupational Therapy,* (Eds. HL Hopkins and HD Smith), (p.9). Philadelphia: JB Lippincott Company.
- Kielhofner G. (1985) *A Model of Human Occupation: Theory and Application.* Baltimore: Williams and Wilkins.
- Levy LL. (1993) Cognitive disability frames of reference. In *Willard and Spackman's Occupational Therapy,* (Eds. H.L. Hopkins & H.D.Smith), (pp.57–69). Philadelphia: JB Lippincott Company.
- Matsutsuyu J. (1969) The interest checklist. *Am J Occup Ther,* 23(4), 323–328.
- Mosey A. (1986) *Psychosocial Components of Occupational Therapy.* New York: Raven.
- Reed K. (2001) Other dementias. In *Quick Reference to Occupational Therapy,* (Ed K. Reed), (pp. 738–742). Maryland: Aspen Publisher, Inc.
- Robichaud L, Hebert R and Desrosiers J. (1994) Efficacy of a sensory integration program on behaviors of inpatients with dementia. *Am J Occup Ther,* 48(4), 355.
- Rogers J C. (1994) Statement: Occupational Therapy services for persons with Alzheimer's disease and other dementia. *Am J Occup Ther,* 48(11), 1029–1031.

- Saha S. (2001) Occupational Therapy. In *Plastic Surgery: Basic Principles and Techniques,* (Ed. P Kumar). Hyderabad: Paras Medical Publisher.
- Schwartzberg SL. (1993) Tools of practice. In *Willard and Spackman's Occupational Therapy* (Eds. HL Hopkins & HD Smith), (pp.270–271). Philadelphia: J.B. Lippincott Company.
- Skolaski-Pellitteri (1993) Environmental adaptations which compensate for dementia. *Journal of Physical and Occupational Therapy in Geriatrics,* 3(1), 31–44.
- Versluys HP. (1989) Psychosocial accommodation to physical disability. In *Occupational Therapy for Physical Dysfunction,* (Ed: Catherine A. Trombly), (pp13-14). Baltimore: Williams & Wilkins.
- Williams CG, Foti D & Covault M. (1998) Dementia. In *Psychosocial Occupational Therapy: A Clinical Practice* (Eds. E Cara and A MacRae), (pp. 328–330). NY: Delmar.

needs to go out to family doctors is that these patients are interesting,
challenging and rewarding to treat, and that a great deal can be done to
help everyone.

16

Care of People with Dementia in the Community

Ian Greaves, Susan M Benbow

Introduction

Most people diagnosed with a dementia are managed in the community.
Many live at home, and only rarely visit health care professionals for
advice or management. Dementias impact not only on the affected
person, but also on their family, friends and society as a whole. Social
pathology can dominate the person's management, and shape their
care plan. The stigma associated with dementia, a chronic debilitating
disease with no cure and very limited treatment, has an enormous
effect on both the public perception of dementia and the attitude of
the health and social care work force (Turner and Benbow, 2002).

Family doctors who are interested in dementia are few and far between.
A United Kingdom survey by the Audit Commission (2000) showed
that over half of the family practitioner workforce admits that they do
not know enough about dementia. Only 48% of those surveyed felt
that they had received sufficient training to help them diagnose and
manage dementia, and only 54% recognised the importance of actively
looking for early signs of dementia. Indeed, some family doctors hold
negative attitudes about giving people an early diagnosis, partly due to
the possibility of distressing people by giving them bad news and partly
because they believe that nothing can be done. The message that

needs to go out to family doctors is that these patients are interesting, challenging and rewarding to treat, and that a proactive caring approach can greatly enhance the person's quality of life.

ROLE OF THE FAMILY DOCTOR IN CARING FOR PEOPLE WITH DEMENTIA

The Audit Commission (2000) report sets out a number of roles. These are summarised below.

Early Identification

Family doctors are well placed to detect cognitive problems early and engage people in further investigations and support systems. For example, under their current terms of service, family doctors are required to offer an annual health check to their patients who are over 75 years of age. This is an opportunity to detect early cognitive impairment. Other opportunities present when people attend for flu immunisations, or screening for coronary heart disease.

Why should family doctors attempt to identify people early? A new range of drugs is available for the treatment of mild to moderate Alzheimer's disease. These are the acetyl-cholinesterase inhibitors, which increase the level of acetylcholine in the brain by blocking the enzyme, which normally breaks it down. Unfortunately, the average time between suspecting that someone may have dementia and making a formal diagnosis may be several years. In the UK, the drugs have been recommended (National Institute for Clinical Excellence, 2001) for use in people who score between 12 and 25 on the Mini Mental State Examination (Folstein et al., 1975), a formal test of cognitive function, which gives a score of up to 30. When people are referred late, they may already score below the recommended treatment range and not be considered for drug treatment. There are other advantages to early diagnosis: it is helpful in planning services for individuals, including treatments for non-cognitive symptoms. These should include psychosocial approaches. Independence can be maintained for as long as possible by environmental manipulation. Social interaction can be improved with activity programmes. People who are given an early diagnosis may be able to make decisions about how they wish to be cared for in the future and whom they wish to make decisions for them when they are unable to decide for themselves. Family doctors are not unique in medicine in being able to cure few but care for many.

Initial Assessments/Investigations

In many areas of the UK, people suspected of having a dementia attend a hospital-based memory clinic (Lindesay et al., 2002) where their illness is investigated and a diagnosis made. Often the necessary physical investigations and formal cognitive testing could be carried out at the general practitioners' (GP) surgery (clinic), which would be less frightening and less disorientating for the person concerned.

Referral to Appropriate Services

Family doctors are well placed to know what services are available locally, within health and social care as well as those run by voluntary organisations, local religious communities etc.

Support, Information and Advice

The GP may act as a source of information, advice and support, but will have links to local and national sources of further help.

Ongoing Monitoring

Often GPs are seeing people regularly in connection with their physical health, which provides an opportunity to reassess and monitor their mental health in familiar surroundings. They may have an established relationship with their patient, which can be built on and which aids the negotiation of future care and support.

Ongoing Physical Health Care

Many older adults with cognitive problems will have concurrent physical illness, which leads to regular contact with the primary care team.

Co-ordination of Care

The family doctor is the person who acts as the central point for information and care coordination.

RECOGNITION OF DEMENTIA

Health care workers who deal with dementia in the community face a series of challenges. 'Dementia' is a syndrome with many causes, not one illness. Some people find it helpful to think of it in terms of 'brain failure'. Health care workers are used to dealing with patients who have heart failure, and most family doctors are happy to diagnose and treat heart failure despite the multiple causes and poor prognosis associated with this condition. Why should the diagnosis and treatment of dementia be different?

Most family physicians in the UK who look after about 2,000 people will have about 1–2 patients a year with a new diagnosis of dementia. For them it is not a common problem. As a rule of thumb, the incidence of dementia in the UK doubles with each increasing decade of life over 60. Only 1% of 60–64-year-olds are affected, whereas dementia can be diagnosed in approximately 30% of all people aged 90 years (Medical Research Council Cognitive Function and Ageing Study, 1998). Increased longevity and changes in social demographics mean that dementia will become more of a problem in the future. Although the incidence is relatively low in comparison with chest infections or cardiovascular disease, patients with dementia cost a lot in health care resources and time. Several agencies are usually involved in their care, and care plans require good communication and multidisciplinary working practices. The first challenge is the recognition of the illness, especially in its early stages.

Be Alert to Early Signs

Dementia is not only a problem, when the patient has memory lapses. Cognitive deficits are often the first indication of change. Patient and/or family may notice a reduction in short-term memory, euphemistically called "senior moments". Most people develop compensation mechanisms such as confabulation, denial, social ritual or bad temper. It can be difficult to spot early changes, but, as the dementia progresses, there may be changes in the ability to function and interact socially. Reduction in verbal reasoning and loss of language skills can result in social isolation.

As the illness progresses, it impacts on activities of daily living and results in dependence on others. The patient presents with difficulties in feeding, dressing, and toileting, as well as more complex activities such as using money, shopping and making telephone calls. Non-cognitive signs and symptoms may develop, including depression, hallucinations, delusions, misidentifications and behavioural disturbances; the latter typified by agitation, aggression, wandering, and sexual disinhibition. Wandering, aggression and inappropriate behaviour usually occur relatively late in the illness and herald a stage when coping at home may become impossible.

Early detection is difficult but not impossible. Firstly, people need to be convinced that early presentation helps. This includes older people themselves. If doctors cannot afford the time, there are plenty of volunteers in the Alzheimer's Society. The message needs to be up beat and positive to combat the existing negative image.

Family doctors are ideally placed to make early diagnoses. Older people are seen much more often than other patients, and, if doctors don't see them, others in the primary health care team do. People aged over 75 get seen by someone at least once a year. It's a case of being alert, having the suspicion and knowing the patients well. What is important is to look for change. Some of the brighter people can cope with a considerable deterioration in their cognitive powers, whilst others may change less but soon become unable to cope. Early detection is an excellent excuse for sitting down and having a cup of tea or a sherry with the retired barrister – how else can one establish a rapport?

The other opportunity for early detection is when seeing people for other reasons, some of which might increase their chance of having a dementia. Family doctors screen everyone now for cardiovascular disease. Those people at high risk of arteriosclerosis are also at high risk of vascular dementia. High-risk patients get examined regularly and have blood taken for renal and lipids levels. They may even undergo an ECG, as it is easy then to spot a change when they have an acute event. It is easy to add a cognitive test to the cardiovascular assessment. Vascular dementia may be particularly challenging for families because it has a pattern of sudden declines and plateaus, whereas Alzheimer's is gradually progressive and perhaps more predictable.

Use Standardised Tests

The Royal College of General Practitioners in Occasional Paper 82 (Williams et al., 2002) strongly recommends that GPs should identify dementia in older patients. In general, they recommend that cognitive function be assessed in a systematic way. They recommend the following but with a warning of cultural specificity:

1. Ask the patient the time to the nearest hour (orientation).
2. Give the patient an address to recall at the end of the test. The patient should repeat the address to ensure that it has been heard correctly (recall).
3. Ask the patient to count backwards from 20–1 (attention).
4. Ask the patient to draw the face of a clock with the fingers pointing to ten to eleven.
5. If the patient fails any of these, go on to a full assessment.

The Mini Mental State Examination (MMSE) is a 30-item standardised test often used in secondary care, but it may be regarded as longwinded for use in primary care. Its advantage is that guidance regarding the use of anti-dementia drug treatments defines the range of people suitable for treatment trial in terms of MMSE score. Some family doctors do use the MMSE, but many find it long and too cumbersome for routine use.

Screen Carers for Depression

The family and carers of people with dementia require special attention. Good communication will involve informing them about the disease, its effects on everyday life and social relations, sources of care, financial benefits and legal issues including that of mental capacity. Advice, signposting and advocacy will help to guide families through the maze of service provision. Intergenerational tensions can obstruct effective care plans, unless handled with delicacy and sensitivity. Early planning to offer carer relief for family holidays and functions, combined with monitoring the impact of the burden of care, can help to prevent carer fatigue. Respite care, day hospital or day centre attendance, befriending and sometimes a shoulder to cry on, all are potentially beneficial. Only the family and person concerned can decide when the time is right to utilise such resources. The voluntary bodies do remarkable work and a close working relationship with the Alzheimer's society and other bodies can be enormously beneficial to the family doctor and to their patients. There is a wealth of information available both in an electronic form and as printed material. Guidelines published by European working groups and American societies may assist practical management.

Link with Old Age Psychiatry for Training and Support

At present most of the people who have been diagnosed with dementia are referred to secondary care, and in the majority of cases the service they get is excellent. Many secondary care services are, like primary care services, stretched to breaking point. Over a third of the family doctors in the Audit Commission survey (2000) felt that they did not have ready access to specialist advice. Specialist teams for older people with mental health problems were fully available in less than half of all areas and partly available in a further third. Most did not have a full complement of recommended core team members. The National Institute for Clinical Excellence put a further burden on these services, when it approved cholinesterase inhibitors for initiation only by specialists in mild to moderate Alzheimer's disease (National Institute for Clinical Excellence, 2001).

The common sense approach to all this would seem to be joint working. The prevalence of the disease does not justify the transfer of memory clinics into primary care. The future of dementia care is likely to involve clearly defined pathways of care. These will serve to break down the tribal barriers of service provision, to improve consistency and rapidity of diagnosis, and to set out best practice for management. This does not necessarily mean doing anything differently – just better.

General adult psychiatrists run outpatient clinics at the surgery in Gnosall. This has reduced stigma and brings services closer to the patient. Failed appointments have reduced from 30% to 1%. Family doctors have gained confidence in the diagnosis and treatment of common psychiatric problems. It is amazing how much diffuses subconsciously into a doctor's brain over a cup of coffee with a consultant colleague. Similarly, the family doctor's background information on patients is vital and much better given verbally than in a 3-page letter of referral. It is easy to help prepare the patient for a consultant opinion, both in the physical work-up with the blood tests and other things that need to be done, and by using our position as the trusted family doctor to help them understand the process and guide them through the multidisciplinary assessments that lie in front of them. Resources are shared – primary care practice nurses, community nurses, and health visitors, are shared with community psychiatric nurses, respite services, day hospitals and other therapeutic options.

The way forward for older people with mental illness must lie in close working between all the agencies and disciplines involved. We could mutually agree pathways of care, with family doctors doing the things they are good at, and consultant old age psychiatrists concentrating on what they are good at. Perhaps particular groups can be targeted to get earlier identification of patients with suspected dementia, and basic investigations can be carried out in primary care to improve the quality of referral. Family doctors could monitor consultant initiated therapies and enact treatment plans: this already happens for diabetics and people with cardiovascular disease. Consultants would see new referrals more quickly and bail out the primary care service when a crisis occurs. Perhaps some of the Community Psychiatric Nurses could regularly visit the nursing homes and help improve the lot of patients with end stage dementia, where the condition is much too severe for them to remain at home.

The social worker who visited the Gnosall practice as part of a pilot scheme was bribed by coffee and compliments to stay on for a few days every week. She now has direct referrals and can sort out problems rapidly, before they become chronic and enduring. Her case management has improved: most problems are dealt with within 2 or 3 days rather than 6–9 months. In exchange, the primary care team gives her nursing and medical input, and, more importantly, has begun to understand her role, and work with her as an integrated team.

In the United Kingdom and elsewhere, government departments are unlikely to commit a lot more funding to care for older people. It is up to health and social care professionals to do the best they can with the resources at their disposal. Examples of best practice abound, and the future of old age psychiatry lies in greater integration with primary care and social services.

Inform Families of Diagnosis

Early diagnosis provides the opportunity to inform families and patients about the illness at a stage when they might be able to make decisions which will influence their future care. This in itself can be challenging as families and doctors often have many concerns about how someone will react to knowing they have Alzheimer's disease or a similar illness (Pinner, 2000).

Provide Information

Once the family and the person with dementia know what the diagnosis is, everyone concerned will need information which is timely, understandable and in a helpful format. Some people can be given suggestions of websites to visit and select topics to read about and later discuss with the health care professionals in contact with them. The Alzheimer's Society website is a gateway to a wealth of useful information. Other families will need a lot of verbal information, sometimes supplemented by information packs. Written information is no substitute for information-giving and discussion, but is a useful adjunct.

Refer to Support Groups (Alzheimer's Society, Age Concern)

Many old age psychiatry services and voluntary agencies run relatives support groups. Some run groups for the people with dementia themselves, and those who have experience of these groups often find them very supportive and gain invaluable information from the others who attend.

COMMON COMMUNITY PRESENTATIONS

A few lucky patients are detected early, either in screening clinics such as the over 75 checks or as part of a routine consultation with their family doctor. Unfortunately, it is not uncommon for concerned relatives or neighbours to present demanding urgent action because the family cannot cope. The phrase that brings a feeling of dread to most family doctors (and old age psychiatrists) is "something must be done doctor". It is often very distressing for relatives to see progressive changes in the cognitive ability and social function of someone they love and admire. Late presentations by relatives who have come to the end of their tether are often associated with complete social breakdown, resulting in a sense of urgency and desperation. The health care worker has to deal with both the person with dementia and the family's feelings of guilt, despair and fear. This presentation may come through other members of the primary health care team, such as health visitors or practice nurses. Wardens who look after people in sheltered accommodation may report changes in behaviour, or deterioration in the ability of residents to look after themselves. Sometimes the person may only be drawn to attention with a request for input from another agency, such as social services or a voluntary agency such as the Alzheimer's Society. This could be in the form of a request to complete the medical assessment form for a social care plan or for residential home placement.

Another common presentation is the request to visit patients in residential homes where there has been a deterioration in their mental health. Staff members report that they cannot cope with abnormal behaviour and want referral for psychiatric assessment or prescription of a sedative medication.

Nighttime wandering is one of the most difficult presentations, when the police phone a family doctor whose patient has been found wandering. The relatives and police see this as urgent, and it is often time consuming and difficult for the GP to impress the same view on the other agencies. In situations like this, team work helps to overcome everyone's frustrations and fears.

Why do Patients Present Late?

Despite the introduction of anti-dementia drug treatments many people are still referred late in the course of their illness. There are many factors in this:

1. Fear – there is nothing more frightening at any stage of life than the fear of losing one's mind.

2. Futility – nothing can be done. There are no treatments that work. Those who don't want to know the answer, don't ask the question.
3. Social isolation – elderly people who only see their relatives on limited occasions may quietly deteriorate and this is only picked up at Christmas or family functions.
4. Fear of nursing homes – 'If I go to the doctor they will say I have got to go into a nursing home … I would rather die'.
5. Stigma – 'I don't want the social round here. What will people say?'
6. Cost – 'I have worked all my life to save something for the kids … I am not losing it all now'.
7. Intergenerational tensions – 'It's not fair on my children … they have their own lives'.
8. Senior moments and denial –'everyone gets forgetful as they get older, it's normal.'
9. Stubbornness – 'You can't make me. I was born here and I will die here'.
10. Not too bad – 'I am all right, I don't believe that I left the cooker on … I can't remember that'.

AFTER DIAGNOSIS: WHAT NEXT?

The facilities for looking after older people and especially those with dementia vary across the world. In rich countries the state offers both financial and physical help through social services agencies. This can range from care plans, designed to keep the patient at home, through to some form of assisted, residential or nursing home accommodation.

The type and level of community care provided depends as much on the beliefs and values of individuals and community as on the availability of service provision. In poorer countries the responsibility for care of elderly relatives falls entirely on the family. It is perceived as a family responsibility to look after relatives, and this can cause enormous strain. As long as there are sufficient number of younger family members, families may be able to support their elders. Unfortunately, there is a marked change in social demography: the population is living longer and the burden of elder care falls onto a dwindling workforce. We have yet to face the consequences of the one child policy of China.

Similarly, the effect of community responsibility is illustrated by the story of a man with profound dementia who was cared for in a small village near Cork in Southern Ireland. He remained in the community where he was born and had lived all his life. He received state benefit of about 200 euros, and once a week was transported to Cork for a bath and change of clothes. The community as a whole accepted the responsibility of looking after him. He was known as "Psycho" — more a term of endearment than a term of abuse. He spent his days propped up in the corner of one or other of the local bars, where the landlord provided and regulated his consumption of Guinness beer and bar food. He was liable to explosive outbursts of bad language and wandering. The community accepted him and tolerated his outbursts and he continued to function, albeit at a lower level, in familiar surroundings.

Unfortunately, the community spirit that sustains this level of social and family care is often missing in some of the richer western societies. Intergenerational tensions arise as families struggle with the competing demands of a busy work life, childcare and eldercare. As a result, there is a greater need for state provision and a complex series of care agencies are often involved.

Care in the community requires a considerable amount of teamwork, with each agency understanding and respecting the other's expertise. Leadership of community teams can be difficult. There is a presumed hierarchy in the service professions where traditionally the senior medical consultant is seen to be the co-ordinator of the care plan. This model can create difficulties as the patient may not be reviewed regularly or by the same person, and outpatient clinics are not the best places to assess an individual's needs. Some services carry out all follow up visits in the community (Benbow, 1990), but this may be more appropriate in high-population urban areas than dispersed rural communities. In some services the person who is providing the bulk of the support assumes the leadership role and co-ordinates reviews of the client's needs. This Key Worker model encourages continuous assessment. It is economical in that the package of care is responsive and appropriate to the patient's needs. Community care should support families and carers and be proactive, in order to prevent the crises that often cause disillusionment, frustration and breakdown of home-based care. The introduction of admiral nurses, whose role is to address and champion the needs of family carers, is one model of sustaining community care. Community care teams, which include mental health nurses, social workers and other support agencies, provide similar patterns of carer support and offer interventions to prevent social breakdown and provide appropriate support to families.

Domiciliary care workers provide practical support to the patients with dementia in the community. They visit the patient in their home to provide essential help with dressing, personal hygiene and other activities of daily living, especially where the family are hard pressed to provide care. One of the problems is that they work for private agencies, and their services are commissioned by social services. They may have many patients to look after in a day, and the patient's needs may not be compatible with the timetable of the agency. The behavioural symptoms of patients with dementia can add to this problem, and relatives frequently complain about the inflexible timing of agency care interventions. Legislation in the UK changed recently and now allows state finance to go directly to the family of the patient so that they can commission the type and level of care required, shifting the focus of responsibility back to families. This has enabled a lot of families of patients with dementia to tailor care plans round the family provision and create sufficient flexibility for people to remain at home for longer.

Care plans should include provision of respite and day care services. Unfortunately, nursing homes have become financially less viable and many have closed, reducing the availability of good respite care. This is short sighted, as the burden of care on relatives, rather than the severity of the cognitive impairment, often determines admission to permanent care.

The voluntary agencies are an invaluable resource in managing the care of people with dementia in the community. They provide a range of services from patient and carer education, support and advocacy, through to befriending and sitting services. Voluntary workers frequently have a wealth of experience as they may have cared for their own relatives with dementia. Charitable societies such as the Alzheimer's Society provide a vast range of skilled and informed people to help people with dementia.

Occupational therapists can assess the homes of people with dementia to provide aids and adaptations that help maintain independence. An enormous amount of research has focussed on the abilities, rather than the disabilities, of people with dementia. They do best in a friendly familiar environment. Simple measures, such as good lighting and primary colour decoration, can make life less stressful for people with dementia and their carers. Familiar furniture, contemporary with the time that the patient was at the peak of their performance, is also helpful.

Although written and verbal communication is reduced, people with dementia can be stimulated with music and other art forms. The brain is a complex organ and there are many ways of compensating for reduced function. Such therapies certainly have a role in the rehabilitation of patients in the community.

Patient Centred Rehabilitation in the Community

Perhaps the best way to illustrate this is to share a personal experience. One family hired the local village hall for a party for mother's 90th birthday. She had about 50 friends who had survived to the fourth stage of life. As a special treat, the George Formby Society was engaged to come and entertain the old folks with some singing. It took an immense effort to get people out of their homes and into the hall and they all sat around with vacant stares, occasionally speaking to one of the family, as they dished out tea and cakes. Then the man from the society started. The atmosphere was transformed as tunes of yesteryear rang out. Feet were tapping and everyone, who half an hour before looked disinterested, joined in with the familiar lyrics. They were laughing and giggling at the saucy bits, and the place and people came to life. They knew all the words, and some even started to give the younger people far too much information about the goings on at the local RAF camp during the war. The lesson here was obvious.

Just as we need to teach the man with one leg to hop, we also need to engage the working portions of the brain in those with dementia. We should engage them in music, art and reminiscence therapies, or what ever else makes people communicate on their own sterms, not those of others. Rehabilitation can be fun if it aims to get people smiling and enjoying themselves.

REFERENCES

- Audit Commission (2000) *Forget Me Not – Mental Health Services for Older People.* London: Audit Commission.
- Benbow SM (1990). The community clinic - its advantages and disadvantages. *International Journal of Geriatric Psychiatry*, 2, 119–121.
- Folstein MF, Folstein SE, McHugh PR. (1975) Mini-mental state: a practical method for grading the cognitive state of patients for clinicians. *Journal of Psychiatric Research*, 12, 189–198.
- Lindesay J, Marudkar M, van Diepen E, Wilcock G. (2002) The second Leicester survey of memory clinics in the British Isles. *International Journal of Geriatric Psychiatry*, 17, 41–47.
- Medical Research Council Cognitive Function and Ageing Study (1998) Cognitive function and dementia in six areas of England and Wales: the distribution of MMSE and the prevalence of GMS organicity level in the MRC CFA study. *Psychological Medicine*, 28: 319–335.
- National Institute for Clinical Excellence (2001) Guidance on the use of donepezil, rivastigmine and galantamine for the treatment of Alzheimer's disease. *Technology Appraisal Guidance No 19.* London: Department of Health.
- Pinner G. (2000) Truth-telling and the diagnosis of dementia. *British Journal of Psychiatry*, 176, 514–515.
- Turner SJ and Benbow SM. (2002) Dementia, stigma and the general practitioner. *Hospital Update*, 64, 45–47.
- Williams EI, Fischer G, Junius U, Sandholzer H, Jones D & Vass M. (Editors) (2002) An evidence-based approach to assessing older people in primary care. *Occasional Paper, 82.* London: Royal College of General Practitioners.

17

Rehabilitation in Dementia: Cognitive Behaviour Therapy for Carers

Ravi Samuel, Shanthini V, Krishnamoorthy Srinivas

Introduction

In the early stage of dementia, primary difficulties are loss of memory, disorientation, restlessness, despondency and anxiety. In this stage, assistance required can be in the form of patiently answering to repeated questions and giving constant reassurance. However, in later stages, physical assistance can be overwhelming to provide help in activities of daily living, managing incontinence, wandering and co-morbid neurological, psychiatric and cardiovascular conditions (Rajkumar and Samuel, 1996). Carers experience mixed emotions about their increasing responsibility and the sight of a loved member of the family suffering from a debilitating condition (Acton et al., 2001). Hence, a rehabilitation approach in which the primary focus is on the carer with the objective of reducing their emotional problems and increasing their efficacy in dealing with the challenges of care giving is discussed in this chapter.

The Process of Care Giving

A patient with dementia will require increasing levels of assistance all through the day necessitating one person to devote all his/her time. With the family system moving towards nuclear family from the concept of joint family, traditional values of filial obligations and responsibility get altered. Hence, quite naturally, the spouse has to take the primary responsibility for the patient. In a joint family, though the primary responsibility of caring is on the spouse, daughter or daughter-in-law and other members of the family contribute directly or indirectly (Rajkumar and Samuel, 1994). In homes where daughter-in-law is not working, she takes the primary care of the patient. When a family can afford to keep a paid assistance, the intensity of caring is shared with the formal carer; but the patient may have difficulty in relating to a new acquaintance for tasks, which are personal in nature. However, a vast majority of Indian population falls into middle class and lower class bracket and keeping a paid assistance may not be quite feasible due to financial constraints. In addition, shame due to patient's behaviour and stigma associated with mental illness, can be barriers to using paid services. Further, geriatric services are in their infancy in India; consequently, there are no respite care centres, dementia nursing homes, institutional care and hospice (Cohen, 1999). So, it is the family members who necessarily have to take care of the patient in their residence with occasional hospitalisation for medical problems. The cost of hospitalisation may also prevent the carer to have the patient in the hospital for long periods.

Care giving with increasing responsibilities can lead to the carers developing interpersonal problems, stress, burden and even physical and mental exhaustion (burn-out) (Samuel, 2000). Carers can experience such negative emotions either due to practical or perceived problems. Assuming over responsibility for the patient; in spite of having done their best, feeling guilty that they have not done much; attributing the patient's illness to his/her previous habits or behaviour are some of the common emotional triggers that the carers individually or collectively experience. Managing certain tasks like cleaning after incontinence, experiencing physical and verbal aggression, searching for the patient if he/she is into the stage of wandering, can lead to extreme negative emotions like anger, frustration, disgust etc. The increase in the symptoms such as incontinence, combativeness, crying, wandering can be influenced by the carer's reaction; a calm response from the carer is likely to make the patient relax unlike an agitated response.

Stigma is accentuated by neuropsychiatric symptoms in the patient. The families can face ridicule among neighbours especially if they think that the person has become insane. Cognitive impairment, particularly poor memory, inability to make decisions, inability to speak coherently are all associated with ageing process; so, families normally do not experience difficulty in the initial stages of the illness (Samuel, 2001).

It is Not Just Burden

The family members of patients with dementia have been referred to as 'hidden' victims (Zarit et al., 1985). Mace and Rabins (1991) used an expression '36 hour day' to signify the kind of schedule a carer is likely to have caring for a dementia patient. Factors such as the carer's personal character, coping repertoire, duration of care, knowledge of the disease and nature of previous relationship, will influence subjective perception of care giving. It is not that all carers report their whole experience of caring just as 'burden' (Dias et al, 2004). They take their responsibility as their chance to contribute to the patient's well being. Carers' emotional experiences can range from feeling guilty of not providing sufficient care to extreme frustration of caring. Carers experience negative emotions when they have poor mastery and control over the situation.

Carers Problems

Directly Related to Patient
- Debilitating cognitive and functional decline.
- Expenditure incurred directly for medical and non-medical purposes.
- Loss of income of the patient.
- Emotional strain of witnessing gradual deterioration of a loved one.

Indirectly Caused by Patient
- Compromising on caring of other elderly and small children at home.
- Since caring leads to physical and emotional strain, carers have an increased risk of developing serious physical and mental health problems.
- Carers' loss of income if they have to give up their job to care.

Independent Problems

- Carers will be unable to pursue their jobs, studies, own interests and pleasurable activities.
- Unemployment, other's illness, sudden death of a family member etc.
- Interpersonal conflicts among family members.

COGNITIVE BEHAVIOUR THERAPY

Cognitive behaviour therapy (CBT) is an integration of cognitive and behavioural approaches. Client is helped to recognize patterns of distorted thinking and dysfunctional behaviour. Systematic discussion and carefully structured behavioural assignments are then used to help carers evaluate and modify their distorted thoughts, faulty interpretations and behaviours (Hawton et al., 1998).

Cognitive Distortions

Cognitive distortions are habitual thought patterns used consistently by an individual to interpret reality in an unreal way. Distortions are a matter of style and may be based on deeply held unrealistic beliefs. Distorted thinking styles are hard to diagnose and treat because they are bound up tightly with an individual's way of perceiving reality. Distorted thinking styles cut off an individual from reality in several ways. Distortions are judgemental; automatically apply labels to people and events before one gets a chance to evaluate them. They also tend to be inaccurate and imprecise and are invariably general in scope and application, failing to take special circumstances and characteristics into account. They give unbalanced view of the world and are based on emotional rather than rational processes.

The Most Common Distortions

Overgeneralization

Instead of taking all the factors into consideration before reaching a conclusion, in overgeneralization the person takes a few factors into consideration and makes a conclusion. The key words used in overgeneralization are: *never, always, all, every, none, no one, nobody, everyone* and *everybody*. For example: the carer thinks, "I should *always* be there for the patient"; "*Nobody* else will be able to care for the patient like I do"; "Nobody wants to help me in caring for the patient".

Filtering / Selective Attention

In filtering, only certain things are heard or seen. Only a particular kind of stimuli is paid attention to, e.g., loss, rejection, unfairness etc. When the patient abuses, carer can think that the patient is 'ungrateful', 'difficult to care for' and may not appreciate moments in which the patient was quiet or was co-operative for other activities.

Self-Blame

Self-blame is a distorted thinking style in which carers blame themselves for everything. Self-blame blinds a person to his/her good qualities and accomplishments.

Personalisation

All events are interpreted to have to do with the person and there is very little sense of control of events. It feels more like the person is under pressure, under siege or under observation by everyone around. Carers can blame themselves for all that goes wrong: patient's wandering, aggression, financial problems etc. Personalisation makes one react inappropriately and create emotional problems for themselves and those around them.

Emotional Reasoning

An emotional universe is chaotic, governed by changeable feelings instead of rational laws. The distortion in this thinking style is to interpret reality and react according to the emotion. Combativeness during bathing or feeding can make the carer break down or start yelling, if he/she interprets that the patient is being difficult with him/her. In reality, it may just be that the patient may not feel like taking a bath at that time of the day.

The Therapy

The client should be informed that cognitive behavioural approach is largely self-help, and that the therapist aims to help the client to develop skills to overcome not only current problems but also any similar ones in future. The therapist should emphasize the role of homework assignments, clearly indicating that major part of the therapy takes place in everyday life, with the client putting into practice what has been discussed in treatment sessions. The collaborative nature of the therapeutic relationship should be discussed; the client is expected to participate actively by collecting information, giving feedback on effectiveness of techniques, and making suggestions about new strategies. Information about the structure of treatment should also be given as to how many treatment sessions will be needed, how long each session will last and where the treatment will take place.

In cognitive behaviour therapy, considerable emphasis is placed on expressing concepts in operational terms and on empirical validation of treatment. Much of the treatment is based on here-and-now, and there is an assumption that the main goal of therapy is to help clients bring about desired changes in their lives. Thus, the treatment focuses on the opportunity of new adaptive learning, and on producing changes outside the clinical setting. Problem solving is an integral part of treatment. All aspects of therapy are made explicit and the client endeavours to work in a collaborative relationship in which they plan together strategies to deal with clearly identified problems. Therapy is time limited, and has explicitly agreed goals.

CBT can help facilitate the process of reducing strain of care giving by changing faulty conceptualisation of problems; intrapersonal, interpersonal and problem focused coping and enabling carer to seek commonsense solutions to problems, which they may be unable to think on their own, due to preoccupation with various activities (Samuel, 2000).

In CBT, antecedent events, problematic behaviour and consequences of such behaviour on patient and family are elicited and then based on systematic discussion; carefully structured behavioural assignments are used to help carers modify their response. Here follows an example: quite frequently the carers report that the patient tries to go out of the house, saying that he/she wants to go to 'his/her house'. If any attempt is made to prevent him/her from going out, he/she is only likely to become aggressive and abusive! Instead if he/she is taken out of the house for a walk, the family can avoid the patient getting aggressive.

Thus CBT enables the carer to develop mastery over symptoms over which they are distressed.

CONCLUSION

Much of the distresses experienced by the carer can be due to their perception of the situation. The demanding task of caring for a person with dementia can impair perception and lead to cognitive distortion. CBT aimed towards minimising if not eliminating cognitive distortions and helping to schedule care giving activities will enable carer to reduce distress, thereby avoiding experiencing the feeling of burden and burn out. The quality of life of the carer has to be good if he/she has to provide optimal care to the person with dementia (Samuel, 2001). An agitated carer can adversely affect the mood of the already confused patient. Hence, it would be beneficial to have CBT as an intervention for the carers in rehabilitation of the patient.

REFERENCES

- Acton GJ and Kang J. (2001) Interventions to reduce the burden of care giving for an adult with dementia: a meta-analysis. *Research in Nursing and Health,* 24(5), 349–360.
- Cohen L. (1999) *No Ageing in India: Modernity, Senility and the Family:* New Delhi: Oxford University Press.
- Dias A, Samuel R, Patel V, Prince M, Parameshwaran R and Krishnamoorthy ES. (2004) The Impact Associated with Caring for a Person with dementia. A report from the 10/66 Dementia Research Group's Indian network. *International Journal of Geriatric Psychiatry,* 19, 182–184.
- Hawton K, Salkovskis P M, Kirk J, and Clark M D. (1998) *Cognitive Behaviour Therapy for Psychiatric Problems: A Practical Guide.* Oxford: Oxford University Press.
- Rajkumar S & Samuel R. (1994) Planning of services. In *Trends in the Management of Dementia.* (Eds. Rajkumar S and Samuel R), p38–39. Madras: Alzheimer's Disease and Related Disorders Society of India.
- Rajkumar S, Samuel, R, and Sahabdeen M. (1996) Burden in caregivers of Alzheimer's disease patients. In *Ageing: Indian Perspective and Global Scenario.* (Ed. Vinod Kumar) P: 249–252. New Delhi: All India Institute of Medical Sciences.
- Samuel R. (2000) Rehabilitation of patients with Alzheimer's disease: An Indian perspective. *In Creative Care: Proceedings of World Alzheimer Congress,* Washington D.C.

- Samuel R. (2000) The role of social worker in rehabilitation of dementia patients. In *Gernotological Social Work in India.* (Eds. Desai M and Raju S) P: 341–352. New Delhi: B.R. Publishing Corporation.
- Samuel R. (2001) A study on well-being of male elderly persons and burden experienced by carers. Master of Philosophy Dissertation, Madras University.
- Samuel R, Rajkumar S and Prabhu R. (1994) Quality of life of the elderly. In *Quality of Life in Health: A Modern Concern.* (Eds. Rajkumar S and Kumar S), p 96–105. Chennai: Madras Medical College.
- The 10/66 Dementia Research Group. (2004) Care arrangements for people with dementia in developing countries. *International Journal of Geriatric Psychiatry,* 19, 170–177.

18

Update on Research in Dementia

Anthony James Elliott

Introduction

Research in dementia is continuing at a tremendous rate, spurred on by the desire for new treatments and the demographic of an ageing population across the world, as by 2025, the world's population 65 years of age and above will be more than double what it is now. The financial and social costs of Alzheimer's disease are staggering. In the United States, the disease accounts for about $100 billion per year in medical and custodial expenses, with the average patient requiring an expenditure of about $27,000 per year for medical and nursing care. In addition, 80 percent of caregivers report stress, and about 50 percent report depression (Small et al., 1997).

As a consequence, research into the causes, effects and treatments of dementia are extremely important. Developments are diverse and a comprehensive review is out of the scope of this chapter. Therefore, this chapter will review important aspects of dementia research, including current thinking relating to the genetics and pathophysiology of Alzheimer's disease, the evidence for the efficacy of various pharmacologic treatments, the concept of 'Mild Cognitive Impairment' (MCI), the ethical issues relating to disclosing the diagnosis of dementia, and finally an update on dementia research initiatives taking place in the developing world.

Genetics of Alzheimer's Disease

In terms of genetics, Alzheimer's disease (AD) is a polygenic, complex disorder in which more than 50 genetic loci are involved. A combination of genetic predisposition and environmental influences is probably responsible for the phenotypic expression of the disease (St George-Hyslop, 2000). It appears that AD patients show about 3–5 times higher genetic variation than the control population (Cacabelos, 2003).

To date, mutations in three genes have been shown to lead to AD: the amyloid precursor protein gene (APP), presenilin 1 (PSEN1) and presenilin 2 (PSEN2). PSEN1 is the most frequently mutated early onset AD (EOAD) gene with a mutation frequency of 18 to 50% in autosomal dominant. In addition, the epsilon 4 allele of the gene encoding apolipoprotein E (ApoE) has been identified as a risk factor for both late onset and early onset AD. Many studies have reported other susceptibility genes, but the ApoE epsilon 4 alelle has been the only risk factor that has been consistently replicated in all AD populations (Rademakers et al., 2003). Extensive cell biology research in the past ten years has led to the hypothesis that the 4 EOAD genes lead to AD through a common biological pathway resulting in abnormal APP processing by subtle different mechanisms.

The Pathophysiology of Alzheimer's Disease

Two microscopic changes occur in the brain in Alzheimer's disease: senile plaques develop between neurons, and neurofibrillary tangles develop within neurons. These changes are thought to be intricately related to the cause, development, and course of the disease. Researchers have speculated that inflammation around plaques destroys neighbouring neurons. Plaques, which are composed of β-amyloid polypeptides, seem to form as a result of disorders in processing β-amyloid and its precursor protein. A further influence may be subclinical ischaemia, because patients with high blood pressure and elevated cholesterol levels tend to have an increased risk for Alzheimer's disease (Kivipelto et al., 2001).

Neurofibrillary tangles are made up partly of a protein called tau, which links together to form filaments. The density of these filaments within neurons in the brain is directly related to the severity of dementia. It is unclear why tangles form, but different alleles of a gene are known to create forms of tau that are more likely to tangle. It is also unclear whether tangles are linked to plaque formation. The ultimate effect of the tangles, however, is compromise of microtubular function, with eventual destruction of the neuron.

Involvement of cholinergic neurons causes levels of acetylcholine within synapses to decline. Levels of acetylcholinesterase also drop, perhaps to compensate for the loss of acetylcholine. While no drug has been shown to completely protect neurons, agents that inhibit the degradation of acetylcholine within the synapse are the mainstay of treatment for Alzheimer's disease. Their use and the research relating to other more controversial treatments will now be reviewed.

The Evidence for Acetylcholinesterase Inhibitors

The acetylcholinesterase inhibitors donepezil, rivastigmine, and galantamine have been proved to be beneficial in patients with Alzheimer's disease in clinical trials (Rosler et al., 1999). They appear to be effective to a greater or lesser degree in the areas of cognition, behaviour, and functional ability.

All 24 to 26 week clinical trials showed statistically significant benefit against recognized cognitive assessment scales such as the ADAS-cog. Cognitive benefits were sustained over 1 to 2 years, and deterioration of cognition will be delayed by one year in about 20 percent of treated patients (Clegg et al., 2001).

A galantamine trial reported statistically significant improvement in behavioural disturbance assessed by the Neuropsychiatric Inventory (NPI) (Tariot et al., 2000). A subsequent trial of donepezil also suggested benefit. It is important to note, however, that these trials routinely excluded patients with severe behaviour disorders, or minimised the number of such patients in the trial, which may have resulted in an overstatement of the benefits of drug therapy.

Apart from benefits to the clinical state of the patients, there is some evidence that these drugs may reduce the need for care. One trial of the first acetylcholinesterase inhibitor, tacrine, showed a reduced risk of future nursing home placement (Knopman et al., 1996). Statistical extrapolations from completed trials of donepezil have also showed a 12 to 21 month delay to nursing home placement.

Although clinical trials have shown benefits, these benefits may not apply to all patients with Alzheimer's disease. For example, patients might be excluded from studies if they have significant coexisting illnesses with symptoms that could be confused with drug side effects. Consequently, the study population might consist of patients who are more likely to respond to the drug.

Acetylcholinesterase inhibitors must be taken regularly and in a dosage sufficient to benefit the patient. Moreover, prolonged interruptions of therapy have been associated with sustained and irreversible cognitive decline (Cummings et al., 2002).

The drugs are associated with typical cholinergic side effects such as nausea, anorexia, vomiting, and diarrhoea, but tolerance to these side effects often develops. However, if therapy with an acetylcholinesterase inhibitor is interrupted for more than several days, drugs need to be restarted at the lowest dosage and retitrated, because of renewed susceptibility to side effects.

Other Treatments

The other recently approved medication for AD is memantine, which is an N-methyl D-aspartate (NMDA) antagonist. It is licensed for the treatment of moderate to severe AD. It is believed to work by regulating glutamate, another important brain chemical that, when produced in excessive amounts, may lead to brain cell death. Because NMDA antagonists work very differently from cholinesterase inhibitors, the two types of drugs can be prescribed in combination.

Studies have shown that the main effect of memantine is to delay progression of some of the symptoms of moderate to severe AD, and allow patients to maintain certain daily functions a little longer (Reisberg et al., 2003).

Vitamin E, an antioxidant, is thought to mitigate the inflammatory effects of plaque formation in the brain. In vitro, vitamin E protects nerve cells from the effects of β-amyloid, but it does not protect against other central nervous system diseases such as Parkinson's disease, in which oxidation is thought to play a part in neuronal destruction (The Parkinson Study Group, 1993).

The argument for the use of vitamin E comes from the Alzheimer's Disease Cooperative Study, which evaluated the effects of 10 mg of selegiline once daily and/or 1,000 IU of vitamin E twice daily as treatments for Alzheimer's disease. The researchers concluded that these agents delayed disability and nursing home placement but not deterioration of cognitive function (Sano et al., 1997). The study population appeared, however, to be highly selected. The subjects were younger but had more severe dementia than control patients and were not taking psychoactive medication. Consequently, there have been questions about whether the results of the study are applicable to a clinical setting.

A recent review (Tabet et al., 2003) concluded that after adjusting for differences between patient groups in the Alzheimer's Disease Cooperative Study, there was insufficient evidence to recommend vitamin E. The review also found weak evidence of side effects associated with the use of vitamin E. The risks may be higher in the general population, in which many patients with Alzheimer's disease also have serious coexisting illnesses.

A number of studies have examined evidence for the use of selegiline, a selective monoamine oxidase inhibitor, in the treatment of AD. Most of these studies have shown some improvement in cognition, behavior, and mood, but little evidence of a global benefit in cognition, functional ability, and behaviour. A recent meta-analysis of 15 clinical trials concluded that there was not enough evidence to recommend selegiline as a treatment for Alzheimer's disease (Birks and Flicker, 2003).

Several descriptive studies have shown that postmenopausal women who take oestrogen have a lower incidence of Alzheimer's disease (Tang et al., 1996). In addition, a recent review of oestrogen and neuroimaging studies demonstrated improved cerebral metabolism in women taking oestrogen (Maki and Resnick, 2001). Although oestrogen may have a neuroprotective effect (Goodman et al., 1996) it does not, however, appear to improve cognition or function in patients with Alzheimer's disease (Mulnard et al., 2000). Moreover, the combination of oestrogen and progesterone actually may increase the risk for dementia and stroke (Wassertheil-Smoller et al., 2003).

Inflammation surrounding beta-amyloid plaques with resultant destruction of neurons is thought to be a key factor in the pathogenesis of Alzheimer's disease. Observational studies have found that persons who regularly use non-steroidal anti-inflammatory drugs (NSAIDs) have a decreased incidence of Alzheimer's disease (Veld et al., 2001). Thus, NSAIDs are likely having some neuroprotective effect. Several studies of anti-inflammatory drugs, however, have not shown a benefit for treatment (Aisen et al., 2000).

A recent review of four trials using ginkgo biloba in the treatment of AD found a modest therapeutic benefit (Oken et al., 1998). There have been, however, several reports of serious side effects associated with commercially available ginkgo, including coma, bleeding, and seizures (Galluzzi et al., 2000).

About 45% of Alzheimer's disease patients have disruptions in their sleep and sundowning agitation, and melatonin secretion is greatly inhibited in AD patients. It has been postulated that melatonin may constitute a selection therapy to ameliorate sundowning and to slow evolution of cognitive impairment in AD. Recent studies have shown that using doses of between 3–9 mg of melatonin at night significantly reduces sleep disturbance and may stabilise behavioural and cognitive symptoms (Cardinali et al., 2002). Unfortunately, these studies have been open label on a small number of patients and more rigorous research is needed in order to confirm these findings.

Treatments for AD – The Future?

As the number of cases of Alzheimer's disease rises in all developed countries, the unmet medical need for disease-modifying pharmacotherapy continues to grow. While acetylcholinesterase inhibitors may have intrinsic disease-modifying activity, this is yet to be proven, and strategies to alter the fundamental neuropathological changes in AD continue to be sought. Much of the evidence suggests that the accumulation of amyloid-beta may play a pivotal role, with research focused on the amyloid cascade hypothesis, and possible intervention along the amyloid pathways. The hypothesis states that amyloid-beta-42 (A-beta-42), a proteolytic derivative of the large transmembrane protein amyloid precursor protein (APP) plays an early and crucial role in all cases of AD. Consequently, blocking the production of A-beta-42 by specific inhibition of the key proteases required for A-beta-42 generation is a major focus of research into AD therapy. The identification of beta-secretase, the aspartic protease that generates the N-terminus of A-beta-42, has triggered a race to develop drug-like inhibitors of this enzyme, which has become one of the major AD targets (Citron, 2004). Although the biology of beta-secretase holds great promise, it will be challenging to generate drug-like inhibitors of this unusual enzyme. The abnormal phosphorylation of tau, however, is also a reasonable target and as the molecular basis of AD is better delineated, more targeted treatment approaches are being proposed (Bullock, 2004).

Although clinical trials have led to the development of several licensed medications for AD, other non-pharmacological approaches may be useful, and one area, which has been researched, is the use of memory aids and retraining.

Memory Training in Dementia

Following a multi-centre trial in the US, known as the Advanced Cognitive Training for Independent and Vital Elderly, or ACTIVE, it was reported that training sessions for 2 hours a week for 5 weeks, improved the memory, concentration and problem solving skills of healthy independent adults aged 65 years and older. The improvement was sustained for 2 years after the training (Ball et al., 2002).

The 2,802 participants were divided into four groups: three groups that received either memory training, reasoning training, or speed of processing training, and a fourth group that received no training. The three types of training were chosen because they showed the most promise in small laboratory studies and were related to tasks of daily living such as telephone use, shopping, food preparation, housekeeping, laundry, transportation, medication use, and personal finances. The improvements in memory, problem solving, and concentration following training were sizeable, and would approximately counteract the degree of cognitive decline that would be expected over a 7 to 14 year period among older people without dementia. No change, however, occurred in the actual, daily activities of the participants, but the authors considered that the training ultimately might be applied to tasks that older people do everyday, such as using medication or handling finances. The effectiveness of memory training in patients with AD has also been studied. Thirty-four patients, who were all taking donepezil throughout the 6-week intervention, were randomly assigned to a cognitive intervention group or a control group. Patients were assessed on neuropsychological tests before the 6-week training programme, immediately after the training, and 8 weeks after completion of the training (Cahn-Weiner et al., 2003). The patients demonstrated modest improvement on recall and recognition of test material presented during the training sessions. No significant effects, however, were observed on any outcome measures, nor were any significant interactions found. These results suggest that although modest gains in learning and memory may be evident in AD patients who are taught specific strategies, the benefits do not generalise to other measures of neuropsychological functioning after a brief intervention.

The Concept of Mild Cognitive Impairment

The advent of symptomatic treatments for Alzheimer's disease has spurred interest in the identification of disease along a spectrum of aging-related cognitive disorders. Several terms have been used to describe the intermediate state between normal aging and dementia, including 'Age-Associated Cognitive Decline', and 'Senescent Forgetfulness'. Particular attempts have been made to profile patients at an increased risk of dementia, which has led to the development of the concept of 'Mild Cognitive Impairment' (MCI) (Peterson, 2000).

MCI has been proposed to identify individuals functioning reasonably who are at higher risk for developing Alzheimer's disease, and are defined as having a complaint of defective memory, normal activities of daily living, normal general cognitive functioning, abnormal memory function for age, and an absence of dementia (Peterson et al., 1997). There are, however, other definitions of MCI, which either incorporate or exclude subjective memory impairment and functional impairment. Unsurprisingly, changes of definition may change prevalence estimates, from 1% for the narrowest, to 3% with the most liberal definition (Fisk et al., 2003).

Many studies have shown increased rates of progression to AD in such individuals compared to individuals with no cognitive impairment (Morris et al., 2001). Rates of cognitive decline from MCI to Alzheimer's disease may vary considerably, however, from between 60.5% to 19.9% over 5 years, and a recent follow-up report suggested that it was very difficult to predict rates of decline between individuals presenting with similar clinical pictures and tests scores (Storandt et al., 2003).

Much focus has been placed on whether MCI is in fact a discrete entity, distinct from both no cognitive impairment and early dementia. The results are so far inconclusive. It has been suggested that MCI may represent early AD, which would be revealed with a sufficiently long period of follow-up. If this were the case, then the frequency of neuropsychiatric symptoms would be expected to be intermediate between normal and that of dementia. Some studies have shown this (Lyketsos et al., 2002).

Alternatively, perhaps MCI represents a heterogeneous group of individuals, within which there are some at increased risk of dementia and others who have a more non-progressive form of cognitive impairment. Supporting the latter is the as yet unexplained finding that some patients initially diagnosed with MCI appear to improve over time (Ingles et al., 2003).

Between the states of no cognitive impairment and dementia exists a wide range of states at least some of which properly can be construed as illness on the grounds that they adversely affect individuals in living their lives, as they would wish. Future research will require both clinical and population based studies of samples, which include considerable heterogeneity, the employment of potential biological markers, measurement of the duration and change in symptoms, and sophisticated modelling techniques, which allow these many considerations properly to be assayed, and not be assumed (or defined) away.

The Diagnosis in Dementia – To Tell or Not to Tell?

With the development of new drug treatments, effective in the earlier stages of dementia, and concepts of MCI leading to patients being seen very early in their illness, there has been an increased urgency and a great deal of research into the better understanding of the issues concerned with giving the diagnosis in dementia.

Controversy exists as to whether dementia patients should be told their diagnosis and prognosis. Arguments in favour of telling are that people have a 'right to know', and that knowing the diagnosis may enable them to make plans for the future. The most common argument made by professionals and carers against disclosing the diagnosis is that it will cause undue distress.

A questionnaire was used to survey the current practice and attitudes of old-age psychiatrists and geriatricians in Nottingham, UK (Johnson et al., 2000). The results of this pilot study suggested that only 40% of respondents regularly told patients the diagnosis. Although physicians were aware of many benefits in disclosing, they had concerns regarding the certainty of diagnosis, the patient's insight, and potential detrimental effects. Similar results were found in a study of primary care physicians (Milne et al., 2000).

Researchers have asked normal older people what information they would wish to receive if they were dementing. These people can be seen as "proxies" for patients with AD. In one study, two hundred patients, 65 years or older, completed a questionnaire assessing opinions about being told the diagnoses of AD versus cancer (Turnbull et al., 2003). Amongst them, 92% responded they wanted to be told if they had AD. Those with personal experience with AD, however, were significantly less likely to want to know themselves if they had AD than were those without personal experience. A variety of reasons were given for not wanting to be told the diagnosis of AD, including a small minority (1.7%) who would consider suicide.

Another study examined the experience of patients and families when a diagnosis of dementia is given (Holroyd et al., 2002). Fifty-seven family members from community dementia support groups answered a questionnaire regarding the diagnosis of dementia in a family member. Half of the families felt they were not given enough information regarding dementia. Interestingly, the majority of family members believed patients should be told their diagnosis and prognosis, yet about half had reported that informed patients had reacted poorly to being told their diagnosis and only about a third felt it was helpful to the patient. Others have also found that families may be ambivalent about their relatives receiving a diagnosis of dementia (Maguire et al., 1996).

Some studies have looked to explore the views of people with dementia themselves. Research has focussed on people's views of the way they were told their diagnosis and the opportunities and limitations offered by receiving an early diagnosis (Fearnley et al., 1997).

Studies have found that participants experienced a range of feelings when first told the diagnosis, including shock, anger, depression, and fear. However, the inappropriate withholding of the diagnosis also caused distress. Some participants felt that the diagnosis helped to explain and validate their own observations. Most participants identified a range of positive opportunities gained by knowing the diagnosis, including planning, accessing appropriate support, and making the most of one's time. They identified few limitations from knowing the diagnosis.

The experience of diagnosis was also affected by medical practice, carer attitudes, availability of information, and social stigma. Some participants who knew their diagnosis felt that in principle, people with dementia should be told as soon as possible. However, they also emphasised the person's need to choose how much information they wished to receive at any given time (Pratt and Wilkinson, 2003).

In general, it appears that results demonstrate wide variability in all aspects of disclosure, although current guidance from the US and UK is that patients should be told their diagnosis (Department of Health, 2002). Further research is needed to develop guidelines for physicians in disclosing dementia diagnoses that includes outcome studies of disclosure to patients.

Research in Dementia in the Developing World

Dementia is an extremely important public health problem, across the world but particularly in developing countries. Epidemiological research in these settings, however, is scarce and presents additional methodological difficulties, mainly regarding the sociocultural adequacy of instruments used to identify cases of dementia.

As a result of these concerns, the 10/66 Dementia Research Group was founded to fill this gap. This is an international network of investigators, mostly from developing countries, and the group's name was based on the paradox that less than 10% of the population-based studies on dementia are directed to 2/3 or more cases of people with dementia living in developing countries; hence the term "10/66".

The 10/66 Group aims to redress this imbalance, encouraging active research collaboration between centres in different developing countries and between developed and developing countries. The group consisted initially of researchers attending a symposium on dementia research in developing countries, at the annual conference of Alzheimer's Disease International held in 1998 at Cochin in Kerala, India. They noted a growing interest in this area, with many active researchers and others wishing to start new studies. Research needed quantifying prevalence and incidence, exploring regional variations in international collaborations using harmonized methodologies, describing care arrangements for people with dementia, quantifying the impact on caregivers and evaluating the effectiveness of any newly implemented services. Methodological problems needed to be addressed, particularly the development of culture- and education-fair dementia diagnostic procedures. It was hoped that good-quality research would generate awareness, pioneer service development and influence policy (Prince, 2000).

In the developing world there is a low level of awareness regarding dementia as a chronic degenerative brain syndrome, and often an absence of supportive health and welfare services. It is the case that families and other informal caregivers are the mainstay of support (Shaji et al., 1996). Descriptive studies have shown that levels of caregiver distress are at least as high as in the developed world, and that many have to cut back on work to care (The 10/66 Research Group, 2004).

A study in South India revealed that the majority of caregivers were young women, often daughters-in-law of women with dementia. The principal sources of caregiver strain were behavioural problems associated with the dementia syndrome, and incontinence. Strain was exacerbated by the lack of supportive response by local health services, and by lack of support and, sometimes, criticism from other family members. There is a clear need for more education, advice and support for families affected by dementia. The authors concluded that community services in developing countries should consider training existing domiciliary outreach services, the community-based multi-purpose health workers, to identify and support family caregivers (Shaji et al., 2003).

An essential part of research into this area has been the development of culturally sensitive dementia assessment scales appropriate for use in developing countries. It has been shown that it is possible to develop a one stage culture and education-fair diagnostic protocol for population-based research (Prince et al., 2003). The Mini Mental State Examination has been developed for use in many countries, one example being a Sinhalese version for use in Sri Lanka (de Silva and Gunatilake, 2002). Activities of daily living scales have also been developed to enable screening for dementia in illiterate rural older populations (Fillenbaum et al., 1999).

The 10/66 Group has expanded significantly over recent years, and research in the developing world continues, although funding of such research remains a major difficulty.

Conclusion

The World Health Organisation and the World Psychiatric Association have recognised that stigma and discrimination against older people with mental disorders such as dementia is widespread and their consequences are far-reaching (WHO and WPA, 2002). It is hoped that continued research in the area of dementia will help to bring about not only greater knowledge, but also bring about lasting reductions in stigma and discrimination.

REFERENCES

- Aisen PS, Davis KL, Berg JD, et al. (2000). A randomized controlled trial of prednisone in Alzheimer's disease. Alzheimer's Disease Cooperative Study. *Neurology,* 54, 588–93.
- Ball K, Berch D, Helmers K, et al. (2002) Effects of cognitive training interventions with older adults: a randomized controlled trial for the ACTIVE Study Group. *JAMA,* 288, 2271–2281.
- Birks J, Flicker L. (2003) Selegiline for Alzheimer's disease: *Cochrane Database Syst Rev* CD000442.
- Bullock R. (2004) Future directions in the treatment of Alzheimer's disease. *Expert Opin Investig Drugs,* 13(4), 303–14.
- Cacabelos R (2003). The application of functional genomics to Alzheimer's disease. *Pharmacogenomics,* 4(5), 597–621.
- Cahn-Weiner DA, Malloy PF, Rebok GW, et al. (2003) Results of a randomized placebo-controlled study of memory training for mildly impaired Alzheimer's disease patients. *Appl Neuropsychol,* 10(4), 215–23.
- Cardinali DP, Brusco LI, Liberczuk C, et al. (2002) The use of melatonin in Alzheimer's disease. *Neuroendocrinol Lett,* 23, Suppl, 1, 20–3.
- Citron M. (2004) Beta-secretase inhibition for the treatment of Alzheimer's disease—promise and challenge. *Trends Pharmacol Sci,* 25(2), 92–97.
- Clegg A, Bryant J, Nicholson T, et al. (2001) Clinical and cost-effectiveness of donepezil, rivastigmine and galantamine for Alzheimer's disease: a rapid and systematic review. *Health Technol Assess,* 5, 1–137.
- Cummings JL, Frank JC, Cherry D, et al. (2002) Guidelines for managing Alzheimer's disease: part I. Assessment. *Am Fam Physician,* 65, 2263–72.
- Cummings JL, Frank JC, Cherry D, et al. (2002) Guidelines for managing Alzheimer's disease: Part II. Treatment. *Am Fam Physician,* 2525–34.

- Department of Health (2002) *Shifting the Balance of Power: The Next Steps.* London: NHS Executive.
- Fearnley K, McLennan J, Weaks D. (1997) *The right to know? Sharing the diagnosis of dementia.* Edinburgh: Alzheimer Scotland - Action on Dementia.
- Fillenbaum GG, Chandra V, Ganguli M, et al. (1999) Development of an activities of daily living scale to screen for dementia in an illiterate rural population in India. *Age Ageing,* 28, 161–168.
- Fisk JD, Merry H, Rockwood K. (2003) Variations in case definition affect prevalence but not outcomes of mild cognitive impairment. *Neurology,* 61, 1179–1184.
- Galluzzi S, Zanetti O, Binetti G, et al. (2000) Coma in a patient with Alzheimer's disease taking low dose trazodone and gingko biloba. *J Neurol Neurosurg Psychiatry,* 68, 679–80.
- Goodman Y, Bruce AJ, Cheng B, Mattson MP (1996) Estrogens attenuate and corticosterone exacerbates excitotoxicity, oxidative injury, and amyloid beta-peptide toxicity in hippocampal neurons. *J Neurochem,* 66(5), 1836–44.
- Holroyd S, Turnbull Q, Wolf AM (2002) What are patients and their families told about the diagnosis of dementia? Results of a family survey. *Int J Geriatr Psychiatry,* 17(3), 218–221.
- Ingles JL, Fisk JD, Merry HR, et al. (2003) Five-year outcomes for dementia define solely by neuropsychological test performance. *Neuroepidemiol,* 22, 172–178.
- Johnson H, Bouman WP, Pinner G (2000) On telling the truth in Alzheimer's disease: a pilot study of current practice and attitudes. *Int Psychogeriatr,* 12(2), 221–229.
- Kivipelto M, Helkala EL, Hanninen T, et al. (2001) Midlife vascular risk factors and late-life mild cognitive impairment: a population-based study. *Neurology,* 56, 1683–1689.
- Knopman D, Schneider L, Davis K, et al. (1996). Long-term tacrine (Cognex) treatment: effects on nursing home placement and mortality, Tacrine Study Group. *Neurology,* 47, 166–177.
- Lyketsos C, Lopez O, Jones B, et al. (2002) prevalence of neuropsychiatric symptoms in dementia and mild cognitive impairment: results from the cardiovascular health study. *JAMA,* 288, 1475–1483.
- Maguire CP, Kirby M, Wen R, et al. (1996) Family members' attitudes towards telling the patient with AD their diagnosis. *BMJ,* 313, 529–530.
- Milne AJ, Woolford HH, Mason J, et al. (2000) Early diagnosis of dementia by GPs: an exploratory study of attitudes. *Ageing and Mental Health,* 4(4), 292–300.

- Morris JC, Storandt M, Miller P, et al. (2001) Mild Cognitive Impairment represents early stage Alzheimer's disease. *Arch Neurol,* 58, 397–405.
- Mulnard RA, Cotman CW, Kawas C, et al. (2000) Estrogen replacement therapy for treatment of mild to moderate Alzheimer disease: a randomized controlled trial. Alzheimer's Disease Cooperative Study. *JAMA,* 283,1007–15.
- Oken BS, Storzbach DM, Kaye JA. (1998) The efficacy of Ginkgo biloba on cognitive function in Alzheimer disease. *Arch Neurol,* 55, 1409–15.
- Peterson RC. (2000) Mild cognitive impairment: transition between aging and Alzheimer's disease. *Neurologia,* 15(3), 93–101.
- Peterson RC, Smith GE, Wearing SC, et al. (1997) Aging, memory, and mild cognitive impairment. *Int Psychogeriatrics,* 9 (Suppl.1), 65–69.
- Pratt R, Wilkinson H. (2003) A psychosocial model of understanding the experience of receiving a diagnosis of dementia. *Dementia,* 2, 181–191.
- Prince M. (2000) Dementia in developing countries. A consensus statement from the 10/66 Dementia Research Group. *Int J Geriatr Psychiatry,* 15(1), 14–20.
- Prince M, Acosta D, Chiu H, et al. (2003) Dementia diagnosis in developing countries: a cross-cultural validation study. *Lancet,* 361, 909–917.
- Rademakers R, Cruts M, Van Broeckhoven C. (2003) Genetics of early-onset Alzheimer dementia. *Scientific World Journal,* 16(3), 497–519.
- Reisberg B, Doody R, Stöffler A, et al. (2003) Memantine in moderate to severe Alzheimer's disease. *New England Journal of Medicine,* 348, 1333–1341.
- Rosler M, Anand R, Cicin-Sain A, et al. (1999) Efficacy and safety of rivastigmine in patients with Alzheimer's Disease: international randomized controlled trial. *BMJ,* 318, 633–640.
- Sano M, Ernesto C, Thomas RG, et al. (1997) A controlled trial of selegiline, alpha-tocopherol, or both as treatment for Alzheimer's disease. The Alzheimer's Disease Cooperative Study. *N Engl J Med,* 336, 1216–22.
- Shaji KS, Smitha K, Lal KP, et al. (2003) Caregivers of people with Alzheimer's disease: a qualitative study from the Indian 10/66 Dementia Research Network. *Int J Geriatr Psychiatry,* 18(1), 1–6.
- Shaji S, Promodu K, Abraham T, et al. (1996) An epidemiological study of dementia in a rural community in Kerala, India. *Br J Psychiatry,* 168(6), 745–749.

- Small GW, Rabins PV, Barry PP, et al. (1997) Diagnosis and treatment of Alzheimer disease and related disorders. Consensus statement of the American Association for Geriatric Psychiatry, the Alzheimer's Association, and the American Geriatrics Society. *JAMA, 278,* 1363–71.
- St George-Hyslop PH. (2000) Piecing together Alzheimer's. *Sci Am,* 283,76–83.
- Storandt M, Grant EA, Miller JP, et al. (2002) Rates of progression in mild cognitive impairment and early Alzheimer's disease. *Neurology,* 59, 1034–1041.
- Tabet N, Birks J, Grimley Evans J et al. (2003) Vitamin E for Alzheimer's disease. *Cochrane Database Syst Rev,* CD002854.
- Tang MX, Jacobs D, Stern Y, et al. (1996) Effect of oestrogen during menopause on risk and age at onset of Alzheimer's disease. *Lancet,* 348, 429–32.
- Tariot PN, Solomon PR, Morris JC, et al. (2000) A 5-month, randomized, placebo-controlled trial of galantamine in AD. The Galantamine USA-10 Study Group. *Neurology,* 54, 2269–76.
- The 10/66 Research Group (2004) Care arrangements for people with dementia in developing countries. *Int J Geri Psychiatry,* 19, 170–177.
- The Parkinson Study Group (1993) Effects of tocopherol and deprenyl on the progression of disability in early Parkinson's disease. *N Engl J Med,* 328, 176–83.
- Turnbull Q, Wolf AM, Holroyd S. (2003) Attitudes of elderly subjects toward "truth telling" for the diagnosis of Alzheimer's disease. *J Geriatr Psychiatry Neurol,* 16(2), 90–3
- Veld BA, Ruitenberg A, Hofman A, et al. (2001) Nonsteroidal anti-inflammatory drugs and the risk of Alzheimer's disease. *N Engl J Med,* 345, 1515–21.
- Wassertheil-Smoller S, Hendrix S, Limacher M, et al. (2003) Effect of estrogen plus progestin on stroke in postmenopausal women: The Women's Health Initiative: a randomized trial. *JAMA,* 289, 2673–2684.
- World Health Organisation and World Psychiatric Association (2002) *Reducing stigma and discrimination against older people with mental disorders. A technical consensus statement.* Geneva: WHO/MSD/MBD/02.3.

19

Dementia and Dementia Care: An International Perspective

David Jolley

Introduction

It is sobering to remember that when I began to work in the university departments of Psychiatry and Geriatric Medicine in Manchester in 1975, one of our Senior Lecturers had recently published a learned review, which questioned the concept of late onset dementia (senile dementia) as illness (Hanley, 1974). An alternative assessment of the facts proposed that the changes of function and histology occurring in some older people represent simply the extreme consequences of normal ageing. We were about to establish the first special service for older people with dementia and other mental health problems in the North West of England, one of about twenty in the world at that time. Only three decades later, we are looking at dementia, especially late onset Alzheimer's disease, as a worldwide phenomenon (Prince, 2002).

Demography of Old Age

Old age is a personal construct. For many it caries an implication of deterioration of function, accumulation of pathology and symptoms, dependency upon others and the approach of death. Some people feel, look and behave old from their forties onwards. Stigmata of early ageing were common in previous generations in the UK, most commonly amongst the poor. There remains a wide spectrum of personal and biological attributes associated with advanced years within individual countries and this is extended by addressing the international scene. Chronological age is easier to define than biological age status and a threshold of 65 years (60 in some countries) is usually taken to delineate old age. These operational definitions are based in an historical appreciation that the adverse attributes of later life had begun to be evident amongst many people of these ages in the UK and other developed countries by the middle of the twentieth century. At the time that old age pensions were introduced, many people were forced to stop work by illness and incapacity before reaching their sixtieth birthday.

Roughly six percent of the world's current population is aged 65 years or older. This mean figure is bracketed by extremes from low numbers (three percent in Africa, five percent in South East Asia and Latin America) to higher numbers (16 percent and more in parts of Europe). Within countries there are communities with concentrations of older people, products of survival compounded by migration of old people into the community or migration of younger people away from it.

Though, hitherto, most interest has been taken in old age in the developed world of Europe, North America, Japan and Australasia, the size of populations in the Third World means that they are home to two thirds of the world's elderly (65 years plus). This proportion is projected to increase very rapidly as improvements in life expectation occur in these countries. Improvements, which took a hundred years to achieve in the UK, are being surpassed within two or three decades (Grundy, 1983; Prince, 2002).

Within this overall pattern of change, the shift toward more very old people (75 years plus and 85 years plus) in both the developed and developing world, means that the number of people with dementia will rise disproportionately. European studies find dementia to be six times more common in people over 75 years than amongst those in their early sixties and more than twenty times more common amongst those surviving beyond eighty-five years.

Thus it is that more and more individuals and families around the world have a personal interest in dementia. Governments, health care and other care agencies are being encouraged to consider plans in anticipation of the predicted needs. In this, the work of Nori Graham in her role as Chairman of Alzheimer's Disease International has been most extraordinary in its importance and impact (Prince et al., 2004).

Dementia Defined

Historical descriptions of the syndrome, we now call dementia, had been available from classical times. Individual case histories and descriptions of the gross and histopathology of the main dementia illnesses began to appear from the beginning of the twentieth century. Nevertheless, it was not until Roth undertook his careful investigation of the clinical characteristics and outcomes of subgroups within a cohort of old people admitted to an English mental hospital (Graylingwell) in the 1940s–1950s, that the dementias were clearly differentiated from within the portmanteau of 'Senile Psychosis' (Roth, 1955). These clinical studies prepared the ground for epidemiological enquiries in Newcastle-upon-Tyne (Kay et al., 1964) and elsewhere in the UK, Europe and North America. The condition had been defined; from that point onwards it could be identified, counted and mapped within populations.

Its biological substrate has been investigated by Corsellis (1962) in London, by Roth and his teams in Newcastle and Cambridge (Roth and Wischik, 1985) and by an increasing number of laboratories around the world. Roth's concept of Senile Dementia has become known as late onset Alzheimer's disease. It remains the most common of dementias. Vascular dementia has been sustained as a separate diagnosis, quite common but varying in frequency (Leys et al., 2002). Lewy body dementia was not described by Roth, but has emerged as a consequence of clinical and pathological approaches from Nottingham and Newcastle (Byrne et al., 1989; McKeith et al., 1992), while the less common Pick's disease is now usually termed frontal lobe dementia (Neary et al., 1998).

Interest in Care

Interest in the academic and biological enquiries into the distribution and nature of the dementias has been sustained and sponsored as a consequence of the clinical and service imperative presenting from the large numbers of old people with dementia encountered by health and social care systems in the UK and elsewhere in the developed world. Aubrey Lewis was amongst the first to observe the threat to the competence of the passive care regimens of the UK asylum system (Lewis, 1946). Simply taking people away from home to await death in inappropriately designed, poorly equipped, ill-staffed, 50 bedded, single sex dormitories was neither acceptable nor a workable solution.

Social psychiatry's successes from the 1930s and 1940s predated the influence of effective physical treatments for the major psychoses and its principles could be applied to any condition, including the untreatable dementias, with the hope of some success. Thus it was that the UK Psychogeriatric Movement (latterly, Old Age Psychiatry) began in the 1960s and 1970s. It followed closely a similar movement providing care for the elderly frail, 'Geriatric Medicine', and the two disciplines worked collaboratively (Pitt, 1974). Their mission was, and is, to bring good practice in the mental health care and physical health care of older people to older people wherever they are living; to work with families and other agencies to promote good health and function, to identify and correct reversible pathologies and to minimise or avoid secondary and tertiary disability, which might follow from removing the older individual from his or her place within their local community. Hence the essence was, and is, to work with respect for the individual and all components, especially the family, friends and other helpers, of their personal world. The first task is to recognise and differentiate the health and mental health problems bringing difficulties to the individual. This remains a task-demanding skill based on training and experience. Alzheimer's dementia is common, especially in people beyond their eightieth year, and its cardinal symptoms well characterised. Yet its differential diagnosis from normal ageing, depression, exhaustion, deafness, other physical illness or symptomatic confusion, within the multiple pathology environment of late life requires care and expertise.

Pioneering psychogeriatric teams in the UK worked from a secondary care base and employed Community Nurses, Occupational Therapists, Clinical Psychologists, Social Workers and sometimes other specialist therapists. Yet they had the advantage of functioning within a comprehensive National Health Service, every patient subject to support from their General Practitioner and Primary Health Care team together with Social Service support, if needed, provided by or commissioned by the Local Authority (Jolley and Arie, 1978). Thus they added expert knowledge and the potential for access to additional resources to a community service designed to be easily available to individuals in difficulty and to have knowledge of them through a life-long commitment. Despite these advantages, services often found there to be lack of knowledge and of sensitive resources to respond to the needs of individuals and families. Indeed, it remains a cause for concern that, even now, Primary Health Care practitioners (and their equivalents in General Hospitals) lack confidence and competence in identifying and caring for common mental health problems in older people (Audit Commission, 2000). Nevertheless, the UK Psychogeriatric experience has been seen to be successful in bringing a positive and useful approach to a previously neglected phenomenon. Under its wing, other initiatives have flourished and progress made beyond what could have been dreamed of in the 1960s.

Early practitioner-academics were invited to lecture in North America, Europe, Australasia, Japan and elsewhere, so that these countries might borrow what was of interest and adapt it to their own needs and tastes. Individual professionals spent time to study and work with the UK pioneers and took back their knowledge and skills to use in their homelands. From the late 1970s Professor Arie's Department of Health Care of the Elderly in Nottingham (Arie, 1981) organised regular international training courses in association with the British Council. These achieved more than a simple exchange of knowledge, for friendships were forged which have endured. National, international and worldwide organisations have been created and these foster good practice in service delivery and research and have influenced government policies. Conferences are held all around the world and journals and latterly web sites have grown to make knowledge and ideas readily available. What began in humble circumstances in the UK, now has benefits from generative centres in every continent.

Their greatest impact has been within the field of dementia, though older people with mood disorders, paranoid disorders, addictions, neuroses and long-standing psychoses have fallen within their remit

(Jolley and Arie, 1992). It is only dementia, which has generated such a massively effective voluntary organisation response. The Alzheimer (Disease) Society has celebrated its silver anniversary and is active in most countries of the globe. Its contribution to improving popular understanding of the condition and the need for research and investment cannot be overstated. Through Alzheimer's Disease International, a visionary programme of research is being sponsored by the 10/66 research group (Dias et al., 2004; Prince et al., 2004; Shaji et al., 2003; The 10/66 Dementia Research Group, 2004). From the early 1990s a network of Dementia Service Development Centres (DSDCs) has been supported from its original base in Stirling, Scotland (www.dsdc.stir.ac.uk), a product of the heroic contributions of Professor Mary Marshall to help professionals care most effectively for people with dementia. This movement has links already with centres in Europe and Australia and will surely be of great help in the developing world.

Concepts of Dementia in Differing Cultures

Enquiries under the auspices of 10/66, using qualitative and quantitative approaches, reveal that the symptoms of dementia and other serious psychiatric disorders are recognised and described within all cultural groups. Yet they are commonly not given a name, nor are they recognised as illnesses. Dementia is likely to be lumped together with other mental problems, nerva frak or nervachem in Goa (Patel and Prince, 2001), and attributed to wearing out with age or a consequence (punishment) arising from misdeeds earlier in life or evidence of misuse or neglect by the family. Alternatively, the syndrome may be described as a return to childhood: for example, Chinnan of Kerala (Shaji et al., 2003) and 'Once a man, twice a child' amongst West Indian elders (Dementiaplus, 2002). In association with such labels and descriptions of the state, explanations of causality, attributing change to the intervention of spirits or the invocation of witchcraft, may be integral to its understanding.

Such concepts are not far removed from lay beliefs in the developed world only a few decades ago. Indeed, there remains within these countries a persistent folklore, of alternative wisdom, its stronghold firmer amongst those with less exposure to, and confidence in, modern education.

Where immigration rules have encouraged the development of multi-cultural cities, knowledge and conceptualisation of dementia and Alzheimer's disease may remain culture-bound, though likely to be transformed in future generations as a consequence of shared education and language (Ayalon and Arean, 2004).

Biological Insights

International studies have been greatly assisted by the development of standardised interview and assessment schedules, validated against clinical diagnosis. In work with older people with mental health problems, the Geriatric Mental State Schedule has been immensely important, translated into numerous languages and linked to a simple AGECAT algorithm (Copeland et al., 2002; Kim et al., 2003). Other instruments have also been translated and validated in several languages (Verhey et al., 2004). Thus it has become possible to investigate differences of psychopathology, prevalence and incidence and associated factors across cultures and in different parts of the world. It is fascinating to find that most studies identify syndromes, with very similar characteristics and very similar rates of age-related incidence and prevalence, across cultures and throughout the world (Prince, 2002). Small area studies have detected differences in incidence and prevalence between communities and one persistent thread is the suggestion that rural populations are less prone to dementia than people who live their lives in cities. This may have implications for an understanding of underlying mechanisms or causes. At a national level, the prevalence of dementia in Southern India and in Nigeria appears to be about half that found in other countries, age-controlled (Ogunniyi et al., 1992; Shaji et al., 1996; Rajkumar et al., 1997; Baiyewu, 2002). It is possible that these findings reflect technical errors in the research, though this seems unlikely. It could be that fewer people are developing dementia in these populations. This would be helpful in understanding aetiology and might have practical importance in suggesting preventive programmes. Another possibility is that people with dementia do not survive for very long within these populations because of susceptibility to other serious illnesses and/or lack of suitable care for them in their dependant and vulnerable state.

Chromosome mapping identified the ApoE gene as a risk factor for dementia and Alzheimer's disease in Caucasians (Saunders et al., 1993). This association is not found to be so strong in Africans or Asians (Farrer et al., 1997; Osuntokun et al., 1995). In Nigerian and Kenyan populations, ApoE is found in a higher proportion of people, yet dementia occurs at about a quarter of the rate recognised in Europe and North America. This encourages the belief that the gene is not itself a direct cause of dementia, but acts via an environmental factor, which is absent in Africa but present in North America. Again, this knowledge may lead toward preventive strategies.

Patterns of Service

The patterns of specialist psychogeriatric services described above and whose influence has encouraged biological, clinical and international research, were developed from the mature population structure and service configuration of the UK of the 1960s and 1970s. Fifteen percent of the population was aged 65 years or older and a healthcare and welfare system, designed to complement the care available from families, was failing under the pressures from the changing shape and volume arising from dementia. The response came from Social Psychiatry, with ready support from Geriatric Medicine, Social Services, voluntary and independent sectors. Only latterly, and with considerable encouragement (Audit Commission, 2000; Department of Health, 2001), has primary health care taken a high profile interest (Greaves, 2003). Contributions from general hospitals have not been notable and may be less sympathetic as shifts to bigger, high-tech institutions with rapid turnover of patients becomes the vogue (Change Agency Team, 2003). Yet in the UK and in Europe and North America, neurologists and other physicians play a very significant part in assessment, investigation and research in dementia. In many countries, clinical practice is based in outpatient clinics, offices or surgeries and has not involved doctors, certainly specialists, in the home-visiting format which is the hallmark of the UK system (Arie and Jolley, 1982; Hemsi, 1982). Much has been learned about the way that families come to understand and conceptualise the problems and needs arising from the syndrome we call dementia. Within the Third World, almost all people with dementia live within their families who will accommodate their needs for understanding, care and supervision as well as they can. There has been little or no expectation of medical or nursing input and little available infrastructure of care beyond the family. The tradition of respect, even reverence, for older people has been seen to be their insurance of safekeeping. Yet the picture is more complex than this and is changing rapidly. Even within traditional systems, it is understood that caring for people with dementia causes a great deal of strain to some families (Patel and Prince, 2001; Liu et al., 2002; Huang et al, 2003; Ngoma et al., 2003; Shaji et al. 2003; Dias et al., 2004; The 10/66 Dementia Research Group, 2004). Although responsibilities may be vested in the male offspring, actual care is usually provided by daughters and grand-daughters-in-law, though older relatives, as in the UK, increasingly play their parts. Where care is given, it is not always freely given and may be contingent upon expectations of material gain by inheritance. This may be a source, as in the UK, of potential conflict between siblings and between generations.

As younger generations become involved with increasingly lucrative commercial work, competitive in the world market, balancing their use of time for family care in contrast to generating income, becomes a matter for consideration. With increased affluence, the attractions of respite care, day care and residential care for older people with dementia become more apparent. Thus it is that that institutions offering this are gaining ground within the Third World, replicating, on a massive scale, the progress seen within the UK whereby people with dementia were much more likely to be found at home (at considerable risk) in the 1960s (Kay et al., 1964) than in the 1980s and beyond (O'Connor et al., 1991). This is a natural evolution of care patterns, yet we hope that the errors encountered in the institutional care sector of the developed world can be avoided in these new ventures (Commission for Health Improvement, 2004). It is important that care and funding systems become more aware and sympathetic toward the needs of families arising from dementia. Many systems are sensitive to physical dependency, and all-but blind to the severity of stress arising from behavioural changes (Arai et al., 2003). The mainstream for the present is, and will be, care at home. The 10/66 group have begun a refreshingly ambitious but practical programme designed to complement local care with improved knowledge of effective care technique (Huang et al.,

2003; Dias et al., 2004; Prince et al., 2004; The 10/66 Dementia Research Group, 2004). Key to the introduction of awareness, investigation and treatment programmes will be the utilisation of non-medical primary health care workers within local health care teams and the progressive strengthening of primary health care input (Liu et al., 2002; Ngoma et al., 2003). In this, those countries facing the prospects of dementia and other age-related illnesses for the first time in large numbers, look likely to produce a more logical and economic system of health and social care than that which has grown in the UK, Europe and North America. It is felt that those of us experienced in dementia care in the UK can provide helpful and relevant teaching and training with colleagues in the Third World. The process is unlikely to prove a one-way exchange, for we have much to learn.

While approaches to clinical assessment and care may be well conducted through community contacts, more sophisticated investigations require access to equipment and expertise inevitably located within acute hospitals. Perversely, it may be easier for people to access modern scanning equipment through clinics associated with university services in India and Africa than is the case within routine services in the UK. This is, no doubt, a function of numbers and priorities. For most patients, scanning provides little information beyond confirmation of a clinical impression and contributes nothing to the reality of care-work. Nevertheless, there are patients in whom the differential diagnosis is not easy and can be resolved by high-tech investigations. This is particularly likely amongst younger people with dementia. Collaboration with neurologist and/or medical geneticist yields the best results in these circumstances.

Prescription of cholinesterase inhibitors and monitoring of response to them and other therapeutic initiatives, have become the remit of Memory Clinics in the UK and elsewhere (Lindesay et al., 2002). Holmes and Lovestone (2003) doubt the logic of such restrictive practice, which was motivated in the first instance by fear of the cost implications. If these medicines uphold the promise to reduce the rate of progress of Alzheimer's disease, then they can play a useful role in reducing the impact on lifestyle and economy, which the expanding numbers of people with dementia threaten. Once again, it seems likely and sensible, that most countries will replicate the work of Memory Clinics within a model of primary care supported by specialists and using specially trained non-medical primary health care staff.

Within the large cities of the developed world, communities with differing histories, cultures and languages live and work alongside each other, work together and grow old together. Sometimes the working generation welcomes mother and/or father in their failing years, to live out their last days within a culture and range of services which is new to them (Dementiaplus, 2002). Awareness of this phenomenon and preparedness by style, inclination and equipment, to cater for the special needs of minority groups, is essential in all dementia services.

Prospects for the Future

Dementia has been opened up as an illness and associated problems that are relevant to the whole world. Knowledge and skills are being shared between professionals, individuals and families internationally. There is an extraordinary fellowship of purpose. This is fostered by ADI and API as well as WHO and WPA (Chiu, 2002). It is doubtful whether there is any other condition, which benefits from such generous and altruistic collaboration.

There is little doubt that governments will continue to be impressed and moved to action. Dementia is an illness of Everyman, as more people survive to experience later life, more families come to know its nature and its needs. Understanding and education will be dispersed and good practices encouraged and must attract appropriate resources. An international network of DSDCs for professionals would complement the work of ADI and facilitate the spread of information and facilitate mutual support on the ground.

Research into its basic biology has been rewarded by extraordinary advances in knowledge over four decades. Efforts and expenditure are being intensified and it seems likely that both preventative and treatment options will become available as a result of these. This work is conducted on a truly international platform. Insights gained anywhere in the world are shared instantly with colleagues who may be able to confirm or modify findings and take part in the next stages of advance.

The pharmaceutical industry has invested in this work and is beginning to realise dividends. It is likely to press on in expectation of further rewards and with an eye to the expanding world market for effective products.

The care industry has developed from roots in family care and local provisions, sometimes organised by religious or voluntary organisations. Small private initiatives still compete with national and, latterly, international organisations, to establish best quality, best value, culturally sensitive, comprehensive programmes of support at home, respite and residential care. The latter is likely to spread as a world phenomenon despite improvements in community care and despite the advantages which will be derived from specialised housing for older people.

Older people themselves are becoming more confident and effective advocates for their own needs. Swept aside into a subculture of pensioned retirement and anticipated dependency for three or four generations within Europe and North America, old people in these countries have become better informed and learned to re-evaluate their position and worth. They know about the illnesses of late life, most certainly about dementia, and can now speak to the approaches these challenges require. The eminence and respect given to elders of the Third World, may have become less robust than it was, but looks likely to be replaced by the assurance coming from knowledge and issues shared in common with other old people around the world.

Public health initiatives designed to improve health in all age groups through lifestyle and diet together with early diagnosis and treatment of pathologies are likely to delay and reduce the incidence of dementia of the Alzheimer type as well as vascular dementia. Increased consumption of alcohol and misuse of other substances may have a contrary effect to increase the incidence of dementia. Let us hope that individuals and governments will see the hazard and take appropriate action. In similar vein, the spread of sexually transmitted diseases, including HIV and syphilis, threaten to add an infection dimension to the epidemic of degenerative dementia.

Clinical activity in the field should see a spread of community-based practice and increased confidence and competence in primary care in both the developed and developing world. It is to be hoped that students in all the health care professions will be taught about dementia and its best management. The only effective mode of work is, and will be, multi-disciplinary with close partnership between agencies and families.

We need to remain open-minded and to learn from our patients and their families and from colleagues in every country, including our own.

Conclusions

- Dementia is established as a serious worldwide health and social care phenomenon.
- Most people with dementia live in developing countries, even though such countries contain relatively few old people.
- The next 30 years will see a dramatic increase in the proportion of people surviving to experience dementia in the developing countries.
- Initiatives taken in the UK, Europe and North America from the 1960s onwards have led to scientific, clinical and service discoveries in dementia, which are now being shared to the benefit of the whole world.
- Further progress is being made in a spirit of mutual respect and reciprocal learning.

REFERENCES

- Arai Y, Zarit SH, Kumamato K and Takeda A. (2003) Are there inequities in the assessment of dementia under Japan's LTC insurance system? *International Journal of Geriatric Psychiatry*, 18, 346–352.
- Arie T. (1981) *Health Care of the Elderly*. London: Croom-Helm.
- Arie T and Jolley D. (1982) Making services work: organisation and style of psychogeriatric services. Chapter 8, p 222–251 in: Levy R. and Post F (eds) *The Psychiatry of Late Life*. Oxford: Blackwell Scientific Pubs.
- Audit Commission (2000) *Forget-me-not. Mental Health Services for Older People.* London: Audit Commission UK
- Ayalon L and Arean P. (2004) Knowledge of Alzheimer's disease in four ethnic groups of older adults. *International Journal of Geriatric Psychiatry*, 19, 51–57.

- Baiyewu O. (2002) Dementia and depression in Africa. In: *Principles and Practice of Geriatric Psychiatry,* (eds. Copeland J, Abou-Saleh M and Blazer D), 2nd edition, p 649–650. Chichester: John Wiley and Sons Ltd.
- Byrne J, Lennox G, Lowe J and Godwin-Austen R. (1989) Diffuse Lewy-body disease: clinical features in 15 cases. *Journal of Neurology, Neurosurgery and Psychiatry,* 52, 709–717.
- Change Agency (2003) Getting it right for dementia in acute hospitals. Available at: www.doh.uk
- Chiu E. (2002) Organisation of service for the elderly with mental disorders. In: *Principles and Practice of Geriatric Psychiatry* (eds. Copeland J, Abou-Saleh M and Blazer D), 2nd edition, p 664–665. Chichester: John Wiley and Sons Ltd.
- Copeland J, Prince P, Wilson K, Dewey M, Payne J and Gurland B. (2002) The Geriatric Mental State Examination in the 21st century. *International Journal of Geriatric Psychiatry,* 17, 729–732.
- Corsellis J. (1962) Mental illness and the ageing brain. *Maudesly Monograph No. 9.* London: Oxford University Press.
- Dementiaplus (2002) Twice a Child. Research report available at: www.Dementiaplus.org.uk.
- Department of Health (2001) *National Service Framework for Older People.* London: Department of Health UK.
- Dias A, Samuel R, Patel V, Prince M, Parameshwaran R, Krishnamoorthy ES. (2004) The impact associated with caring for a person with dementia: a report from the 10/66 Dementia Research Group's Indian Network. *International Journal of Geriatric Psychiatry,* 19, 182–184.
- Farrer L, Cupples LA, Haines JL, et al. (1997) Effects of age, sex and ethnicity on the association between apolipoprotein E genotype and Alzheimer's disease. *Journal of the American Medical Association,* 278, 1349–1356.
- Greaves I. (2003) A GP's view of treating people with dementia in nursing homes. *Dementia Bulletin,* (autumn), 1–4.
- Grundy E. (1983) Demography and old age. *Journal of the American Geriatrics Society,* 31(6), 325–332.
- Hanley T. (1994) Neuronal fall out in the ageing brain: a critical review of the quantitative data. *Age and Ageing,* 3(3), 133–151.
- Hemsi L. (1982) Psychogeriatric care in the community. In: *The Psychiatry of Late Life,* (eds. Levy R. and Post F), Chapter 9, p 252–287. Oxford: Blackwell Scientific Pubs.

- Holmes C and Lovestone S. (2003) Long-term cognitive function and decline in late-onset Alzheimer's disease: therapeutic implications. *Age and Ageing,* 32, 200–204.
- Huang H, Shyu Y L, Chen M, Chen S and Lin L. (2003) A pilot study on a home-based training programme for improving care-giver self-efficacy and decreasing the behavioural problems of elders with dementia in Taiwan. *International Journal of Geriatric Psychiatry,* 18, 337–345.
- Jolley D and Arie T. (1978) Organisation of psychogeriatric services. *British Journal of Psychiatry,* 132, 1–11.
- Jolley D and Arie T. (1992) Developments in Psychogeriatric Services. In: *Recent Advances in Psychogeriatrics 2.* (ed. Arie T), Chapter 11, p 117–136. Edinburgh: Churchill Livingstone.
- Kay D, Beamish P, and Roth M. (1964) Old age mental disorders in Newcastle upon Tyne. *British Journal of Psychiatry,* 110, 146–158.
- Kim J, Stewart R, Prince M, Shin I, and Yoon J. (2003) Diagnosing dementia in a developing nation: an evaluation of the GMS-AGECAT algorithm in an older Korean population. *International Journal of Geriatric Psychiatry,* 18, 331–336.
- Lewis A. (1946) Ageing and senility. A major problem for psychiatry. *Journal of Mental Health,* 92, 150–170.
- Leys D, Engulund E and Erikinjunti T. (2002) Vascular Dementia. In *Evidence Based Dementia Practice* (eds. Qizilbah N et al.), p 260–287. Oxford: Blackwell Science, www.ebdementia.info.
- Lindesay J, Marudkar M, van Diepen E and Wilcock G. (2002) The second Leicester survey of memory clinics in the British Isles. *International Journal of Geriatric Psychiatry,* 17, 41–47.
- Liu SI, Prince M, Blizard B, and Mann A. (2002) The prevalence of psychiatric morbidity and its associated factors in general health care in Taiwan. *Psychological Medicine,* 32, 629–637.
- McKeith IG, Perry RH, Fairbairn AF, Jabeen S, Perry EK. (1992) Operational criteria for senile dementia of the Lewy Body type. *Psychological Medicine,* 22, 911–922.
- Neary D, Snowden JS, Gustafson L, et al. (1998) Frontotemporal lobar degeneration: a consensus on clinical diagnostic criteria. *Neurology,* 51, 1546–1554.
- Ngoma MC, Prince M and Mann A. (2003) Common mental disorders among those attending primary health clinics and traditional healers in urban Tanzania. *British Journal of Psychiatry,* 183, 349–355.

- O'Connor D, Pollitt P, Brook C, Reiss B and Roth M. (1991) Does early intervention reduce the number of elderly people with dementia admitted to institutions for long term care? *British Medical Journal,* 302, 871–875.
- Ogunniyi A, Osuntokun BO, Lekwauwa UB, Falope ZF. (1992) Rarity of dementia as measured by the DSM-III-R in an urban community in Nigeria. *East African Medical Journal,* 69, 64–68.
- Osuntokun B, Sahota A, Ogunniyi AO, et al. (1995) Lack of association between the e4 allele of APOE and Alzheimer's Disease in a community study of elderly Nigerians. *Annals of Neurology,* 38, 463–465.
- Patel V and Prince M. (2001) Ageing and mental health in a developing country: who cares? Qualitative studies from Goa, India. *Psychological Medicine,* 31, 29–38.
- Pitt B. (1974) *Psychogeriatrics.* Edinburgh: Churchill-Livingstone.
- Prince M. (2002) Epidemiology. In Jacoby R and Oppenheimer C (eds) *Psychiatry in the Elderly,* 3rd edition, Chapter 4, 80–101. Oxford: Oxford University Press.
- Prince M, Graham N, Brodaty H, et al. (2004) Alzheimer's Disease International's 10/66 Dementia Research Group: one model for action in developing countries. *International Journal of Geriatric Psychiatry,* 19, 178–181.
- Rajkumar S, Kumar S and Thara R. (1997) Prevalence of dementia in a rural setting: report from India. *International Journal of Geriatric Psychiatry,* 12, 702–707.
- Roth M. (1955) The natural history of mental disorders in old age. *Journal of Mental Science,* 101, 281–301.
- Roth M and Wischik C. (1985) The heterogeneity of Alzheimer's disease. In Arie T. (ed) *Recent Advances in Psychogeriatrics,* Chapter 6, 71–92. Edinburgh: Churchill-Livingstone.
- Saunders A, Strittmatter WJ, Schmechel D, et al. (1993) Association of apolipoprotein E allele with late onset familial and sporadic Alzheimer's disease. *Neurology,* 43, 1467–1472.
- Shaji KS, Smitha K, Lal KP and Prince P. (2003) Caregivers for Alzheimer's disease: a qualitative study from the Indian 10/66 Dementia Research Network. *International Journal of Geriatric Psychiatry,* 18, 1–6.
- Shaji S, Pramodu K, Abraham R, Roy KJ, Varghese A. (1996) An epidemiological study of dementia in a rural community in Kerala, India. *British Journal of Psychiatry,* 168, 745–749.

- The 10/66 Dementia Research Group (2004) Care arrangements for people with dementia in developing countries. *International Journal of Geriatric Psychiatry,* 19, 170–177.
- Verhey FR, Houx P, Van Lang N, et al. (2004) Cross-national comparison and validation of the Alzheimer's Disease Assessment Scale: results from the European Harmonisation Project for Instruments in Dementia (EURO-HARPID). *International Journal of Geriatric Psychiatry,* 19, 41–50.

Appendix 1

....

Outline of Clinical Assessment for Dementia

....

HISTORY

History from Patient and Carers

- Cognitive decline: onset and course
- Noncognitive symptoms: including change in personality
- Biological functions: sleep, appetite, excretory functions, mobility
- Activities of daily living: abilities, inabilities: managing hygiene, money; ability to use household instruments, gadgets, machines

Physical Disorders, Impairments

- Physical disorders as probable aetiology
- History of head trauma, exposure to hypoxia (cardiovascular diseases, surgery, anaesthesia), metals associated with dementia
- Impairments that may mask or aggravate cognitive dysfunction

Current Medications and Substance Use

- Medication side effects or toxicity that may impair cognition (e.g., benzodiazepine, neuroleptics, lithium, SSRIs, TCAs, antiepileptics)
- History and current use of substances like alcohol, LSD, cocaine, amphetamine

Family History

- Dementia
- Disorders aetiologically associated with dementia
- Neurological disorders

Carer's Stress

MENTAL STATUS EXAMINATION

Consciousness

Attention and Concentration

- Assessed by clinical behaviour
- Days of the week backwards
- Digit forward and digit backwards: present digit in a monotone one second apart; a forward span of 5 or more is normal
- Months backwards
- Spelling 'world' backwards
- 20 – 1, 40 – 3, 100 – 7 serial subtractions
- Vigilance is tested by 'A' test with finger tapping

Orientation

- Assessed by clinical behaviour
- Time: current time, day, date, month, year, sense of passage of time
- Place: room, ward, hospital, place, village or city nearby, etc.
- Person: self and others

Language

Phonation, articulation, fluency, comprehension, naming, repetition, reading, writing and prosody are assessed.

- Observing spontaneous speech helps establish fluent and non-fluent aphasias
- Comprehension: Respond to verbal commands, to 'yes or no' questions, one step commands for body movements are used to study comprehension (e.g., 'show me your tongue', 'nod your head', 'touch your right knee', 'is it raining outside', 'is this place a temple')

- Fluency: 'tell me as many words as you can think of starting with letter s', 'tell me as many animals as you can think of'; I will count them for one minute.
- Expression: This can be assessed by asking open ended questions, allowing the person to talk on a subject; it can also be done by observation of his spontaneous speech ('what are the uses of table', 'what is a station' 'what is morality')
- Repetition of words, phrases and sentences
- Naming is assessed by asking the patient to name everyday objects and their parts
- Reading aloud and explaining a passage of appropriate difficulty. These two aspects may be impaired independently. Comprehension of reading material is tested by asking the patient to follow what is written, e.g., 'raise your left hand' or to read and fill in the blanks, e.g., 'a man who repairs cars is known as ____'. (Adequate vision must be present before considering alexia, the inability to understand the meaning of written words)
- Writing. Assessed by asking to write a complete sentence. Impoverished agrammatic output or fluent paraphasic writing similar to the errors noted in verbal output may be reproduced here. (Consider mechanical agraphias due to limb paresis, movement disorders, limb apraxia)
- Articulation: Asking to repeat a difficult phrase: elicits dysarthria

Memory

- Impairments are often evident during interaction, history taking
- New learning, recall of recently and remotely learned information are assessed, confabulation (filling in the gaps of memory by imagined or untrue experiences that the patient believes but that has no basis in fact) is checked.
- Both verbal and non-verbal domains are to be tested.
- Remote: apparent from history, personal events (childhood data, dates of marriage, birth dates of children) and impersonal events (historical events), topographic memory and memory of skills
- Recent past memory: events of past few months

- **Recent:** personal orientation is one means of assessing recent memory. Recall of items and events up to last few days; address test with five facts, object test with five unrelated objects and verbal story; reproducing unrelated words after registering.
- **Immediate** (or short term memory: that lasts for 30 seconds): registration ('I am going to tell you three words, please repeat them after I finish'. Take one second to say each word), digit forward and backward; verbal immediate recall; memory for designs tests (drawing designs after they have been removed from view).
- **Non-verbal memory:** Asking patient to reproduce a clock-face showing a specific time, after a five-minute interval.

Praxis

Apraxia is the failure of the ability to carry out well-organised voluntary movement correctly despite the fact that motor, sensory and co-ordinative functions are not significantly impaired (Bickerstaff and Spillane, 1989).

- *Constructional praxis:* copying of figures (two and three-dimensional), drawing a clock and setting the asked time; arranging objects into patterns (arranging match sticks into triangle or square or copying it)
- *Dressing apraxia:* observable by informants or by asking the patient to dress or take off shirt
- *Gait apraxia:* tandem gait test
- *Ideomotor apraxia:* There is an inability to imitate or mime an act involving use of objects. Patient performs automatic acts normally, such as shaking hands and is able to formulate the idea of an act and to describe how it should be done, but when it comes to carrying out the movement on command, he is unable to do it correctly. It is assessed by asking the patient to hold out his arms, put out his tongue, show the teeth, to show how to brush, use scissors, wave goodbye, etc.
- *Ideational apraxia:* The formulation of carrying out a complex act with multiple components is defective; though the execution of different parts of the complete act may be normal. For example, when told to do each of these actions separately the patient will be able to take a match box, hold it correctly, open it correctly, take out the match correctly and do the same with a cigarette packet

but when told to go through a motion of lighting a cigarette, will be unable to do so. This form of apraxia is recognised by the patient's inability to use objects properly and not tested for by imitation or miming (Bickerstaff and Spillane, 1989). Example of a test: 'I am going to give you a paper, take it in right hand, fold it, and put it on the table'.

Agnosia

It is the inability to understand the significance of sensory stimuli even though the sensory pathways and sensorium are intact.

- *Astereognosia:* failure to identify from the feel of three-dimensional form and is tested by placing a familiar object in the patient's hand with his eyes closed.
- *Visual agnosia:* It is assessed by placing some common object and colours in front and asking the patient to name objects, describe their use, and pick out ones mentioned; picking out objects of same colours, arranging objects in shades of increasing lightness.
- *Visual object agnosia:* inability to name or describe the use of the objects shown, but is able to identify them when he touches them or by their characteristic noise or smell (a patient with nominal aphasia will be unable to find the exact name, which ever sense is used)
- *Visual agnosia for colours:* inability to identify, match or arrange colours.
- *Visuospatial agnosia:* (visual agnosia for space): inability to judge one's own position in relation to other objects). It is assessed by asking the patient to walk towards a particular point, having placed some chairs in the way; it is observed whether he is able to find his way towards the correct place and around the obstructions.
- *Environmental agnosia:* inability to recognise familiar places
- *Prosopagnosia* (impaired recognition of familiar faces): assessed by asking to identify familiar or famous faces or match similar faces from a number of photographs
- *Agraphaesthesia (agraphognosia):* Assessed by writing letters on palm or skin; and asking the patient to recognise.

- *Auditory agnosia:* First it is determined that the hearing is normal. Patient, with eyes closed, is asked to recognise sounds like, ringing bell, shaking coins, tearing paper, etc. If there is associated aphasia confusing the answers, he is asked to illustrate the sound himself, if he recognises it.
- *Phonagnosia:* inability to identify familiar voices

Calculation

- Assessed by verbal and written, addition, subtraction, multiplication and division
- Example: 'One and two step problems', 'how much money do these coins make', 'if you buy two books worth 7 and 4 rupees (currency) and give the shopkeeper 20 rupee note, how much you will get back'
- Mental calculation is assessed, paper and pencil not required.
- Premorbid mathematical abilities are taken into consideration

General Information

- Assessed with reference to subject's background
- Geographical information, current events, major common historical facts, famous personalities

Judgement

- Assessed from clinical behaviour
- Personal judgement: assessed mostly from history, self care, etc.
- Test judgement: response to solve a problem in a given situation: e.g., 'what will you do if you see smoke in your house'
- Social judgement: assessed mostly from history

Abstract Ability

- Similarities, dissimilarities: by asking to explain the similarities and dissimilarities among objects, e.g., 'apple and banana', 'chair and table', 'car and bus'
- Proverbs: by asking to explain (hidden) meanings (it is better to record verbatim responses)

Executive Function

- Motivation to attempt, goal setting and planning, capacity for concept formation are observed.
- Errors of judgement, failure to anticipate, poor problem solving techniques, lack of flexibility and perseveration are checked.
- Colour form sorting test: The patient is presented with a random array of forms (square, circle, triangle) of different colours (blue, yellow, green, red) and asked to 'put those together that belong together'. It is assessed whether or not the patient is able to sort the forms according to a clear principle, that is, by shape or colour. If the patient succeeds, the forms are once again presented in a random array, and the patient is asked to 'sort them in another way'.

Thought

- Document verbatim samples of speech and when relevant, written samples
- Stream, form, possession and content of thought are commented

Mood

- Affect, quality, intensity, appropriateness, fluctuations, range, reactivity, communicability, catastrophic responses

Perception

- Hallucinations, illusions, imagery

Insight

- Insight into their own condition, understanding their own limitations

PHYSICAL EXAMINATION

General Examination

Systemic Examination

Detailed Neurological Examination

- Lobe functions

- Cortical sensations: stereognosis, tactile localisation, tactile discrimination, figure writing, sensory inattention
- Frontal lobe tests: primitive reflexes: grasp, pout, palmomental; alternate tapping: finger tapping, foot tapping; perseveration, reciprocal coordination
- Neurological soft signs

ASSESSMENT SCALES USEFUL IN CLINICAL SETTING

- Mini Mental State Examination (Folstein, et al., 1975)
- Temporal Orientation Test (Benton et al., 1994)
- Blessed Dementia Scale (Blessed et al., 1968)
- Brief Cognitive Rating Scale
- Memory for Design Tests
- Abbreviated Mental Test Score (AMTS) (Qureshi and Hodkinson, 1974)
- Activities of Daily Life Scales (Fillenbaum et al., 1999)
- Bayer activities of daily living scale (B-ADL)
- Manchester and Oxford Universities Scale for the Psychopathological Assessment of Dementia (MOUSEPAD) (Allen et al., 1996)

INVESTIGATIONS

Routine

- Complete blood cell count
- HIV
- Thyroid profile
- MRI brain (CT may not be helpful in many cases)
- EEG (abnormalities in many dementias, classical triphasic sharp wave complexes in Creutzfeldt-Jakob disease)
- B_{12} level
- RBC folate level
- Anti-nuclear antibody (ANA) (for systemic lupus erythematosus)
- Fluorescent treponemal antibody test (FTA) (VDRL may be normal in neurosyphilis)
- Serum electrolytes, proteins, liver function tests, blood sugar, urea, serum creatinine (abnormalities, might be complicating a dementing illness)

If Indicated by Clinical Reasons

- Chest X-ray (tumours: primary site or secondaries)
- Genetic testing (for Huntington's disease)
- Copper and ceruloplasmin levels (for Wilson's disease)
- Metal levels (arsenic, thallium, mercury, lead, manganese)
- Anti-Borrelia antibodies (for Lyme disease)
- 'Wet prep' for acanthocytes (for neuroacanthocytosis)
- Antineuronal antibodies (for paraneoplastic limbic encephalitis)
- Leukocyte arylsulfatase A level (for metachromatic leukodystrophy)
- Very-long-chain fatty acid level (for adrenoleukodystrophy)
- Cerebrospinal fluid (CSF) examination (through lumbar puncture): CSF VDRL, evidence of chronic meningitis like tuberculosis, cryptococcal infection, for antibodies, immunoassay for 14-3-3 protein for Creutzfeldt-Jakob disease
- Angiography (for granulomatous angitis)
- Skeletal muscle biopsy for the possibility of Kuf's disease
- Lymph node or jejunal biopsy to help rule out Whipple's disease
- Tonsillar biopsy for ruling out CJD

FURTHER READING

- Allen NHP, Gordon S, Hope T, Burns A. (1996) Manchester and Oxford Universities Scale for the Psychopathological Assessment of Dementia (MOUSEPAD). *British Journal of Psychiatry,* 169, 293–307.
- Benton AL, Sivan AB, Hamsher K deS, Varney NR, Spreen O. (1994) *Contribution to Neuropsychological assessment: A Clinical Manual,* ed 2, New York: Oxford University Press.
- Bickerstaff ER, Spillane JA. (1989) *Neurological Examination in Clinical Practice.* 5th Edition. Delhi: Oxford University Press.
- Blessed G, Tomlinson BE, Roth M. (1968) The association between quantitative measures of dementia and of senile changes in the cerebral gray matter of elderly subjects. *British Journal of Psychiatry,* 114, 797.
- Fillenbaum G, Chandra V, Ganguli M, et al. (1999) Development of an activities of daily living scale to screen for dementia in an illiterate rural older population in India. *Age and Ageing,* 28, 161–168.
- Folstein MF, Folstein SE, McHugh PR. (1975) "Mini-Mental State": A practical method for grading the cognitive state of patients for the clinician. *Journal of Psychiatric Research,* 12, 189–198.

- Goldberg D (1997) *The Maudsley Handbook of Practical Psychiatry.* Chennai: Oxford University Press.
- Levin HS, Soukup VM, Benton AL, Fletcher JM, Satz P (1995) Neuropsychological and intellectual assessment of adults. In *Comprehensive Textbook of Psychiatry,* (eds. Kaplan HI, and Sadock BJ) 6th edition. Baltimore: Williams and Wilkins.
- Qureshi K, Hodkinson M. (1974) Evaluation of a 10 question mental test of the institutionalised elderly. *Age and Ageing,* 3, 152–157.

Note: This outline has been prepared to help clinicians for history taking and evaluation for persons suspected to have dementia. This is not an exhaustive account of all the clinical tests, scales, procedures or examinations that are used for evaluation of dementia. Clinicians are encouraged to adapt according to clinical situations and choose appropriate methods of evaluation.

- Kar N (2004) *Outline of Clinical Assessment for Dementia.* Occasional Paper, Geriatric Care and Research Organisation.

Appendix 2

....

Legal Issues in Dementia Care

....

Specific laws differ in different countries and in different states even in the same country. The practitioners should orient themselves to the prevailing legal provisions in the s⁺ates they practice. Here a few relevant legal concepts are mentioneᴅ This is not an exhaustive account of all legal issues that may arise in connection with the care of dementia patients.

Competence

Competence is the capacity to understand the nature and the consequences of an intended act.

A person may be legally competent to perform one particular act and not another.

It is assumed that all adults have legal competence.

Capacity

A person lacks capacity in relation to a matter if at the material time he is unable to make a decision for himself in relation to the matter because of an impairment of, or disturbance in the functioning of the mind or brain.

Loss of capacity can be temporary. Capacity at this particular time for this particular issue is tested. Person's ability to make decisions generally is not relevant. Cause of incapacity is immaterial.

A person is 'unable' to make a decision for himself if he is unable:
  i. to understand the information relevant to the decision,
  ii. to retain that information,
  iii. to use or weigh that information as part of the process of making the decision, or
  iv. to communicate his decision (whether by talking, using sign language or any other means).

Informed Consent

A valid informed consent requires three elements: information disclosure, competence, and voluntariness.

Disclosure involves a process of explaining to the patient in lay language the essential components of the medical transaction: the nature of the illness; the purpose of the proposed treatment; all reasonable alternatives to that treatment, including the option of no treatment; and the possible benefits and risks of the proposed treatment and its alternatives.

Competence concerns whether the patient has sufficient mental capacity to make a personal, reasoned choice among the various treatment options, including those not recommended by the physician.

Voluntariness concerns process of decision making that occurs in the absence of undue influence.

Testamentary Capacity

It is the competence to execute a will. It presupposes that the person making a will knows (1) that he or she is making a will, (2) the nature and extent of his or her property, (3) who are his or her natural heirs, and (4) the effects of the manner in which his or her property will be disposed.

Mental impairment is a ground for legal challenge. Other issues that affect the validity of a will are undue influence on the free will of the will maker and sometimes mental disorders with delusions that are influencing this decision taking process.

Competence to Contract

It requires that the person understands the nature and the consequences of the contract and that the decision to contract was not the direct result of undue influence.

Competence to contract in demented patients can be legally challenged.

Guardianship

Global incompetence in several areas of functioning like incapacity to manage personal matters, self-care, and lack of capacity to manage even rudimentary financial transactions, may necessitate the appointment of a guardian or conservator to ensure the person's well being.

Living Will

It is a revocable written document prepared by a competent adult and specifying the circumstances under which that person will consent to the cessation of specific treatments.

Durable Power of Attorney

It is a written document that permits another person to act on behalf of the declarant in the event of the declarant's decision-making incapacity.

Laws and Policies in India Related to Older People

- Children Act, Section 2, (k): regarding guardianship
- Code of Criminal procedure, 1973, Section 125 (1) (d) for maintenance of elderly parents.
- Finance Act, 1992, Section 88B: regarding income tax rebate
- Hindu Adoption and Maintenance Act, 1956 Section 20(3) for maintenance for aged and infirm parents.
- Indian Constitution, Article 41: States role in providing social security to the aged.

- Indian Contract Act, Section 13: regarding consent
- Indian Evidence Act, Section 92: regarding capacity
- Indian Penal Code, Section 466: regarding capacity
- Industrial Finance Corporation Act, Section 10A (4) regarding competence
- National Policy on Older Persons, 1999
- Transfer of Property Act, Section 102; Section 7: regarding durable power of attorney

REFERENCES

- Children Act, 1960. (1960) *Bare Acts.* New Delhi: Universal Law Publishing Co
- Indian Contract Act, 1872. (1998) *Bare Acts.* New Delhi: Universal Law Publishing Co
- Indian Evidence Act, 1872. (1998) *Bare Acts.* New Delhi: Universal Law Publishing Co
- Indian Penal Code, 1860. (1986) *Bare Acts.* New Delhi: Universal Law Publishing Co
- Industrial Finance Corporation Act, 1948. (1998) *Bare Acts.* New Delhi: Universal Law Publishing Co
- Leong GB, Eth S (1995) Medico-legal issues. In *Comprehensive Textbook of Psychiatry;* Eds Kaplan HI, Sadock BJ, 6th Edition. Baltimore: Williams and Wilkins.
- Transfer of Property Act, 1882. (1998) *Bare Acts.* New Delhi: Universal Law Publishing Co

Note: It is emphasized that the readers should check for the exact laws and acts operative in a particular region. The definition, interpretation and application of various legal concepts may vary. It is useful to consult legal professionals if there is need.

Prepared by the contributions of Dr Raveesh BN, MD, Assistant Professor of Psychiatry, Department of Psychiatry, JSS Medical College and Hospital, Mysore, India, through his article 'Legal issues for patients with dementia', Occasional Paper, Geriatric Care and Research Organisation, 2004; and Dr Vivek Pattan, MD, Department of Psychiatry, Gwent Health Care NHS Trust, Newport, South Wales, UK.

Index